SPORTSWRITING

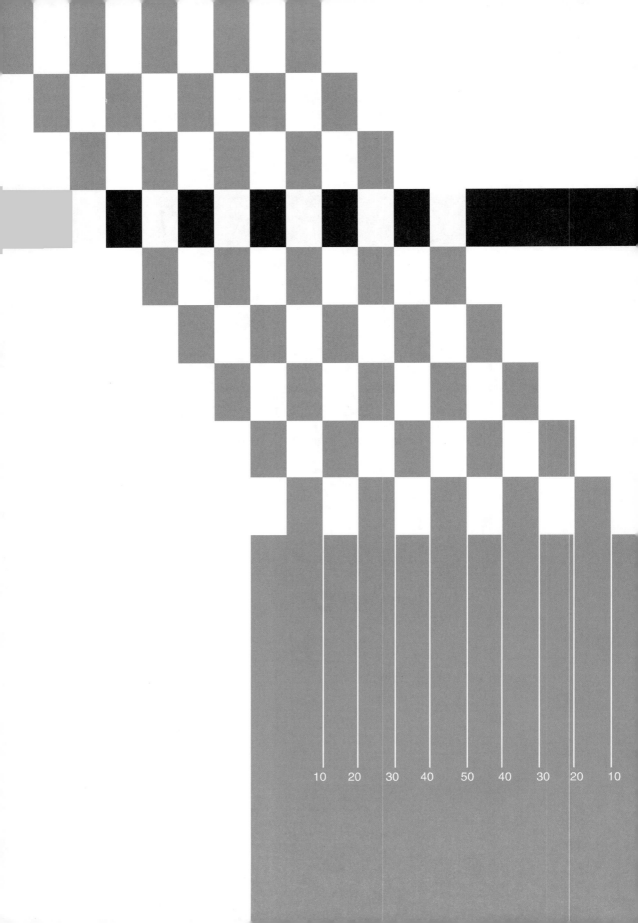

SPORTSWRITING

THE LIVELY GAME

CONRAD C. FINK

IOWA STATE UNIVERSITY PRESS / AMES

Conrad C. Fink is the William S. Morris professor of Newspaper Strategy and Management at the Henry W. Grady College of Journalism and Mass Communication, and director of the James M. Cox Jr. Institute for Newspaper Management Studies, University of Georgia, Athens. He was a reporter, editor, foreign correspondent and vice president of The Associated Press before becoming an award-winning teacher. Professor Fink has written seven other books on journalism.

Iowa State University Press
2121 South State Avenue, Ames, Iowa 50014

Orders: 1-800-862-6657
Office: 1-515-292-0140
Fax: 1-515-292-3348
Web site: www.isupress.com

♾ Printed on acid-free paper in the United States of America

First edition, 2001

Library of Congress Cataloging-in-Publication Data
Fink, Conrad C.
   Sportswriting: the lively game/Conrad C. Fink.
     p. cm.
   Includes index.
   ISBN 0-8138-2246-7 (alk. paper)
   1. Sports journalism. 2. Sports journalism—Vocational guidance.   I. Title.

pn4784.S6 F56 2001
070.4′49796—dc21   00-063472

The last digit is the print number: 9 8 7 6 5 4 3 2 1

This book is dedicated to my students,
from whom I have learned much.

Contents

Preface

You of course recognize these names: Joe DiMaggio, Ted Williams, Steffi Graf, Joe Louis, Chris Evert, Mickey Mantle, Monica Seles, Red Grange, Martina Navratilova, Ken Griffey Jr.

They're sports *heroes* all—athletes whose feats on the field and the court are woven into the American fabric, implanted in our public consciousness.

How about these names? Red Smith, Frank Deford, Heywood Broun, Grantland Rice, Stanley Woodward, Jim Murray, Tom Boswell, Mike Lupica.

Sportswriters all—writers whose bylines are admired throughout American journalism, writers whose keyboard feats are to journalism what the home run is to baseball, the slam dunk to basketball, the hole in one to golf.

Sports heroes, sportswriters ... their fortunes and fame are intertwined in what can only be termed as America's passionate love for the spectacle of men and women testing the barriers, fighting against the clock and striving to overcome the limitations of their own bodies and minds—and each other.

That has been the romance and adventure of sports since the Greeks and Romans, and as you move ahead in this book, studying how to report and write about it, I urge you to enjoy yourself and plunge into its reality.

But, you must accept another reality: From pee-wee leagues to big leagues, sports in America can be hard-headed big business, at times so tawdry—sordid even—that you'll have difficulty seeing the romance and adventure.

As a sportswriter sorting through those conflicting characteristics and, perhaps, your own mixed emotions, your first duty is to your readers—always, the readers. And that will require reporting and writing that, yes, applauds, cheers and marvels as warranted but also probes and examines objectively and questions dispassionately. And, when the truth requires an honesty that is embarrassingly revealing or even cruel, you must deliver it—at times with a loud and raspy Bronx cheer.

Not all sports-writer heroes of the past did that. But the sports-writing game has changed. Of the many differences between sportswriting today and the writing of yesteryear, this is most striking: Whether you are writing for newspapers, magazines, broadcast or the electronic services of cyberspace, the essentials of sports journalism today are those of *all* journalism—detailed, careful and *honest* reporting delivered through accurate, fair and colorful writing.

Consequently, the best sportswriting measures well against the best writing on any subject, whatever the medium. Indeed, sportswriter bylines grace some of the greatest reporting and, certainly, some of the best writing in all journalism. Red Smith won a Pulitzer Prize not for *sportswriting* but for *essays* on sports—graceful, beautiful essays that will stand against any in literature (Lord, how that man could write!); Frank Deford, Jim Murray, Tom Boswell, Mike Lupica and others would be in anybody's Writers' Hall of Fame.

Fans and editors agree.

As in no other sector of journalism, reader-fans identify with sportswriters, seeking out particularly the bylines of skilled columnists who work their way up the reporting ranks until they're permitted to call it as *they* see it, to write it in highly personalized styles as *they* think it should be written.

Knowing the insatiable interest of fans, editors throw enormous resources into sports coverage.

Newspapers devote huge staffs and newshole (space for news) to sports. Most magazines offer at least some sports coverage and, of course, many are devoted exclusively to sports. Television pays billions of dollars for sports programming, and Internet services, in their infancy and only now struggling toward first base, offer you great career potential. And books? As the new millennium dawned, Amazon.com alone listed *32,000* on sports!

So, move ahead in *Sportswriting: The Lively Game*, aware that sportswriting is fun, yet serious, offering you thrills and adventures, yet laying on you all the obligations inherent in principled, ethical and professional journalism.

As a student of sportswriting, you're launched on a journey of discovery. Start the trek with fresh eyes, an open mind and adventurous spirit and you'll have a wonderful time.

Here is a route I've mapped out to, I hope, ease your journey.

Organization of This Book

Part One: The Kickoff

Every game has a necessary beginning, and so does *Sportswriting: The Lively Game*. To set the scene for what follows, this book begins with two chapters aimed, first, at showing you how sports coverage fits into the overall journalistic mix in America and, second, what you, as a sportswriter today, owe your ever-more sophisticated and demanding readers.

Chapter One, The Writer's Arena, examines how your sports coverage must fit into the marketing mix and overall news strategies of newspapers, magazines, broadcast and electronic media. Understand your medium, its strategic business objective, your audience and your competitors—or you'll fail in sports, as in any other sector of journalism.

Chapter Two, What You Owe Your Readers, illustrates there is more to sportswriting than covering games. Off-field stories about drugs, violence and cheating can overshadow those about struggles on the gridiron or basketball court, and that can force you to decide where your allegiance lies. Does it lie with the sport? The athlete? Your employing medium? Your readers? Discard the "homeboy" philosophy, disdain boosterism—and do the job *for your readers* with ethical integrity. Also, learn libel law!

Part Two: Our Blocking and Tackling: Strong Reporting

Strong reporting is a key to success in sportswriting. Like any athlete, you need solid fundamentals. Journalism's five Ws and How are to us what blocking and tackling are to football, a smooth backswing to golf and flawless fielding to baseball. But in sports reporting, as in sports, there's more to it—much more.

Chapter Three, Reporting the Key Elements, discusses capturing for your readers the factual context of the event—turning points, star performances, the statistics and, always, the look-ahead angle, answering the "what's next?" question that all fans ask.

Chapter Four, Reporting the Wider Picture, turns to more broadly reporting sports as a societal phenomenon and how you must illuminate off-field angles—the business, legal and societal issues of sports. Know something about drug rehab? Knee reconstruction and contract negotiations? You must.

Part Three: Making the Writer's Muse Move

There is writing *genius* in sports pages. Some of journalism's best writers hang out there, and if you want to join them remember this: Strong reporting skills get you a job; adding strong *writing* skills gives you a career.

Chapter Five, Writing It Straight, covers writing the basic news stories so essential to grasp before you move your writer's muse too far, too fast. Learn first to do straightforward game stories and basic interviews—how to write *breaking news*. Then (*only* then) should you move on to writing sports poetry!

Chapter Six, Taking Readers Beyond the Score, turns to writing that's analytical and interpretive—but still aimed at the *news* pages of your sports section. Analytical writing of spot news is necessary in sports (as in most journalism) to lead readers through the complexities and to what really happened and what it really means.

Part Four: Covering the Majors

So avid are sports fans that I will get an argument merely by stating here that the "major" sports are football, baseball and basketball. In the North (and, increasingly, elsewhere), hockey fans will scream; in the South, stock car racing fans will shake their heads sadly. Nevertheless, the constraints of book writing dictate that I turn in Part Four to three "major" sports, then to others later.

Chapter Seven, Covering Football, addresses reporting and writing tips peculiar to covering the game that has helmets colliding throughout America, from pee-wee leagues to the NFL.

Chapter Eight, Covering Baseball, looks at reporting and writing for the bat-and-ball crowd.

And Chapter Nine, Covering Basketball, reports on what the writing pros do from courtside.

Part Five: Covering the Others

For many reader-fans, the "major" sports are almost irrelevant; for them, the action is in hockey, tennis, soccer or golf. We'll look at writing careers in those sports sectors in Chapter Ten, The Wider World of Sports.

Part Six: Columns: The Winner's Circle in Sportswriting

More than any other newspaper or magazine department, sports offers enormously attractive opportunities in column writing. In television, sports commentators star. Opinion writing floods cyberspace. Columnists indeed are very popular. But as at the Kentucky Derby, only the very best make it into the winner's circle—and then only after solid experience on the spot-news firing line.

Chapter Eleven, Writing Game Columns, looks at how columnists cover sports events with a finely balanced mix of old-fashioned spot-news reporting and *informed* (note, *informed*) opinion. After many events, the principal or "lead" story is accompanied by a column of game narrative and analysis—the "how" and "why" of winning and losing—plus other "sidebars," such as dressing room stories or coach interviews.

Chapter Twelve, In This Corner ..., studies those regular columnists whose writing is "anchored" in a fixed position—an upper corner of a sports page, perhaps—but who are freed to roam wherever the writer's muse moves. It's a coveted spot in journalism, one *you* legitimately can strive for during a career of covering *the lively game*.

Addendum

Want to label yourself an amateur? Let your writing demonstrate you don't know style. All aspiring journalists must learn The Associated Press style, which most newspapers use. You'll need to obtain and learn *The Associated Press Stylebook and Libel Manual*, but meanwhile I've created an addendum as a handy reference to highlights of AP style.

Acknowledgments

For years, my students, to whom this book is dedicated, clamored for a book on sportswriting. When I could turn to it, the idea caught the fancy of Judi Brown of Iowa State University Press. To them, to her and to E. Anne Bolen, editor and project manager of this book, and Kristen Kertz, copy editor, go my thanks.

Thanks also to Tom Russell, a sports fanatic who took time out of his duties as dean of the University of Georgia's Henry W. Grady College of Journalism and Mass Communication to serve as consultant and copy editor.

Sophie Barnes, also a sport expert, applied her expertise to the manuscript, along with superb keyboarding skills that rescued the manuscript from my old-newspaper-guy's typing and editing.

Lou Boccardi, president of The Associated Press, my old regiment, graciously permitted me to include as an addendum extracts from *The Associated Press Stylebook and Libel Manual.*

Finally, to all sportswriters quoted in this book, a salute: As a group, you're among the most talented journalists in the business.

PART ONE

The Kickoff

W ell, you're a lifelong sports fan, a passionate and knowledgeable reader of sports pages ... and you and your laptop are ready for the opening whistle in any stadium, at any courtside and on any athletic field.

Right?

Not so fast.

If you want to be there for a newspaper, magazine or broadcast medium—and get paid for it—you must grasp two realities not particularly bothersome for your predecessors in the press box, those marvelously free-wheeling sportswriters of yesteryear.

First, understand that sports coverage today must fit into the overall journalistic *and marketing* mix of your medium. Sports coverage, like coverage of any other subject, is planned carefully by editors—whether in print or broadcast—to fit their overall news strategies. Sportswriters must dovetail into that.

So, we'll open Chapter One, The Writer's Arena, by discussing how sports coverage is planned. Then we will turn to how you must write your stories to fit into your editor's pursuit of a chosen audience and your medium's competitive stance and strategic business objective.

Second, we will discuss how you'll find only *part* of the sports story in the stadium or arena. Many important stories break off-field, sometimes in the *un*heroic actions of sports heroes involved in drugs, violence or cheating. Other important stories flow from the sometimes tawdry action in the hard-headed, dollar-oriented business arena of big-time sports.

That is, sports lover, early on you'll face the reality that much in sports isn't lovable, and you'll have to reexamine any romantic notions you have about the world of games. Simply put, your loyalty to the ideals of sports and loyalty to your hometown team inevitably will clash at times with your responsibilities as an ethical *journalist*. Boosterism and uncritical adoration are out; hard-eyed but fair reporting is in, and that, the ethics of sports journalism, is the subject of Chapter Two, What You Owe Your Readers.

1

The Writer's Arena

LET'S SAY it's your first day on the job in a small-town newsroom (where it all begins for most journalists) and sports stories are erupting everywhere—local peewee leagues are hard at it, your town's high school football team is in action and 16 other high school football teams in nearby counties are gearing up. Major college and pro stories are breaking in a nearby city.

Which assignment will be yours?

It depends, of course, on your editor's assessment of your abilities: Are you still a peewee reporter, or are you an experienced college newspaper reporter who now can handle something more complex?

Just as importantly, however, your editor will assign you within an overall operational plan laid down to use efficiently the sports department's reporting resources—you and your staff colleagues plus nonstaff, part-time "stringers" and The Associated Press and other news services that bring huge national and international reporting resources to sports.

How can your editor sort through all that and make the appropriate assignments? Only by knowing, intimately, the newspaper's overall journalistic objectives and how sports coverage fits into the total news effort to attract the right audience of readers in the correct geographic market.

And, when you eventually draw your assignment, how do you proceed? Where *is* the story? What *is* the news? How will you "angle" it, and how will you write it?

First, understand that what you're doing has enormous importance to your newspaper's overall success. Research reveals this pattern of adult readership of a newspaper's various sections:

Weekday Adult Readership

General news	95%
Entertainment	79
Sports	78 (Men, 88%, women, 68%)
Editorial	76
Business/finance	75
TV/radio listings	74
Food/cooking	73
Classified ads	73 (tie)
Comics	72
Home (local)	71[1]

Second, you obviously must take a deeper look at the planning behind the newsroom effort before you grab your laptop and rush for the door.

You, Your Editor and Media Strategy

The fundamental *business* objective of all news media is to gather readers, viewers or listeners who can be "sold" profitably to advertisers. It is advertisers who pay most bills in our free-enterprise, market-driven media.[2]

For newspapers, advertisers deliver about 80 percent of total revenue. For many papers, reader contribution of 20 percent in subscription fees and single-copy sales doesn't cover even newsprint costs.

Magazines pull about 50 percent of their revenue from readers. Obviously, that other 50 percent must come from advertisers.

Broadcast TV and radio both depend 100 percent on advertisers. Cable TV relies principally on subscriber fees, although advertiser revenue increasingly is important.

Internet news services—their types, styles and importance—still are in a shakedown period, and we don't yet know precisely what role they will play in the media mix or, indeed, what advertiser interest will be in using them.

But, increasingly in cyberspace and, certainly, in the major media, the game plan is to build news content that captures audiences for advertisers.

Just any audience anywhere? No.

From all media, advertisers demand audiences with certain *demographic characteristics* (age, income, education) within a relevant *geographic market* (a city and surrounding counties for most newspapers and local TV stations, for example).

Your Demographic Target

It's a given: Americans who are upscale in education and income generally read newspapers, magazines and books. The strongest TV viewing habit is in low-income groups of lesser education.[3]

Advertisers, therefore, turn particularly to newspapers and magazines to reach *demographically attractive* readers able and willing to buy consumer goods and services.

And, driven in major part by that advertising consideration (*your* salary, however small, has to be paid, after all), print media formulate news content to deliver the "top" of the demographic market. And they succeed.

Newspapers boast many college-educated readers. *The Atlanta Journal* and *Constitution*, for example, claim to reach about 78 percent of college graduates in the Atlanta market and 84 percent of those who have done post-graduate work. The papers' "reach" is only 38.6 percent of adults with less than a high school education.[4]

Newspapers score impressively among high-income adults. The *Journal-Constitution* claim to reach 71 percent of households with $35,000 to $49,000 in annual income and 83.4 percent of households with $100,000 or more.[5]

Some newspapers—the *New York Times, Wall Street Journal, Los Angeles Times*, among them—claim audiences heavy with millionaires, as do magazines such as *Forbes, Fortune* and *Business Week*.[6]

Readers of such demographic quality don't just fall into newspaper or magazine laps. Editors court, woo and entice them with news content shaped, toned and presented to pull them in. If you're working for a newspaper, take that drive for demographic quality as your first clue about what your editor is thinking while sorting through all those peewee league games and assigning priorities to coverage of high school, college and pro sports.

Also, take that strategic news mission as a personal clue about how you must develop news values and judgments *and* reporting and writing abilities to support the mission.

For example, should you land at *Forbes* or *Fortune* (both of which cover sports, despite their business orientation), come equipped with story ideas on polo, yachting and rich man's golf, not mud wrestling or peewee baseball.

Your Geographic Target

To most advertisers, even wealthy readers are not truly valuable unless they live nearby, within shopping distance.

Think about it: Why would any advertiser in Atlanta pay to reach a *Journal-Constitution* reader, no matter how wealthy, who lives 350 miles away? That reader won't drive to Atlanta to buy groceries!

The relevant *geographic market* normally is a city plus nearby counties for most of the 1,500 U.S. dailies, more than 9,700 weeklies and many city magazines and other local publications.[7]

Of course, for national newspapers—the *Wall Street Journal, USA Today, New York Times*—and many magazines, geography is less important than demography: Their advertisers sell goods and services nationwide, and they willingly "buy" readers nationwide, as long as they meet demographic standards.

So, in that small-town newsroom of yours, a new factor enters the editor's equation: The sports-writing team must create news content to pull in demographically attractive readers, but *also* ensure that most of them are in the geographic market defined by advertisers.

Don't misunderstand: With a cruel deadline a few hours off, your editor won't be pawing through mounds of marketing research to decide your first assignment. The news business is much too rushed and chaotic for that, and overburdened editors quickly make hundreds of news judgments daily on instinct born of experience.

Anyway, of all news departments in a newspaper, sports may pay the least daily attention to that marketing-driven campaign for *just* the right readers in *just* the right place. Editors and publishers generally look upon their sports sections as hugely successful reader attractions—the sections that pull in and hold persons who otherwise might not read newspapers. And with "churn," or turnover, of newspaper subscribers very high (exceeding 100 percent annually for some newspapers), those loyal reader-fans are highly valued regardless of their demographic quality.[8]

Indeed, they are so valued that many newspapers give sports more newshole than any other single hard-news category—21 percent of total newshole for sports in one study, compared with 15 percent for business, 14 percent for local nonsports news and 7 percent for national. Only "features" got more newshole—26 percent total in all sections of the newspapers studied.[9]

Sports editors clearly are given the freedom to deploy their reporting resources and independence to run successful sections.

Nevertheless, sports editors *are* part of a newspaper-wide strategic effort and over time, through custom and with smart use of modern marketing research, sports editors *do* reach detailed understanding of their newspapers' business objectives in the advertiser-driven marketplace and *do* develop journalistic tactics their departments must follow to help newspapers reach those objectives.

To succeed in sportswriting today, you must understand why varying news values are assigned news stories and how judgments are made on whether, how—and by whom—they will be covered.

News Values in the Sports Arena

Finally! Your wait is over. Today's reporting assignments are passed out.

- The sports editor is taking the pro story in a city 50 miles away.
- The assistant sports editor will cover the major college story.
- The most senior staff writer on duty today will take your town's high school story.
- The three other local sports reporters—including you—will cover the most significant of those 16 other high school teams in nearby counties.
- Stringers (journalism students from a local university) will take the remaining area high school stories, and one part-timer will come in to write a peewee league wrap-up from telephoned reports by coaches and team managers.
- The Associated Press will be the source for all other major stories.

Now, why were those assignments parceled out that way?

Well, the sports editor and assistant editor took the pro and college stories because many local readers follow those teams closely. They are *big* news. Anyway, that's the way it is in the newspaper business: Writers atop the pecking order get the day's best assignments (although your editors better not grab too many or they'll have a staff revolt). Also, although you may not want to admit it, those two editors are the most experienced reporters and best writers in the department.

The most senior staff writer gets your town's high school story because prep sports are enormously important to local readers—and thus to the newspaper. Senior writers accept prep assignments willingly because they'll get major (probably section-front) "play" for their stories and plenty of reader-fan reaction.

Your assignment to that area high school story is important, too. Reader interest extends far beyond local preps, to even distant high schools, because so many states have statewide championships and age-old rivalries. Anyway, the outlying high school you'll cover plays your town's local team next week, and readers will expect "scouting" details from your story.

For Love of the Game

Cal Powell is a sports reporter and columnist for the *Ft. Walton Beach (Fla.) Daily News* who prefers covering high school sports above university and pro sports. Why? *For love of the game.*

BY CAL POWELL

I get asked the question at least a couple times a week ... why I want to cover high school sports.

Why not colleges, or better yet, why not pros? That's what it's all about, they tell me. That's the pinnacle.

And that's when I laugh.

Simply put, I cover high school sports because I enjoy it.

Isn't that a good enough reason?

Some of my earliest memories in life are of sitting with my brother in the back of a school bus late at night as the heroes that were my father's football players danced and sang in the aisles after a big road win.

Then they'd all cheer their good fortune ... a large part of the reason I still love high school athletics is rooted in one word: pride.

High school sports are driven and sustained by kids, coaches and teachers with pride.

Pride in their work, in their school and in themselves.

It's seen in the 140-pound noseguard. The slow-footed, but tenacious point guard.

Kids who would do anything just to be on the field, on the court.

Just to be playing because it's fun and rewarding ...

There's just a purity that still exists in high school athletics. When you see it, you know it. It's beautiful.

I covered the University of Georgia football team for three years in college ... but when things reach that kind of grand scale, a lot of the purity, the simplicity, the beauty of sport, is lost.

It's just not the same.

Cover the pros? I have nothing in common with a millionaire defensive back ...

The sport itself is secondary at the higher levels of competition. It's more about money and fame ...

That's not to romanticize (high school sports) too much, though. There is corruption in high school athletics, for bad people can ruin even the finest of things.

But the beauty still exists.

It perseveres, thrives even, despite the crooked coach and the dishonest administrator.

It's seen in the faces of every kid who's ever picked up a ball. Every coach who's ever picked up a whistle ...

Excerpted with permission from, "For Pride, Love of Prep Games," a column published by the *Fort Walton Beach (Fla.) Daily News,* July 2, 1999, p. C-1.

Stringers and part-time staffers are needed because *no* newspaper can afford to staff all sports stories. Every sports department has an elaborate web of stringers to cover minor and, sometimes, major stories.

The Associated Press is the single-most important external resource for most newspapers. The AP covers (literally) the world of sports, and, depending on which level of service your newspaper takes, can pour hundreds of thousands or *millions* of words into your newsroom daily. Many major newspapers—*Los Angeles Times, Washington Post, New York Times*, among them—operate news services that add to the worldwide coverage.[10]

So, that's how the first news judgments are made: Editors frantically try to cover the sports waterfront with limited reporting resources and use diverse values—including assessment of your capabilities—in passing out assignments.

Now, what values do *you* take to reporting and writing in the sports arena?

News Judgment: A Checklist

Driving to that outlying high school, reflect on why your editor decided its football game tonight is news and why a valuable staffer (you) should cover it (at a cost in your salary and travel expenses) instead of some other sports event.[11]

In analyzing this, use—but modify—standards of news judgment we use in all journalism:

Proximity

For all but national newspapers, establishing a strong franchise in *local news* is the principal journalistic objective. Why?

First, of course, our advertisers demand local audiences of readers and, in all news categories—general news, business, politics and government, as well as sports—readers deem local news most important. Alternative sources of all kinds—television, radio, magazines and the Internet—offer your readers international, national and state news. But none matches newspapers in substantive and detailed local news coverage.

And that means, second, that local newspapers have a dramatic *competitive edge* in the unceasing battle against other media for the allegiance of readers and advertisers alike.

So, as you plan your reporting and writing "attack" for tonight, think of how your story can meet the *proximity test* by focusing on local angles (the team plays your hometown team next week) and how you can present factual substance, color and analysis that no competing medium can match.

Now, a necessary modification of "proximity":

Sports reader-fans have wider interests in their news specialty than do many readers who focus on other types of news. Not to oversimplify, but many sports fans follow a wide variety of sports, local or not. Not many readers principally interested in, say, local education want to read about a routine school board meeting in a town 200 miles away. But many local sports fans *will* be interested, for example, in that distant town's star quarterback—and they'll track him through college into the pros. East Coast readers follow West Coast games and vice versa. Local readers wear caps bearing the insignia of distant colleges or pro teams.

So, define "proximity" broadly: Local news in sports is any story anywhere, regardless of where it breaks, if it is of interest to local readers.

Tonight, though, you must focus on *local impact* in the narrowest sense.

Impact

No question: That outlying town is on the periphery of your newspaper's circulation territory, so *some* readers out there will consider your story as local news for their own hometown.

However, your editor's principal consideration in assigning you is that the game tonight will have *impact* on your hometown team next Friday night.

Measure impact by evaluating the *number* of people likely affected by an event and how *deeply* they are affected. On both counts, your story tonight meets the impact test: Reader-fan interest in hometown prep sports runs very wide and passionately deep.

So, (and more on this later), your reporting tonight should highlight angles likely to be important next week. If the defensive line shows weaknesses tonight, point that out as an opportunity for your own team next week. If the quarterback demonstrates a weak passing arm, note in your story that your hometown team can expect to encounter a running game next week.

For reader interest *and* your own career interest, demonstrate in your story a grasp of such subtleties—and shoot for Page One play in the sports section (or, maybe even A-1)!

Timeliness

In all journalism, high priority goes to a spot-news event—something important that's breaking *right now*. That's why we call them *news*papers and *news*casts.

But in sports reporting there is no time out, no off-season. To some reader-fans every development is timely.

We cover the board of education's monthly meeting, and then generally take time out until next month unless something really big breaks. In sports, reader-fans want that spot break—the game story—all right. They also want "precedes" and "follows"—stories that run up to the game and stories that follow it, *even on relatively low-grade news developments*.

Take baseball's spring training: Snow still blankets the Mason-Dixon line, but baseball writers are hard at it with season precedes—contract negotiations, players' health, who's been a bad boy over the winter, trades, coach interviews ... the list is endless. *After* the World Series, the cycle begins again, and reader-fans lap it up, 52 weeks a year.

So, yes, timeliness counts in sports journalism, as in all journalism. But modify timeliness as a measurement of *newsworthiness*. Even low-grade, off-season stories can be timely and newsworthy in sports.

That is, stay focused for the moment on tonight's game, the spot-news story. But soon afterward start thinking of how you can cover this outlying high school in the days ahead as it prepares for *next week's* game against your home-town team.

Conflict

In all media, editors (and readers, viewers and listeners) assign priority to stories of conflict—between armies, politicians, ideas, good guys and bad guys.

In sports reporting, of course, even higher priorities are assigned conflict. However, there are two points to take into consideration.

First, conflict in sports is multi-layered and filled with nuances and subtleties. Tonight, for example, your story of conflict is not simply 11 young men battling 11 others. Rather, conflict includes a long rivalry between two schools, two coaches who've been trying to out-fox each other for years, a quarterback against a defensive secondary, two opposing lines—heck, even rival bands and cheering sections get into it. Strong reporting and good writing must capture *all* those conflicts.

Second, in sports, probably more than in other sectors of journalism, an aura of *phony* conflict can surround individuals, teams and events. Fight promoters with ringside seats to sell stage weigh-ins featuring two pugs threatening to knock off each other's heads; athletic departments with stadiums to fill advertise "traditional" rivalries between teams that have been playing each other for three or four years—the sales hype never ends. Don't buy into it.

Prominence

The president of the United States is more prominent—and thus more newsworthy—than a low-ranking Agriculture Department bureaucrat.

So, too, is a head coach more prominent (and, thus, more newsworthy) than an obscure assistant coach. A star quarterback is more newsworthy than an interior offensive lineman who labors dutifully but relatively obscurely in the mosh pit of the middle.

Just as your Washington colleagues assign high priorities to individuals prominent in government and politics, so must you ensure strong coverage of sports figures in whom the public has great interest.

Neither in Washington nor on the playing field, however, should journalists forget that low-ranking bureaucrats make things go in government on a day-to-day basis or that the quarterback is a star in large part because his relatively anonymous line keeps sack-minded defensive players off his back.

That is, balanced and truly meaningful sportswriting avoids granting god-like status to individuals just because they can run faster, hit harder or throw balls farther than most of us. *Prominence* goes into your news judgments; just keep it under control.

So, tonight, if that star quarterback passes for great yardage and runs for even more, give him the prominence he deserves. But weave into your writing the contributions by those guys in the mosh pit. Discerning readers will applaud you.

The Off-Beat and Unusual

You'll also make readers (and your editors) happy if you seek stories with off-beat angles.

Life sometimes gets very ordinary. Much of what happened yesterday, happens today, and probably will happen tomorrow. So, there is real news value in the unexpected edging out the expected, in departures from the norm—the underdog team that wins, the unknown quarterback who stars, the second-string lineman who causes a game-turning fumble.

And for goodness sake, if you see a funny story, *lunge* for it. The whole world is desperate for a laugh.

Competition (Yours) in the Sports Arena

Think it's competitive only down on the playing field where they knock heads?

Look over your shoulder in the press box: Somebody likely is trying to knock off *your* head.

Despite the smiles, the backslaps and the camaraderie of the press corps, every reporter there—in print, television and radio—is plotting to get the edge on you, to find an exclusive reporting angle you don't have and to write with a dash and vigor you lack.

Nothing personal, you understand. It's just business.

Competition for readers, viewers and listeners is fierce in all media. Any newspaper or broadcast station that lags, soon fades. The push for ever-improved marketplace position is unrelenting.

Beyond that, however, is an enormously strong tradition of personal competition in reporting. It's *fun* to beat competitors, to out-report and out-write everybody in the press box.

Editors are watching, too. For them, winning is a matter of pride—and job security, both theirs *and yours*.

That's right, we're talking here about *your* survival in the sports arena. Miss important reporting angles too often or get out-written regularly and you may find yourself invited to consider another line of work.

Don't assume such competitive pressures exist only in big league reporting.[12] Even if your newspaper is the only daily in your small town (as is likely), you are under a competitive microscope tonight. Note:

- *Nearby metros* cover prep sports for the same reason your small daily does: Readers love it. And, many of *their* readers take two newspapers and are *your* readers—subjecting you to *competition by example.* Two-buy readers will compare your reporting and writing to that of metro staffers perhaps much more experienced than you.
- *Weekly newspapers* in your paper's circulation territory will cover tonight's game as high-priority local news. They'll *vacuum* the stadium for game details, color and names, names, names—a staple of community journalism. Weekly reporters may not out-write you, but they'll have *columns* of newshole for a story you may have to do in 300 to 400 words. Choose your words carefully.
- *Television*—especially local cable TV—regards prep sports among its biggest viewer attractions. Many of your readers will *see* tonight the game they'll *read* about in your story tomorrow. See the pressure that puts on you?
- *Local radio* considers prep sports inexpensive yet popular programming. And that means even more of your readers tomorrow will have a framework of understanding they'll use to judge your story.

So, never forget that in small-town journalism you're writing for an audience that 1) might be in the stadium tonight with you and 2) is very passionate about games and how reporters write about them.

No matter where you go eventually in journalism, you'll likely never be closer to readers than you are now, in local sports, or be more subject to their criticism (or, less frequently, the recipient of their praise).

Add to your list of pressures the expectations of fans and their sometimes insanely partisan critiques of your writing. (My favorite example comes from a small-town editor who was telephoned by a woman complaining his newspaper had given the "other" team *28 words* more coverage than the hometown team!)

Know Thyself and Thy Competitors

Is your task of being competitive against other media hopeless when you're working for a newspaper that still puts ink on paper, as Gutenberg did in the 1400s?

Not at all.

In fact, newspapers give you distinct competitive *advantages* even in this electronic era of instantaneous communication.

And, if you play the reporting game smart, you can work around your competitive *disadvantages*.

Understand the strengths and weaknesses of your medium and your competitors if you hope to labor effectively—and win—in the sports-writing arena.

Newspaper Strengths (and Weaknesses)

Here's your basic competitive weakness:

The game ends tonight at, say 9 p.m., and if you're working for a *morning* paper, you have just minutes to write and "file" your story.

You must write quickly because back in the newsroom, editors must process your story along with scores of others that pour in before their first-edition game night deadline of about 11 p.m. to 11:30 p.m.

Presses will roll shortly after midnight so papers can be loaded into trucks and sped toward readers' driveways for arrival, ideally, at about 6 a.m.

That is, you must write at 9 p.m. to 9:30 p.m. tonight, a story that will "stand"—be journalistically valid—at breakfast tables tomorrow morning!

And, at those breakfast tables by the way, reader-fans already may be discussing the game that they attended or saw on television or heard on radio.

If you're working for an afternoon paper, your competitive problem is even worse: What possible angle do you have on a game already seen on television or heard on radio *and read about, as well, in the morning newspaper?*

Much of this book focuses on how you can report and write your way around the terrible time disadvantages suffered by newspapers. For now, keep in mind that newspapers don't try, and haven't for decades, to be first in reporting spot-news details for an event such as a football game. Radio killed that role for newspapers, television put it in a coffin, and the Internet is burying it.

However, newspapers *do* strive—mightily—to report exclusive and unique news angles (which, of course, you'll find only in aggressive off-field reporting, not by simply watching the game from the press box along with all your competitors).

And, importantly, newspaper sportswriting has shifted heavily into interpretive and analytical writing—away from simply who won—and into *why* and *how* they won and deeply into the wider context of what it all means for the game next week or the new season next year.

High premium is put on creative, engaging writing that is *just good reading*—a pleasurable experience for readers even if it takes them back through a game they saw in person or watched on television. Indeed, TV watchers frequently read print versions for something they missed during the telecast or didn't understand at the time, or just to mull over someone else's version of what they saw themselves.

The product of all that—probing reporting and creative, analytical writ-ing—keeps newspapers more than competitive in the sports arena.

There are strengths not to be underestimated: The newspaper is a portable, easily managed and inexpensive compendium that enables you to give readers a principal game story (the "lead" story), "sidebars" (allied stories) of all kinds, plus statistics—long, seemingly unending columns of agate-type summaries, linescores, boxscores, league standings and other esoterica—over which true sports fans pore for hours. Readers don't need a computer to interact with their data source, as a newspaper won't crash. Plus, they can "download" a fully updat-ed version tomorrow for 35¢ to 50¢—less than the cost of a good candy bar!

Finally, for you future sportswriters, the *competition* between print and cyberspace likely will become *cooperation*. Most newspapers (well more than 1,000 of the nearly 1,500 dailies, at last count) publish online services, and it's likely you'll write for both.

Picture it: The game ends and you file urgently a spot-news game story for the Web service—who won, the score and bare highlights. Then you turn to an in-depth analytical piece for tomorrow morning's paper.

Such a combination will give you the best of two worlds, the infinite trans-mission capacity—unlimited newshole—and speed of cyberspace plus the lux-ury of relatively contemplative and insightful writing offered only in print.

Magazine Strengths (and Weaknesses)

Obviously, with newspapers blanketing sports seven days weekly and radio and television leading fans by the hand into the arena, magazines can't offer you a career in competitive sports coverage.

Right?

Wrong.

Magazines, even slower than newspapers in reaching their readers, and near-ly incapable of reporting exclusive angles not already covered by newspapers, radio and television, are *flourishing.*

More than 18,000 magazines are published in the United States, and virtu-ally every one (*Modern Maturity*, included) touches on sports.

Each year, many new magazines devoted exclusively to sports are launched.

In total revenue, *Sports Illustrated*, *Golf Digest*, *Car and Driver* and other magazines devoted exclusively to sports are among the nation's largest, regard-less of content.

Sports Illustrated alone sells more than 3.3 *million* copies weekly (and on average, 4.6 million copies of its annual swimsuit issue). *SI* is the third-largest magazine in subscription revenue (behind only *TV Guide* and *Reader's Digest*).[13]

How can it be, against you-are-there TV coverage and pervasive daily news-paper reporting, that magazines are a major and very competitive sports-news medium?

For these reasons:

- Millions of sports fans, simply put, are insatiable in their interest. Even after watching a game on television tonight, then reading about it in the newspaper tomorrow morning, they'll turn to magazines next week for another sports-writing "fix." Nowhere else in journalism do we enjoy such voracious reader appetites.
- By their very nature, magazines are a perfect "niche" medium that can focus intently on one subject. Magazines don't have the newspaper's responsibility to cover all important news—at home and abroad, in politics and out—in addition to sports. Magazines can go into depth, targeting very narrow reader interests. Note *Guns & Ammo, Backpacker* and *Fur-Fish-Game*.
- Relieved of spot-news missions, magazines also can focus on the truly important element in sports reporting (or any other news sector): people. Magazines are splendid vehicles for 1) colorful profiles of sports figures who do it on field and court, and for 2) how-to-do-it people stories for readers who want to learn how to do it!
- Lacking immediacy and much chance to break hard news, magazines have grown to emphasize excellent writing. They attract some of journalism's best writers, who keep reader-fans panting in anticipation of next week's *SI* or other sports magazines.

Who wouldn't read a magazine that offers this kind of writing, which Mike Lupica delivered in an *Esquire* article on Canadian hockey star Wayne Gretzky at practice:

> Gretzky had come across center ice in his long gray sweat suit, moving like a swan, and had gotten ready to shoot the puck at the goalie. But then, in an instant, the shooting motion was gone, his stick was dropping in front of the puck, Gretzky was making a blind pass behind him, and the man skating on right wing had put the puck into the net. I waited for someone to cheer, the man fixing the boards, or the man behind the skate-rental counter, or the blond girl waiting for the ice so she could become the next Katarina Witt. But it was just Gretzky being Gretzky. ...
> It was like finding Baryshnikov in an Arthur Murray studio.
>
> —Mike Lupica, *Esquire*[14]

Do *you* want to write like that? Well, I can't promise a magic formula, but join me in Chapter Two for more hints on how you can try.

Summary

—To succeed in sportswriting, you must understand how sports coverage fits into the overall news strategy of your newspaper or magazine.

—Sports news follows only general news and entertainment as the news segment most popular with newspaper readers; magazines, radio and television all devote major resources to sports coverage.

—Writers must know their newspaper's *geographic* target, where circulation is concentrated, and the *demographic* target—the age, income and education characteristics of chosen readers.

—To attract readers, sports editors employ staff writers, stringers and The Associated Press, which takes enormous worldwide resources to sports coverage.

—In defining an event's news value, consider *proximity*—whether the event breaks locally *or*, regardless of origin, whether it interests local readers.

—*Impact* is evaluated by the number of people likely affected by an event and how deeply, and is an important yardstick for measuring newsworthiness.

—High priority goes to *timeliness* in evaluating newsworthiness, but in sports modify this as a yardstick because reader-fans have year-round interest in even off-season and relatively low-grade news breaks.

—*Conflict* is one standard for judging newsworthiness in all of journalism, but sophisticated sports reporting goes far beyond the obvious—one team in conflict with another—to find the conflict between coaches, in school rivalries and other forms of competition.

—*Phony conflict* is constructed in sports by promoters and athletic departments eager to sell tickets, but professional sportswriters don't buy into it.

—As in all journalism, *prominence* of individuals in sports adds to their newsworthiness, but keep it under control and don't assign godlike status to athletes simply because they can run fast or throw balls far.

—All of journalism seeks the unusual, off-beat or humorous story; if you see one in sports, lunge for it, and your readers (and editors) will thank you.

—Competition between the media is fierce, and to survive you must learn to use the strengths of your medium and report and write around its weaknesses.

—The newspaper's basic weakness is the time-consuming and cumbersome production and delivery process that forces you to write stories your readers will see many hours hence—well after they've watched on television or listened on radio.

—Your strengths in newspaper sports reporting include the tradition—and newshole—for analytical and interpretive writing that takes readers far beyond who won and into why and how they won and what it all means.

—Because they are even slower in reaching readers, magazines stress thoughtful, insightful reporting and great writing that gives readers with voracious appetites for sports a pleasurable experience.

Exercises

1. Study your local daily newspaper (or a newspaper designated by your instructor) and, in about 400 words, describe the newspaper's apparent overall news strategy and how sports coverage seems to fit into it. Is coverage in the paper predominantly local or does it focus on a wider regional or national picture? Does selection and play of *sports* stories reflect that picture? Judging from newshole and staff writers devoted to sports, does this newspaper regard sports as a principal offering to readers?

2. Study the *front page* of your local newspaper's sports section (or of a newspaper designated by your instructor) and comment, in 350 to 400 words, on how well each story meets the news value checklist described in Chapter One. Do editors and writers seek stories with *proximity*, *impact* and *timeliness*? Do you think *conflict* and *prominence* were among yardsticks used in judging news values? Do you see any *off-beat* or *humorous* stories?

3. Study the sports section of a newspaper designated by your instructor and analyze, in 350 to 400 words, whether writers show awareness of television competition. Do the writers—local and AP—stress analytical and interpretive angles not already explored by the broadcast media? Or do writers stress who won (which TV viewers already know) rather than *why* and *how*—and what it all means?

4. Interview a local sports *editor* (perhaps your instructor will invite one for a classroom interview) on his or her coverage strategies. What role does the editor play in overall news strategies of the newspaper? And in planning sports coverage, what goals are laid down for reporters and writers? Report your interview in about 400 words.

5. Interview a university or local newspaper sportswriter on why he or she entered sports reporting and what career preparation was made. What career hints can the reporter give you and your classmates on *your* career preparation? Be specific in writing guidance the reporter gives. Make your story a how-to-do-it lesson, in 350 to 400 words.

Recommended Reading

Great writers are voracious readers, and an aspiring sportswriter has no better "classroom" than the sports pages of leading newspapers.

Read the sports sections in the *Boston Globe*, all three New York City papers (the *Times*, *News* and *Post*), *Atlanta Journal-Constitution* (one of the nation's best sports sections), *Dallas Morning News*, *Washington Post*, *Philadelphia Inquirer*, *Chicago Tribune*, *Seattle Times*, *Los Angeles Times*, to name a few.

USA Today's sports coverage is so strong that it is among that national newspaper's biggest reader attractions.

Among magazines, you *must* read *Sports Illustrated*, which, even though a weekly, breaks significant sports news in addition to presenting wonderfully insightful essays on subtleties and nuances somehow overlooked in daily journalism. You can spend profitable hours at your local supermarket's magazine rack, feasting in the scores of top-flight sports magazines available.

For a real treat, see David Halberstam, editor, *The Best American Sportswriting of the Century* (Boston: Houghton Mifflin Company, 1999), a superb collection of truly great sportswriting.

News strategies discussed in this chapter for newspapers are covered in depth in Conrad Fink, *Strategic Newspaper Management* (Boston: Allyn and Bacon, 1996) and for magazines in Conrad Fink and Donald E. Fink, *Introduction to Magazine Writing* (New York: Macmillan Publishing Company, 1994).

Also see Douglas A. Anderson, *Contemporary Sports Reporting*, 2nd ed. (Chicago: Nelson-Hall Publishers, 1994) and Heinz-Dietrich Fischer, *Sports Journalism at Its Best* (Chicago: Nelson-Hall Publishers, 1995).

Notes

1. Simmons Market Research Bureau, quoted in Newspaper Association of America's *Facts About Newspapers 1998*, p. 8.

2. I discuss media strategies in depth in Conrad Fink, *Strategic Newspaper Management* (Boston: Allyn and Bacon, 1996), Conrad Fink and Donald E. Fink, *Introduction to Magazine Writing* (New York: Macmillan Publishing Company, 1994), and Conrad Fink, *Inside The Media* (New York: Longman, 1990).

3. For example, Simmons Market Research Bureau noted that of adults earning more than $75,000 annually in 1997, 69 percent read newspapers on weekdays, 78 percent on Sundays. Readership declined steadily with declining income. Details are in *NAA Facts About Newspapers 1998*, op cit.

4. The *Journal-Constitution* made these claims in marketing information quoting Atlanta Consumer Market Study, 1992.

5. Ibid.

6. The *New York Times* and *Journal* aim at readers in the very upper socioeconomic reaches nationwide, as does the *Los Angeles Times*, in Los Angeles County. This nets many readers with $100,000-plus household incomes. All three papers are read by the very wealthiest Americans, as are the magazines cited.

7. Current numbers of dailies and weeklies are available in *NAA Facts About Newspapers*, op cit, for the most recent year.

8. Details of this serious problem of "churn" are available in Conrad Fink, *Strategic Newspaper Management*, op cit.

9. Carl Sessions Stepp, "The State of The American Newspaper," *American Journalism Review*, September 1999, p. 60.

10. The Associated Press, a membership cooperative, offers newspapers a variety of

services devoted exclusively to sports and, for small papers, services featuring carefully selected sports and general news items.

11. I examine news values and judgments in more detail in Conrad Fink, *Introduction to Professional Newswriting* 2nd ed. (New York: Longman, 1998).

12. Operational methods and the competitive status of newspapers, magazines, radio and television are examined in detail in Conrad Fink, *Inside the Media*, op cit.

13. Circulation figures are from "Ticker," *Brill's Content*, June 1999, p. 132; magazine revenue figures are from "Ad Age 300," *Advertising Age*, June 14, 1999, p. S-2, et seq.

14. "Hockey's Only Hope," February 1989, p. 55.

2

What You Owe Your Readers

THE BLOND young woman charged across the soccer field, shouting triumphantly and pumping her clenched fists—then ripped off her jersey and displayed her black sports bra.

On television.

As millions watched.

It was Brandi Chastain, who had just scored the winning penalty kick for the U.S. soccer team in the Women's World Cup.

Was this a beautiful display of youthful exuberance? A joyful, spontaneous celebration of victory?

Or, something more studied?

Across America, sportswriters turned to their keyboards to wonder. Why? Because by taking off her jersey, Chastain revealed not only her bra but also the brand symbol on it—the unmistakable Nike swoosh, known throughout the world as the cutting edge of a multibillion dollar marketing scheme.

Quickly, the debate escalated.

Richard Sandomir of *The New York Times*:

> The sports bra fix had to be in ... Nike stood to gain millions if viewers detected the teensy black-on-black swoosh on Chastain's bra and made the obvious trek to Nike Town. And Chastain *is* a Nike endorser, as are five other teammates.[1]

Noting that Nike denied any conspiracy, Sandomir described the event as "underwear's finest moment."

Which, of course, raised the question of propriety. Sandy Bailey, editor of *Sports Illustrated for Women*, took that on:

> It's perfectly acceptable outerwear. This isn't like men wearing jock straps outside or women wearing thongs in public. A sports bra is a bra in name only. Women wear it outside to jog and to work out in gyms.[2]

Underwear? Bras and jock straps? Marketing conspiracies?

What's going on here?

What's going on is that as a sports journalist today you owe your readers far more than the game story, more than the on-field kick that wins the game or the player error that loses it. And discharging that obligation to readers inevitably takes you deeply into compellingly important questions of fairness and balance, *into the ethics and integrity of journalism.*

Just think of the subcurrents beneath the Chastain story:

- Women's sports struggling for attention from—and fair treatment by—a public and media that historically favor male sports.
- Suggestions of crass commercialism tainting amateur sport.
- Public examination of the motives (and principles) of a young athlete.
- The ethics of highlighting so dramatically the money in women's sports when male-dominated sports have wallowed in marketing money for generations.

It's complicated stuff for reporters to handle, particularly because sports journalists themselves are under scrutiny—as are all journalists—by a public increasingly suspicious of *our* motives, *our* propriety.

Clearly, as you head out to that football game tonight, you need more in your tote bag than reporting and writing skills. You also need a sharply defined personal code of ethics, and that we uncover in Chapter Two, along with a quick look at the basics of libel law.

The Credibility Gap (Yours)

What? *You*, the unknown newcomer to sports journalism, *already* face a credibility gap between you, your work and the reading public?

Yes.

Like it or not, you face, on your first job, an undercurrent of deep unease in public attitudes about the media and those who, like you, report for them.

Researchers funded by the American Society of Newspaper Editors sum up an exhaustive study of public attitudes:

> A probe of the public's mind reveals a troubled image of journalism. The public's fundamental concerns about journalism ... center on accuracy, the newspaper's relationship with its community and perceptions that newspapers too often are biased and tend to over-cover sensational stories.[3]

Further, a concurrent survey of *journalists'* attitudes reveals they agree in large measure with the public's negative assessment!

The research indicates your first goal in delivering what you owe your readers should *not* be trying to emulate the writing magic of Red Smith, Frank Deford, Tom Boswell or any other sportswriter hero you might have.

Rather, you first should turn to five basic considerations.

Accuracy Comes First

The researchers, led by Dr. Christine D. Urban, are blunt:

> The public and the press agree that there are too many factual errors and spelling or grammar mistakes in newspapers. ... Small errors undermine public confidence in the press. ... As far as the public is concerned, there's no excuse for errors.[4]

We journalists blame "deadline pressure" for many of our errors, but the public doesn't buy that excuse. Neither does a huge portion of the public buy into stories pegged to anonymous sources.

Nearly half the readers surveyed in the Urban research say a story should not be published unless sources go on the record and are quoted by name.

Lesson: Readers say the first thing you owe them is an accurate, factual story pegged to identified sources. Your readers are telling you: *Get it right!*

That's not easy in sportswriting.

First, you're dealing with news fully as complex as any in journalism. Writers covering politics, war, business or science don't cover much that's more complicated than football coaching strategy or business management in big-time sports or the psychology of athletes performing under emotional stress.

Second, you're writing for reader-fans fully as expert in your news specialty as are other readers expert in, say, politics, business or science.

Consequently, your reader-fan's *threshold of satisfaction* is very high. To pass the test—to build credibility in your byline—you must avoid errors of fact in statistics-laden writing about who, where, what and when and avoid errors of analysis and interpretation in reporting why and how.

Avoid Harmful Cynicism

Urban's research finds readers complaining that "newspapers don't consistently demonstrate respect for, and knowledge of, their readers and communities."[5]

Translation: Much of the public regards us as cynical, uninformed and quite willing to hurt people in order to get a story.

But, journalists I know make great effort to understand their story and their readers. And, though quite willing to throw a punch if a punch is needed, they do try to avoid harming people needlessly.

So, why the disparity between the public's and press's interpretation of our motives?

Well, Urban, like other researchers, points out that journalists generally aren't representative of the public they serve. That is, you didn't come out of the same starting blocks as your readers. You are younger and better educated than your readers, on average, and even (believe it or not) better paid.

Those disparities, plus your professional culture—the sometimes rough and caustic culture of the newsroom—can yield an approach to the ethical responsibilities of journalism that, put simply, disgusts your public at times.

Think of that tonight in the football stadium as you write about those young men on the field playing their hearts out before adoring parents and fans.

What you owe your readers may well include coverage that is hard-hitting, even cruel in its critique. If so, write it that way. Nothing in this book should make you hesitate before your ultimate responsibility of delivering coverage that is accurate, balanced, fair and at times, hard-hitting.

But write the tough stuff understanding that some reader-fans will conclude angrily that you don't know the game and its larger community of players, parents and fans. They'll conclude you're just trying to sell newspapers.

One good rule to follow: If what you see on the field tonight is a laughable performance, *let your reporting—objective and dispassionate—reveal that*. Don't let your reporting wallow in systemic cynicism; don't let your writing drip with unbroken sarcasm.

Write It Straight, Without Bias

Research shows many of your readers will go through your story tomorrow morning suspecting you of foisting your point of view—your bias—on them. Urban notes:

> The public suspects that the points of view and biases of journalists influence what stories are covered and how they are covered. ...
>
> All we want is fair play and neutrality, and please keep your opinions on the editorial page, Americans say. Don't kid us. We know that journalists write for their editors, not their readers.[6]

Again, in Urban's research, as well as in other studies, it's clear that a majority of Americans think newspapers are concerned principally with making money, not serving the public interest.

However, understand the word "bias" stirs complicated emotions. When he was chairman of Dow Jones & Co. Inc., publisher of *The Wall Street Journal*, Warren M. Phillips, commented:

> Could it be that bias sometimes is in the eye of the beholder? Do we sometimes have slanted readers?
>
> People are so committed, so involved, so agitated in this age of change and controversy and instant communications that many of them look for newspaper accounts of events ... to reinforce and agree with their own views, even their prejudices. If they don't get that, they often feel the press is not credible.[7]

That is, if your reporting tonight reveals that Team A played a lousy game, you're likely to be accused by some reader-fans of being biased toward Team B. Part of becoming a professional in this business is learning to take heat from readers who favor shooting the messenger because they don't like the message.

However, there indeed are special traps in sportswriting that can pull you away from objective writing and into subjective, opinionated writing that some readers will perceive as biased. Note:

- Many sportswriters are fervent sports fans themselves, and many cover sports and teams they've adored since childhood. Thus does "boosterism"—unthinking, uncritical coverage of the home team—raise its ugly head. It's easy to get sucked into the camaraderie of a locker room, easy to get swept along by thousands of fans noisily pulling for the hometown heroes. Stay cool.
- The very nature of modern sportswriting, even on an ostensibly spot-news story such as tonight's football game, can pull you into subjective analysis. It's in reporting the how and why and the look-ahead meaning

of an event, so essential when you're competing against television, that you must analyze and interpret. And that's where you can slip unthinkingly into reporting and writing that may be perceived as biased.

Beware of Sensationalism

An overwhelming majority of Americans tell researchers that journalists sensationalize the news to sell newspapers and, further, that we enjoy doing so.

Add this to what your readers say you owe them: fewer "sensational" stories that, as Urban says, "grind on and on."[8]

This is tricky business.

For example, is it "sensational" to report that a football player is arrested for using illegal drugs? Or, is that information the discerning reader-fan not only wants but *needs* to know?

Is it "sensational" to report the player's second brush with the law? His third? Fourth? Does continuing coverage of his drug problem "grind on and on"? Sure, it does, but isn't it news?

It's often in the eye of the beholder that the line is drawn between "sensationalism" and reporting valid news of compelling importance to readers. But even among journalists there is suspicion that some stories *are* sensationalized and *are* strung out for too long by newspapers that, as Urban says, "are really chasing Pulitzer Prizes or overly aggressive reporters ... trying to make a name for themselves."

Your challenge: develop a balanced sense of news values and judgment that leads you into a full and probing examination of a news event but that stops you short of "milking" it for prize-winning impact beyond its intrinsic news value.

Double-Check and Consider "Privacy"

Readers value investigative reporting, Urban finds, but they want you to:

- hold a story until you've double-checked accuracy.
- withhold suspects' names until charges are filed.
- not report long-ago love affairs ("amorous shenanigans," in Urban's words) of public figures.
- do more to protect the privacy of people in the news.

No principled journalist would publish a story whose accuracy is questionable. Right? Who would short-circuit the legal system and convict people in the press before they have their day in court? Or who would dig through old love affairs or invade someone's privacy?

Well, *you* might be tempted to do so.

Picture it:

You have an extremely important story. And you fear aggressive competitors will scoop you if you hold too long. You're 98 percent certain all facts check out. Are you going to hold for the final 2-percent check?

Or, you learn the star quarterback is swept up in a drug raid—but formal charges aren't filed yet. Are you going to hold that one?

Or, a star third baseman who has risen to fame in part through press coverage of his clean All-American lifestyle, which wins him millions in product endorsements, is revealed to be a secret womanizer. But now, of course, he says his lifestyle is private, none of your business—or the public's. Going to hold?

Now, What to Do?

Are there answers universally accepted among journalists to the ethical questions you'll ask? No.

Is there a rule or a standard procedure to follow on pretrial publicity for the quarterback seized but not charged in a drug raid? No.

Is there a definitive answer to whether you should respect that womanizing third baseman's demand for privacy? No.

No. But there *are* guidelines developed by journalism associations and individual newspapers that will help you develop your personal approach to the ethics and social responsibility of journalism.

Note *personal*. Adherence to a code of ethics or operating standards is not a condition for calling yourself a journalist, as it is if you want to practice medicine or law. Indeed some journalists say even general and voluntary guidelines must be avoided because codes of any sort serve to restrict press freedom and, additionally, could encourage courts and legislatures to convert guidelines into laws, counter to the First Amendment's free press guarantee.

Nevertheless, existing codes can help you sort out your thinking on ethical issues you inevitably will encounter on and off the playing field. Key points:

A Journalist's Basic Responsibility

In its "Statement of Principles," The American Society of Newspaper Editors, a leading professional organization, lays on you what it calls a "particular responsibility":

> Journalism demands of its practitioners not only industry and knowledge but also the pursuit of a standard of integrity proportionate to the journalist's singular obligation. ...
>
> The primary purpose of gathering and distributing news and opinion is to serve the general welfare by informing the people and enabling them to make judgments on the issues of the time. Newspaper men and women who

abuse the power of their professional role for selfish motives or unworthy purposes are faithless to that public trust.

The American press was made free not just to inform or just to serve as a forum for debate *but also to bring an independent scrutiny to bear on the forces of power in the society*, including the conduct of official power at all levels of government (*emphasis added*).[9]

The Society of Professional Journalists, in its "Code of Ethics," puts a sharp point on its definition of your basic responsibility:

The public's right to know of events of public importance and interest is the overriding mission of the mass media.[10]

The Washington Post, like many newspapers, has its own code of ethics, which is a *condition of employment* for all reporters and editors. The *Post* outlines their responsibility:

The Washington Post is pledged to an aggressive, responsible and fair pursuit of the truth without fear of any special interest, and with favor to none.[11]

The *Post*'s code requires reporters to approach "every assignment with the fairness of open minds and without prior judgment" and to routinely search for opposing views and comments from persons accused or challenged in stories—and to do so without "arrogance."

Maintaining Your Independence

In all of journalism—and particularly in sports reporting—you'll walk a fine line between getting cozy with sources to unlock news but not getting so close that you sacrifice your independence.

The American Society of Newspaper Editors takes a hard line on that:

Journalists must avoid impropriety and the appearance of impropriety as well as any conflict of interest or the appearance of conflict. They should neither accept anything nor pursue any activity that might compromise or seem to compromise their integrity.

The Society of Professional Journalists' code puts it this way:

Journalists must be free of obligation to any interest other than the public's right to know the truth.

The Washington Post warns reporters to avoid conflict of interest "or the appearance of conflict of interest" and gets specific: pay your own way, accept no gifts or free tickets and avoid active involvement in "any partisan causes." The code adds:

> We make every reasonable effort to be free of obligation to news sources and to special interests. We must be wary of entanglements with those whose positions render them likely to be subjects of journalistic interest and examination. Our private behavior as well as our professional behavior must not bring discredit on our profession or to the *Post*.

Dedicate Yourself to Fair Play

It comes under many headings in codes of ethics: honest journalism, impartiality and objectivity. The Society of Professional Journalists calls it "fair play" and describes it this way:

> Journalists at all times will show respect for the dignity, privacy, rights and well-being of people encountered in the course of gathering and presenting the news.
> 1. The news media should not communicate unofficial charges affecting reputation or moral character without giving the accused a chance to reply.
> 2. The news media must guard against invading a person's right to privacy.
> 3. The media should not pander to morbid curiosity about details of vice and crime.
> 4. It is the duty of the news media to make prompt and complete correction of their errors.
> 5. Journalists should be accountable to the public for their efforts, and the public should be encouraged to voice its grievances against the media. Open dialogue with our readers, viewers or listeners should be fostered.

So, newspaper and association codes give you general guidance for handling ethical dilemmas. But helpful specifics are in a code drawn especially for sports reporters.

What Sports Editors Say About Ethics

The leading professional organization in sports journalism is Associated Press Sports Editors (APSE), an association of editors drawn from newspapers that are members of The Associated Press.

AP, a news-exchange cooperative, has the largest sports-news service in the world. AP Sports Editors independently monitors AP's sports services and suggests improvements.

Let's examine a code of ethics drawn up by the sports editors:[12]

Pay Your Own Way

The APSE code turns first to "freebies," or free gifts and free food—the "free ride" common in an earlier era of sportswriting when reporters traveled, ate and drank with teams, at team expense.

In those bygone days, ties between reporters, teams and people they covered were close—scandalously close, at times—and conflict of interest, real and perceived, cast doubt on press credibility.

The APSE's code is adamant:

1. The newspaper pays its staffer's way for travel, accommodations, food and drink.
   (a) If a staffer travels on a chartered team plane, the newspaper should insist on being billed. If the team cannot issue a bill, the amount can be calculated by estimating the cost of a similar flight on a commercial airline.
   (b) When services are provided to a newspaper by a pro or college team, those teams should be reimbursed by the newspaper. This includes providing telephone, typewriter or fax service.

Restrict Your Free-lancing

Another tradition of days bygone in sports journalism was permitting reporters to pick up an extra buck or two through free-lancing for virtually any organization. Many writers today free-lance, but the editors' code counsels an important restriction: don't free-lance for the organization you cover.

2. Editors and reporters should avoid taking part in outside activities or employment that might create conflict of interest or even appearance of a conflict.
   (a) They should not serve as an official scorer at baseball games.
   (b) They should not write for team or league media guides or other team or league publications. This has the potential of compromising a reporter's disinterested observations.
   (c) Staffers who appear on radio or television should understand that their first loyalty is to the paper.

Take No Deals or Discounts

Big-time sports *drips* money. Major league franchises are worth hundreds of millions of dollars; athletes are paid tens of millions. Even at the college level, big-time sports equals big money.

With so much money being passed around, sportswriters must beware of being influenced by the rich environment in which they work or engaging in practices that create the perception of conflict of interest.

The sportswriters' code addresses this in no-nonsense language:

3. Writers and writers' groups should adhere to Associated Press Managing Editors and APSE standards: No deals, discounts or gifts except those of insignificant value or those available to the public.
   (a) If a gift is impossible or impractical to return, donate the gift to charity.
   (b) Do not accept free memberships or reduced fees for membership. Do not accept gratis use of facilities, such as golf courses or tennis courts, unless it is used as part of doing a story for the newspaper.
   (c) Sports editors should be aware of standard of conduct of groups and professional associations to which their writers belong and the ethical standards to which those groups adhere, including areas such as corporate sponsorship from news sources it covers.

And That Includes No Tickets

APSE gives separate and special treatment to an old practice in sports: giving free tickets to newspapers beyond press box credentials.

The code states:

4. A newspaper should not accept free tickets, although press credentials needed for coverage and coordination are acceptable.

Beware of Award Voting

It happens frequently, and it's flattering. But think about the implications.

Not long into your sportswriting career you'll be asked to vote in a poll or survey on who is the best athlete or which team is the best. It's flattering because being asked signals that somebody presumes you're an expert.

But, first, the whole process of voting for the All-American this or the All-American that is of doubtful news validity. After all, can a sportswriter in the Southeast really know enough about teams or athletes in the Northwest or Northeast or other distant regions to make sound rankings of national prowess?

Second, voting is a commitment, an investment of sorts in the athlete or team for which you cast your ballot. That, in turn, raises the spectre of unthinking, unblinking boosterism—backing the favored athlete or team, regardless.

APSE's code doesn't counsel outright against participating in polls (fans love them) but it does wave a warning flag.

5. A newspaper should carefully consider the implications of voting for all awards and all-star teams and decide if such voting creates a conflict of interest.

Watch Those Unnamed Sources

For generations, many sportswriters considered themselves different and apart from the rest of journalism.

Even Red Smith, one of our greatest sportswriters, called sports the "toy department," implying sports reporting had a mission different from other forms of news reporting and that sports reporters thus operated under different rules.

Not so, says APSE: Sports reporters must follow their newspaper's code of ethics (and, by implication, industry association codes, if their newspaper doesn't have one).

APSE pays particular attention to unnamed sources:

> 6. A newspaper's own ethical guidelines should be followed, and editors and reporters should be aware of standards acceptable for use of unnamed sources and verification of information obtained other than from primary news sources.
> (a) Sharing and pooling of notes and quotes should be discouraged. If a reporter uses quotes gained secondhand, that should be made known to the readers. A quote could be attributed to a newspaper or to another reporter.

The reference to pooling ties back to the traditional friendships of the press box and what can be dangerous sharing of information among sportswriters. Press box lore tells of reporters even filing dispatches not only for their own newspapers but also for competing papers because reporter-friends for some reason themselves could not write ("some reason" frequently being heavy drinking, another dangerous tradition of the press box).

In such a friendly environment, a practice developed of sharing information: One reporter would visit the winner's locker room, for example, and come back with quotes; another would cover the losers—and quotes and other information would be shared.

Today, intense competition between reporters is the best insurance that readers will receive the best possible reporting and writing. Pooling erodes that guarantee.

Pooling also puts you in the position of reporting information you personally cannot verify. This becomes a serious ethical lapse, particularly if you relay the information as your own.

Sometimes, pooling is inescapable—for example, when only a limited number of reporters can be accommodated physically. In such cases, an AP reporter often is selected because that news service represents thousands of newspaper and broadcast outlets, and two or three other reporters might be picked also. In using such "pool reports," it's an ethical requirement that you explain for readers the circumstances under which you obtained information.

Eliminate Race and Gender Inequities

APSE is adamant:

> 7. Assignments should be made on merit, without regard for race or gender.

APSE speaks like this to the sports world we cover as much as to the editors who assign reporters without regard to race or gender. APSE says teams must give reporters, male or female, equal access to the news.

The most troubling friction point has been ensuring female sportswriters have equal access with male reporters in male-dominated sports, such as football.

For generations, sportswriters (all males) wandered through locker rooms, interviewing athletes before or after their showers (or, *in* the shower, as one of my colleagues did following a heavyweight boxing match).[13] That didn't work when female reporters arrived in sports, and newspapers insisted that teams provide "interview rooms" or other access where presumably fully-dressed athletes could meet reporters of both sexes.

Today, women are succeeding at top newspapers in sports reporting, once almost exclusively male.

Use Common Sense

APSE concludes its code with this:

> Guidelines can't cover everything. Use common sense and good judgment in applying these guidelines in adopting local codes.

The difficulty, of course, is that "common sense" varies among individuals, arising as it does out of different attitudes and life experiences. Obviously, different sportswriters view ethical issues different ways.

Is there a more methodical approach to ethics that doesn't rely on what sometimes is unreliable "common sense"? Yes.

Making Decisions on Your Own

When confronted with an ethical dilemma, you can make decisions based on something more substantial and more reliable than "common sense."

Use a five-step process:

1. Assemble all the facts. This can be more difficult than it looks. For example, deciding how—or whether—to write about a woman soccer player ripping off her jersey and displaying her bra requires assembling facts on her explanation, the sponsoring company's policies, and coach and co-player attitudes. The list of required background facts is long.

2. Identify the ethical issue you face. Is it the reader's right and need to know vs. a young player's right to exuberant victory celebration? Is it news vs. voyeurism? Often, you'll find *several* ethical issues arising out of what might appear to be a simple equation.

3. Consider your alternatives. To write it or not? To write it but in language that makes doffing a jersey spontaneous and joyful? Or to write it as a studied, paid-for TV commercial?

4. Decide what you should do.

5. Do it—write it as you think it should be written, pulling no punches.

But what values and principles go into such judgments? Structured moral reasoning can flow from an approach devised by Dr. Ralph Potter at Harvard University.[14]

Consider Societal Values

Potter's approach, modified and adapted by scholars in ethics, requires journalists to consider societal values generally accepted by a majority of citizens as characteristics important to civilized society.

That is, approaching the jersey-jerking story, you would use a checklist:

- ✓ Truth-telling. It's basic to civilized society, of course, and requires journalists to write the truth. Do not shade it, and do not fabricate it. To lie is to commit cardinal sin in journalism.

- ✓ Justice. That's reward or punishment as deserved, not based on race, color, creed, gender or socioeconomic status. That is, report and write in accordance with a story's news values, dealing even-handedly with people you cover.

- ✓ Humaneness. Don't needlessly harm people; help them when you can and, as a journalist, try to minimize harm to those thrust into the news.

- ✓ Freedom. It's in the American fabric and, certainly, journalism. Stay free of any association, ideology, group or person that might restrict your freedom to cover the news on its merits.

- ✓ Stewardship. If you benefit from a system—freedom of the press, for example—your responsibility is to protect it and extend it to others.

Other societal values include the *Golden Rule* (treat that soccer player as you think you should be treated); the *Golden Mean* (is there a way to write your story without skewering her but not ignoring the news?); *promise-keeping* (keeping your word and fulfilling contracts) and *loyalty* (to self, employers and peers).

But, there's more.

Consider Journalistic Principles

Generations of journalists have developed job-related principles that flow from broader societal values. Consider these:

Serve the public. Among principled practitioners of our craft, this ultimately is what journalism is all about. We are surrogates of the public, serving the needy and the voiceless. We report and write to meet the public's right and need to know. Think first of your public when resolving an ethical dilemma.

Monitor the powerful. It's implicit in the First Amendment and the social contract between the press and public. We are watchdogs of the public interest, and that includes monitoring—and holding accountable—powerful institutions in society. Increasingly, those powerful institutions today include sports organizations.

Be balanced and fair. Equal treatment of all persons in the news, regardless of their fame or wealth (or lack thereof), is implicit in fair journalism, as is reporting all sides of an issue. Many journalists consider balanced and fair reporting and writing attainable, whereas "objectivity" is not because no one, it is argued, can be truly free of his or her own background or attitudes. But objectivity—dispassionate and even-handed treatment of the news—is a very worthwhile goal.

Be compassionate. The media spotlight lands on people in the news. Some seek it and deserve it, some don't. Can you cover the news—the young soccer player—as you must, yet do so with compassion and respect?

Be independent. This requires staying free of influences that might skew your reporting. That's why the Associated Press Sports Editors' code warns so harshly against taking gifts and favors.

Be courageous. There *is* a penalty sometimes attached to doing the right thing. Don't want to embarrass that young soccer player? Wait until your editor sees that incident reported in a competing newspaper but not your own. Jobs can hang in the balance when ethical issues arise.

Consider Your Loyalties

During the decision-making process in ethics, you'll be tugged by conflicting loyalties. To whom, or what, do you owe first loyalty? Self? Public? Employer? Truth? Compassion? Sports?

Three sectors are of particular concern:

Loyalty to self and conscience. If nothing else, codes of ethics written by journalists' associations and newspapers reveal an admirable effort to foster integrity and professionalism in journalism. Principled journalists who accept that spirit develop a *professional conscience*, which you must consult first when ethical questions arise.

Ethics in journalism is highly personal. No written code relieves you of personal responsibility for judgment calls in ethics. So, listen to what your conscience whispers; it might be your first signal that an ethical problem has arisen. Then, make a decision that will make you feel good when you look in a mirror.

Loyalty to society. No problem, right? Journalists serve society. Our readers' interests and needs motivate us. But nevertheless, conflicts abound.

For example, to serve society must you expose an individual in the news to the cruel spotlight of unwanted publicity? Does your responsibility to society ever outweigh responsibility to your employer? Will you refuse to write a story that is ordered by your editor but which you think is contrary to broader societal needs? Will you, that is, put aside loyalty to self and risk your job in a confrontation with your editor over that story? You *do* have a responsibility to your employer.

Loyalty to the hand that feeds you. Must it exist? Or, does your responsibility end with delivering 40 hours or so of honest labor each week in return for a paycheck?

After all, you *were* hired to help get the newspaper out each day. And, whether written or implied, a contract exists under which you agree to work as directed.

Many journalists, however, develop loyalty that goes far beyond job responsibility. Many have enormous pride in the newspapers they work for and perform with loyal intensity and competitive effort not found in many other occupations.

But, again, the potential conflict arises: When ethical dilemmas develop, where does your first loyalty lie? Certainly, the hand that feeds you has strong pull on your loyalty, but does loyalty to public—indeed, to self—ever pull harder?

In journalism, or in books about journalism, writers try to not only pose questions but also provide answers. In ethics, as you've seen by now, there are no rule books and no answers chiseled in stone. That may leave more questions than answers before you right now. But, you *can* develop a decision-making process, based perhaps on the five steps outlined here, and arrive at a principled professionalism that opens for you a career based on journalistic integrity.

Now, Briefly, the Law

First, a warning:

Entire books—*libraries*—are written on press law. Full treatment of the subject is far beyond the scope of this book. And, I am not a lawyer.

So, take what follows as only the beginning of what must be your careful study of relevant press law. As you head to that football game tonight, remember that the legal environment in which you work is, in a word, dangerous.

Here's what's happening:

Many individuals offended by what's written about them want a reporter or editor to *listen* to their complaints but get brushed off far short of a fair hearing, let alone a corrective story. Already thinking, as research shows, that the media are cold, distant and arrogant, many offended individuals then take what they say is the only step open to them: They call a libel lawyer.

In court, a newspaper, or individual reporter, faces an uphill battle. Juries, after all, are drawn from a wider public already suspicious of the press, and by a wide margin they return verdicts against media defendants in libel trials. Juries often make huge awards—in the millions of dollars, sometimes—and in many cases, punish the media, tacking on punitive awards for additional millions.

Upon appeal, many verdicts against the media are overturned. Huge monetary awards often are reduced. *However*, the cost of defending against libel suits is so high that, win or lose, the profit levels of newspapers and careers of individual reporters can be affected.

What's new in all that? This: The parade into court is being joined by public figures and officials once regarded as open to, and accepting of, intense press scrutiny. From the president of the United States and on down the line, public officials and figures are arguing that they, just like private individuals, have the right to unsullied reputations and that whether they seek the spotlight or not, they too have around them a "zone of privacy" the press must not penetrate.

Thus, a former boxer sues *Sports Illustrated* over an article about fixing fights and using cocaine. The jury awards him $8.5 million.

Thus, a professional golfer takes action against a newspaper on grounds he was held in false light.

Throughout sports, athletes serve notice that they will not open some things, including their private lives, to press scrutiny—and will sue trespassers.[15]

So, learn the basics of libel law.

What Is Libel?

Libel is written defamation that, in turn, is *injury to reputation*. It exposes a person, or a *business*, to dislike, hatred, ridicule or disgrace.

In particular, beware any story that alleges criminal behavior, incompetence, inefficiency, immoral, fraudulent or other dishonorable conduct. Particularly dangerous is any story that harms professional reputation and causes financial loss to a person or business.

Your risk is obvious: Modern sportswriting frequently takes you far from the playing field and into the private lives and conduct of athletes. *Our* argument is that the private conduct of public figures can be important news; increasingly, *their* argument is that they deserve off-field privacy.

Your risk increases because of the money in sports. If your story causes financial loss to an individual or business (read that, *sports* business), your risk compounds. Athletes today earn millions in product endorsements, which can be jeopardized by stories on, say, wife abuse, drunk driving or cocaine use.

Libel lawsuits, which are costly to pursue, sometimes are called the "rich man's relief." Many athletes you cover are rich.

Other things to remember:

- A libel must be *published*. But that can be in a memo to your editor or an e-mail message to a friend, as well as in a sports section. A libel may have been published if someone other than the writer and target saw the offending material.
- To prove libel, a person must prove he or she was *identified*. But that doesn't require name, age and address. Identification may have been made if a reasonable person could infer identity from your story. So, being vague, as in "a former linebacker for the Chicago Bears," doesn't protect you if thousands of Bears fans immediately know who you mean.
- Libel doesn't require literal language. The context of a statement or *overall impression* it creates can defame, too. Don't write in indirect nuances and subtleties about that former linebacker if a jury can draw the impression that you are saying he is a wife-beater.

Defending Against Lawsuits

The First Amendment ("Congress shall make no law ... abridging the freedom of speech, or the press.") is the constitutional foundation of the freest and hardest-hitting media in the world—ours.

Subsequent court rulings added protections for the press—but also defined openings for plaintiffs who might want to sue you.

In summary, it's essential in our litigious society that you *write defensively*. Note:

- The *only* absolute defense in a libel action is truth, *but* you must be able to prove the truth of what you write. That includes quotes by or information from sources.
- You have *qualified privilege* in reporting accurately and without malice official proceedings and most official records. But:

✓ What or who is official varies from state to state, so be certain you check local law.

✓ "Malice" is interpreted as publishing information you knew was false *or* publishing it with "reckless disregard" of whether it was true or false. Public officials and figures generally must prove malice and thus carry a heavier burden of proof than a private individual who sues.

"Neutral reportage" is a defense some courts recognize for fair and balanced "neutral" reporting of charges and countercharges made about public officials or figures by responsible individuals and organizations (such as coaches criticizing, say, umpires).

In invasion of privacy cases, your defense is strengthened if there is *current newsworthiness* in the event you're covering. That might cover your story about a famous athlete seized last night in a drug raid; it might not cover dredging up a story about what the athlete did as a teenager 20 years ago.

In writing opinion columns, keep two things in mind:

1. There is strong defense in "fair comment and criticism" *if* you publish opinion and comment on matters of *public interest or importance* and if you *write fairly and with honest purpose.*

2. Your *facts* must be provably true. Courts have held there is no such thing as inaccurate opinion, but they will look carefully at the facts you publish in your opinion piece.

For example, you may be safe expressing this *opinion*: "I think coach Fred Smith does a lousy job of preparing his players academically."

But, unless you can prove it, you're in big danger by writing this as a *factual statement*: "Coach Fred Smith cheats and breaks the rules to gain academic eligibility for players."

To avoid lawsuits:

• Be fair, accurate and balanced in your reporting and writing.
• Have sound journalistic reason for your stories.
• Give all parties a chance to comment.
• Write in objective, nonjudgmental language.
• Be extra careful with any story that harms reputations.

But what if you *still* get a complaint?

How to Handle a Complaint

When the telephone call comes (as it *will* during your career) with the complaint that, "You've libeled me," keep these points in mind:

If it's a lawyer calling, hang up. Only lawyers talk to lawyers. What you say might dig you into a deeper hole. ("Gee, you might be right; that *does* look libelous. Sure didn't when I wrote it last night." Bingo. You've acknowledged error.)

If your caller is not a lawyer, stay cool, courteous and professional. *But listen only.* "Please tell me what offends you," is a good line. Make no comments on the merits (or lack of) in the complaint.

When you have full details, including name and address of the complainant, go immediately to your supervising editor. Avoid the very human impulse to handle this yourself by telling the caller, "I'll write another story tomorrow that will correct this one."

Editors are paid to keep you—and thus the newspaper and themselves—out of trouble. Make *your* problem *their* problem; let the solution be an institutional solution. That may be an attempt by a senior editor to "talk down" the angry complainant or a call for the newspaper's attorney to prepare for battle.

In talking to your editor and attorney, be fully forthcoming. Avoid another very human impulse of disguising any errors in your story. Only with full and frank revelation by you can the newspaper properly assess how to proceed.

Summary

—Research shows deep public distrust of journalists' motives, so even as a beginning sportswriter you have a credibility gap with the reading public.

—Your first requirement is accuracy in your reporting and writing; get it right, readers say.

—Dr. Christine D. Urban, in research for the American Society of Newspaper Editors, finds readers saying we don't respect readers or communities, and we are cynical and out simply to get a story so we can sell newspapers.

—Readers also say they want bias-free reporting, but bias often is in the eye of the beholder.

—Readers complain too many stories are sensational and "grind on and on," which poses problems for journalists covering dramatic but newsworthy stories that indeed do last a long time.

—Readers want us to hold stories until they're double-checked and protect the privacy of people in the news.

—Ethics codes developed by professional journalism associations and individual newspapers lay out voluntary guidelines helpful in resolving ethical dilemmas.

—Codes counsel journalists to serve first the public, stay independent from conflicts of interest and dedicate themselves to fair, balanced journalism.

—The APSE, the leading professional organization of sportswriters, warns particularly against accepting free gifts and free-lancing that creates conflict of interest.

—APSE warns against overuse of unnamed sources and "pooling" (sharing) information with other sportswriters.

—In solving ethical dilemmas, consider societal values, such as truth-telling, humaneness, the Golden Rule and journalistic principles, such as serve the public, monitor the powerful and be compassionate and courageous.
—Understanding libel law is crucial because athletes, like other public figures and officials, increasingly are suing to protect their reputations and privacy.
—Libel is written defamation, which is injury to reputation exposing a person or business to dislike, hatred, ridicule, disgrace; provable truth is the only absolute defense.

Exercises

1. Read the sports section for four consecutive days in a newspaper designated by your instructor and, in about 350 words, describe whether the reporting and writing meet your reader-fan *threshold of satisfaction*, as described in Chapter Two. Do writers exhibit a level of professionalism and expertise that meet the likely needs and wants of discerning readers or, in your opinion, does a credibility gap exist between the newspaper and its reader-fans?

2. Interview a coach or sports official designated by your instructor (perhaps one will be invited to your class) on how sports reporting and writing generally are perceived in the sports (not newspaper) world. Does this subject of our coverage agree with so many in the general public that we often are inaccurate, cynical and quite willing to hurt people to get a story and sell newspapers? In about 300 words, describe what the interviewee says about press coverage.

3. In about 350 words, discuss whether you regard athletes at all levels—high school into the pros—as "public figures" open to intense media scrutiny. Should the private lives of public figures be open to examination? If yes, under all circumstances or just some? If no, why not? Should reporters respect a "zone of privacy" around athletes?

4. Of all the ethical challenges reporters face, as discussed in Chapter Two and the ethics codes therein, which single area of ethics do you think is most crucial for sportswriters? Are you most concerned about freebies or conflicts of interest or privacy or fair play? What must a reporter do to avoid the ethical dilemma that you think is most important? Write this in 250 to 300 words.

5. Interview at least three authoritative sources—reporters, editors, journalism or law professors—on legal *and* ethical implications in use of unnamed sources. In about 400 words, describe what your interviewees say about whether too many anonymous sources are quoted by reporters and whether that practice creates a credibility gap between the press and public. Conclude with *your* opinion. Should unnamed sources ever be used? If yes, under what circumstances? If no, wouldn't many stories that the public needs and want never see light?

Recommended Reading

"Examining Our Credibility," published in 1999 by Christine D. Urban for the American Society of Newspaper Editors, is an enormously impressive examination of public attitudes toward the press. It's available at ASNE Foundation, Publications Fulfillment, 11690B Sunrise Valley Drive, Reston, VA 20191-1409.

I examine ethics in *Media Ethics* (Boston: Allyn and Bacon, 1995); newspaper applications are in my *Introduction to Professional Newswriting,* 2nd ed. (New York: Longman, 1998); ethics from a magazine writer's perspective is studies in *Introduction to Magazine Writing* (New York: Macmillan Publishing Company, 1993). For ethics in advocacy journalism see my *Writing Opinion for Impact* (Ames: Iowa State University Press, 1999) and in business journalism, *Business News Writing* (Ames: Iowa State University Press, 2000).

An excellent working journalist's approach to libel law is in *The Associated Press Stylebook and Libel Manual.* Fuller treatment is in Kent R. Middleton, Bill F. Chamberlin, Matthew D. Bunker, *The Law of Public Communication,* 4th ed. (New York: Longman, 1997).

Other resources:

Student Press Law Center, 1815 N. Fort Meyer Drive, Suite 900, Arlington, VA 22209, (703) 807-1904, splc@splc.org, www.aplc.org.

Reporters Committee for Freedom of the Press, 1815 N. Fort Meyer Drive, Suite 900, Arlington, VA 22209, (800) 336-4243, rcfp@rcfp.org, www.rcfp.org.

Notes

1. Richard Sandomir, "Sports Business," *The New York Times,* July 18, 1999, p. SP-6.
2. Ibid.
3. "Examining Our Credibility," a research report published in 1999 by Christine D. Urban for the American Society of Newspaper Editors, ASNE Foundation, 11690B Sunrise Valley Drive, Reston, VA 20191-1409.
4. Ibid, p. 5.
5. Ibid, p. 5.
6. Ibid, p. 6.
7. See fuller discussion in Conrad Fink, *Media Ethics* (New York: McGraw-Hill, 1988), p. 58.
8. "Examining Our Credibility," op cit, p. 6.
9. For full text see Conrad Fink, *Media Ethics* (Boston: Allyn and Bacon, 1995), p. 305.
10. Ibid, p. 309.
11. Ibid, p. 130-135.
12. Ibid, p. 331.

13. My colleague was Charlie Chamberlain, AP Chicago sportswriter who decided—in the shower—that he would request transfer out of sports and into general news. His request was granted.

14. For details, see Conrad Fink, *Media Ethics* (Boston: Allyn and Bacon, 1999), p. 8.

15. AP dispatch for morning papers of June 11, 1999, which appears in "Boxer Awarded $8.5 Million in Libel Suit," *The New York Times*, that date, p. C-6.

PART TWO

Our Blocking and Tackling: Strong Reporting

L ike the athletes you cover, you need strong fundamentals to play the game—in your case, the lively game of sports-writing.

Of all fundamentals in journalism, strong reporting skills are most important. They are to you what blocking and tackling are to football players, a smooth backswing to golfers and flawless fielding to baseball players.

Become a strong reporter, and you can succeed even if you aren't a great writer. It's worth emphasizing. If Red Smith you are not, and if a great wordsmith you never will be, don't despair.

First, Red wasn't born a great writer, either. He worked *hard* at writing, once likening it to sitting down at a typewriter and cutting open a vein. Developing your writing ability is an unending (and painful) process.

Second, however, many successful careers are built in journalism on strong reporting fundamentals with an overlay of good but not great writing—writing that communicates simply and clearly, even if it doesn't soar or roar.

Reporting is so important that we devote both chapters to it in Part Two.

Chapter Three, Reporting the Key Elements, explores the combination of statistics and factors, such as turning points and star performance, that must buttress any well-reported sports story.

In Chapter Four, Reporting the Wider Picture, we move off-field and into the broader sports story of organized games as a societal phenomenon. In sports reporting, at times you'll think you're covering legal affairs, medical news or the business beat.

3

Reporting the Key Elements

Do you see a striking similarity in the following leads?

NEW YORK—The ball landed long and Serena Williams could not move. Her legs buckled, her arms fell to her side, one hand rose to her heart.

"Oh, my God," she gasped. "I won."

Late yesterday afternoon, the powerful 17-year-old from Compton, Calif., won the U.S. Open when she beat top-seeded Martina Hingis in an emotional second-set tie-breaker.

Frank Fitzpatrick
The Philadelphia Inquirer[1]

OAKLAND, CALIF.—There would be no executioner's song here yesterday afternoon. The Athletics live for another day, and may yet be drawing breath in October.

The Red Sox? On an afternoon in which a killer's instinct would have been as welcome in Boston as it always is here in nearby Alcatraz, the Sox spared the A's, making three errors in a 6-2 loss to Oakland that kept the wild-card differential at three games with 22 left.

"Three errors, five hits—you know it's going to be a long day," said center fielder Darren Lewis, whose fifth-inning overthrow of third base was sandwiched between misdirected offerings from rookie Donnie Sadler in the first and rookie third baseman Wilton Veras in the sixth, the three errors leading to four unearned runs.

"I'm human, I make mistakes," said Lewis, who has made a career of keeping those mistakes to a minimum and has the Gold Glove to prove it. "That's just the way the game goes."

Gordon Edes
The Boston Globe[2]

Steve Young moved slowly through the 49ers locker room yesterday, doing the Fred Sanford shuffle on aching legs, both of which were cut and bandaged. His throwing hand sported a compression wrap. The man looked like he'd been in a train wreck.

Yet the 49ers quarterback, who endured five vicious sacks and a total of 21 ringing hits by Saints defenders in Sunday's 28-21 come-from-behind NFC West victory, was remarkably sanguine. But he is concerned.

The weekly beatings can be considered part of the job description, Young acknowledged. But three weeks shy of his 38th birthday, the cumulative effects of so much pounding can't be dismissed.

Nancy Gay
San Francisco Chronicle[3]

Standing at her locker in Houston's Compaq Center on Sunday evening, a third WNBA championship MVP trophy tucked under her arm and a white THREE-PEAT hat on her head, Cynthia Cooper of the Houston Comets could finally look on the bright side of the New York Liberty's stunning, elimination-foiling victory in Game 2 the day before. She could be thankful that game will be remembered for its finish—Teresa Weatherspoon's Hail Mary heave from half-court with 0.4 of a second left improbably banked off the glass and into the basket to give the Liberty a 68-67 win—and not for the fact that it was one of Cooper's worst games as a pro. "We were fortunate we had another game to play," said Cooper, who went 1 for 12 from the field and had only 12 points in the loss. "I wanted a chance to redeem myself."

Kelli Anderson
Sports Illustrated[4]

First, *dis*similarities in the leads above:

- The leads are about different sports (tennis, baseball, football and basketball).
- They appeared in newspapers on the East Coast, West Coast and a national magazine.

The *similarity*, of course, is that those leads are about *people*—not games, not statistics, but real men and women who, after all, are what sports is all about.

The first rule of strong reporting: focus on people, the principal key element in sportswriting.

Key Element #1: People

If sports is about people—and it is—you can't play the sports-reporting game without your own people skills any more than a hockey player can shoot a goal without a stick or a baseball player can hit one out of the park without a bat.

It's *people skills* you'll need to unlock a story's human element—not computer skills and not skills in navigating the Internet. As valuable as they are, those extraordinarily powerful cyberspace reporting tools won't deliver to you the people story and won't give your writing the people touch.

What will? People *sources*. And how do you develop them? Read on.

Developing People Skills

It was the biggest story in years for New Jersey Nets basketball fans: After a long, tortured search for a new head coach, the Nets decided to continue Don Casey in the job.

Everybody knew that. The Nets had announced it.

But not everybody knew the intriguing story of the deal the Nets made with Casey. Only a few insiders knew for sure.

Insiders *and one reporter*.

The reporter was Chris Broussard of *The New York Times* who led his paper's sports section with the authoritative inside details (emphasis added):

> *A person with knowledge of the contract* said that the deal is worth about $1.4 million during the first year and that the Nets have an option to terminate the contract before the 2000-1 season.
>
> Casey has yet to sign the contract, which will be completed over the weekend.
>
> Neither Casey nor the team's top officials were available for comment, but a *person close to Casey* described his mood as "ecstatic."
>
> Chris Broussard
> *The New York Times*[5]

Big news also was across town, in the New York Rangers' camp. Captain

Brian Leetch had become a free agent and, it was feared, might jump to another hockey team.

Feared by many, that is, but not by sportswriter John Dellapina of *The New York Daily News* or his readers. He broke the news on a Friday (emphasis added):

> The finest player who has ever played the bulk of his career as a Ranger now gets to play out the rest of his career as a Ranger.
>
> Captain Brian Leetch, 31, and still in the prime of his athletic life, has passed up a shot at untold free-agent millions, agreeing to a record-setting, four-year contract worth approximately $35 million.
>
> The agreement, *which won't be formally signed and announced until a Garden press conference Monday*, was reached late Wednesday at the end of the latest in a series of meetings between Rangers' president Neil Smith and Leetch's agent, Jay Grossman.
>
> At roughly $8.75 million per season, it easily will make Leetch both the highest paid Ranger in history (Wayne Gretzky made $6.75 million in '97-98) and the highest paid defenseman in NHL history (Ray Bourque is slated to make $6 million next season).
>
> John Dellapina
> *The New York Daily News*[6]

So, people sources enable two reporters to break big stories (one with attribution to anonymous sources, the other with no attribution).

How can *you* build such sources?

Know Your Sport

Your slick personality or your world's-most-winning smile won't open up a news source if you have to ask what a linebacker blitz is or request translation of, "That guy tends to lose the high ones in the sun."

You'll get nothing at courtside except disdain if you confuse a star's tendonitis with how her racket is strung.

If you don't understand the meaning of those two previous paragraphs, you're not ready to develop reliable sources in, respectively, football, baseball or tennis.

Successful sports reporters are *serious students* of the sport they cover—as serious as any Washington correspondent is about politics or any economics reporter is about international trade.

To coaches, players and business office types, your understanding (or lack thereof) of the game will become apparent the first time you ask a question.

Study your sport, and read about it. Then study and read more.

Randy Moss, of the *Fort Worth Star-Telegram*, studies horse racing and understands it takes more than a fast horse to win a race; it also takes a smart trainer. Understanding that enables Moss to *talk the game* with trainer Tom Bohannan, whose Prairie Bayou won the Preakness Stakes—but only after Bohannan "almost had an anxiety attack" getting the horse ready. That track talk, in turn, draws a key insight:

> A relieved Bohannan explained later that he never felt such pressure.
>
> "I knew the only way Prairie Bayou could get beat was if I screwed him up," he said.
>
> Randy Moss
> *The Fort Worth Star-Telegram*[7]

News breaks that Barry Sanders, the Detroit Lions' running back, wants to be traded. Lions fans are in an uproar—and in the dark. Will Sanders be traded immediately?

Mike Freeman's readers know he won't be. *The New York Times* writer, displaying superb understanding of the game he covers, sheds light:

> A consensus of general managers, coaches and players interviewed since Sanders made his announcement is that the running back will be seen running for yardage on the field again.
>
> The only disagreement is where. Some think he will play with Detroit this season. Others, including one executive with the Lions, think Sanders will sit out this season and then demand a trade in hopes of playing with a contender next year. That scenario is plausible.
>
> Sanders has $18 million left on his deal over the next four years. He has been paid almost one-third of his $11 million signing bonus. If Sanders was traded now, the unpaid portion of the bonus, more than $7 million, would count immediately against the salary cap, which is $57.3 million. As of late this week, the Lions had only $625,000 worth of cap room left. Thus, this year it is impossible for Detroit to trade Sanders.
>
> But the Lions would be able to make a deal next year when the salary cap is expected to increase to about $62 million.
>
> Mike Freeman
> *The New York Times*[8]

Note above that Freeman interviews sources and is able to give his readers a valuable consensus, and, second, Freeman has an insider source ("one executive with the Lions") he taps for his readers.

Inside information plus authoritative insights build credibility in your writing—a confidence factor that brings readers back to your byline day after day.

Incidentally, one inside source on the Sanders story was his teammate,

Herman Moore, a Lions wide receiver. The day Sanders announced his plan Moore received *141 pages* on his beeper from reporters; but Moore talked to Mike Freeman—a byline of integrity in sportswriting.[9]

Build Your Reputation for Integrity

Knowing your sport—*talking the talk*—can get you into the inner circle of sports experts you must develop as news sources. But you need more than encyclopedic understanding of sporting world nuances and subtleties.

You also need a reputation for integrity.

Simply (but crucially), news sources will not open up for a reporter they don't trust. Building trust must be a priority mission, because from your first day on the beat, sources will wonder:

First, can you be trusted to report information—particularly quotes—accurately? Are you *professional*, a reporter who will handle information fairly and with balance? Sports figures who live—or see their careers die—in the public limelight regard reporters who can't get it right as dangerous as dynamite.

Second, is it possible to speak confidentially or off the record with you? If not, the inside stuff so important to enlightened, forward-looking journalism, won't come your way. Beware the anonymous source or, particularly, anyone who demands anonymity in return for information. They may be trying to "spin" you, or to entice *you* into writing something for which *they* don't want to take responsibility. But you'll use unnamed sources on occasion, or stories important to the public won't surface. If you promise confidentiality, you must protect it, no matter what pressure you come under to divulge your source— and your sources must know you will.

Work Hard

There is no substitute for hard work in developing sources. Indeed, walkin' and talkin'—meeting people and interviewing them—is most of what good reporting is all about.

But you can't interview everyone on your beat (although even the bat boy might tip you to a story). What do you do?

Locate—and cultivate—sources who are authoritative and strategically positioned.

Obviously, coaches, general managers and players are positioned to know. And, you've got to "work" them hard as sources. But official sources or spokespersons have two drawbacks:

First, the modern sports organization—amateur or pro—is deep into image-making and highly skilled in controlling (not to say, spinning) the news. Media-savvy politicians have nothing on many coaches and players when it comes to manipulating reporters. Count on it: Team officials will give you *a* story but not often *the* story.

Second, you'll have to share with the entire press corps most anything that does seep out of team officials, and you're after *exclusives*, right? (If not, try another occupation.)

So, of course you must attend all press conferences, sit in on the briefings and be there for "media days," those official smile-for-the-press days highly favored by university athletic departments, when tons of athletic beef are trotted out wearing brand new uniforms for the cameras, then herded behind the public relations screen once more.

But it's *after* such PR shows that a reporter's real work begins. Pointers:

- Think of an "information route" around and through the organization you cover. Where, when and how is information likely to move? In covering a pro football team, for example, you know that money concerns, contracts and trades are handled in the general manager's office; the coaching staff initiates information on game strategies, player assignments and so forth; trainers handle injuries. In that manner you can identify generally where news is located.
- At each location, look for individuals who know what moves along the "information route." Although the head coach is tight-lipped, perhaps an assistant coach (with his or her own career agenda) might open up to you. Will a second-level executive in the general manager's office talk? A trainer might point you to an important story on injuries.
- Prepare to spend most of your working days (and nights) making the rounds, talking to people, telephoning and then making the circuit again.

Work Smart

Unlike survivors a reporter meets at a train wreck or shell-shocked victims of war, many news sources in sports are cool, calculating and media-savvy people cannily experienced in the ways of reporters and the power of the press to help or harm.

Opening up such sources likely depends on your ability to convince them that:

First, the self-interest of the sources themselves, or their teams or their players, will be served by giving you information. Virtually everyone in organized sports, from club owner down to newest rookie, understands the fan support they need comes, in major part, from media coverage. More fundamentally though, it's in the self-interest of a winning coach to exploit victory by talking to you. It's in the self-interest of the loser to explain the loss (and promise fans a better outcome next weekend).

Second, if sources see nothing obvious is to be gained, you must convince them that, at least, their self-interest will not be harmed by talking to you and, anyway, the story should be in print and you're the experienced and trustworthy reporter who can get it there.

A third factor often emerges. Some people enjoy talking to reporters and being part of the exciting process that gets stories in newspapers. It's flattering to be interviewed. Mostly, these sources are not "stakeholders" in the story whose self-interest will be affected by your coverage.

Whatever your sources' motivation, you can improve your chances of success with a few important steps:

- Visit, don't telephone. *Nobody* of consequence in news does business on the telephone with strangers.
- Start low-key. Expecting to score in your first visit with a source is like expecting to find true love on a blind date. It happens only infrequently. And don't whip out your reporter's notebook in the first meeting. Chat 'em up, talk a lot about *them*, a little about *you*.
- Be nice and professional. That's not a contradiction of terms, and you must ensure, through all the smiles and friendly chats, that everyone understands you are there as a reporter who takes down names and facts and puts them in the newspaper. Establishing this up-front can save you much agony in the future if you must do a story harmful or embarrassing to sources with whom you've become too friendly.
- Repeat often. Visit tomorrow, next week and keep visiting. Keep a source notebook of names, addresses, telephone numbers and job responsibilities or news specialties. Be *methodical* in working sources.

Develop Strong Interviewing Skills

Your single most important tool for unlocking the human element is the interview.

People stories are somewhere among the *millions* of words on the Internet and in those *tons* of documents stored by every university athletic department and pro team. But you find the true human element, or at least get pointed at it, in interviews.

A few hints:

First, develop variable interview techniques.

You can use a direct, let's-get-to-the-point approach with those "media-savvy" sources we've discussed. For example, coaches who have been around a while will understand even before you ask that what you want to know is why the second-string forward was put in the game in the final minute or why the fake punt was called on fourth and 15, on the team's own 20-yard line. So ask, and don't dance around the question.

However, you'll also interview the "media innocent," the inexperienced freshman quarterback or 18-year-old pitcher in the bush leagues. For such innocents, you need an entirely different technique, one that is gentler and more indirect. Hard direct questions frighten them to death.

Second, the success of your interview likely will be determined *by you well before the interview begins.*

Prepare well. Brief yourself thoroughly on the interviewee, the story at hand and its background. Begin with the advantage of knowing more than the interviewee thinks you know.

And, although you must listen to the "rhythm" of an interview and let it flow naturally, have a list of prepared questions in your notebook. Ask closed-end questions that require a specific answer ("Will Jones start at quarterback?") to steer the interview in newsy directions. Ask open-ended questions ("What's new?") and you'll go where the interviewee wants you to go (which often is *away* from the news)!

Third, go into the interview as the real you—a well-briefed reporter who is friendly but is a professional in search of news—on the record, for publication.

Don't attempt, as so many beginners do so disastrously, to be somebody you aren't—a comedian, for example—unless you truly are a great joke teller. Play to your own strengths and your personality, not somebody else's.

And, fourth, don't be awed by the Great One. Whatever your experience (or *inexperience*), you are a journalist on a legitimate news-gathering mission. Be proud of that.

Being able to stay cool and going into an interview with confidence in yourself flows from two things: a) being thoroughly prepared in advance, and b) practice.

Try this approach:

Entering the room, quickly judge whether your interviewee has limited time (signaled, perhaps, by fidgeting or frequent looks at the wall clock) or more time (signaled, maybe, by offering coffee). Adjust your pace accordingly.

Some reporters favor a direct opening: This is an interview, on the record, and here's my tape recorder to prove it.

With a "media innocent" (and even some media-savvy pros) that bluntness causes immediate freeze-up. A better approach is to open with chatty informality, then gently lead the conversation where you want it to go.

Wait until a pertinent fact emerges, then say something like, "That's interesting. Let me take a note to make certain I quote you correctly."

With that, you can pull out notebook and pen in a nonthreatening manner. And, importantly, you've made clear the interview is on the record.

It's at this point that some reporters also pull out tape recorders. But recorders frighten many people (although the *real* media-savvy sources may have their own recorders in action already)!

Don't forget the point of the interview: The source has facts; you will pull them out.

Begin with an open-ended question that lets the interviewee go in directions of his or her choosing. This sets an advantageous tone: It isn't a one-sided torture session and *both* sides will be able to hold a reasonable conversation. (You sometimes can *see* sources relax when they realize this.)

Each interview has its own rhythm, so there is no formula for success. But keep other things in mind:

First, go in with a specific story in mind *but* listen carefully for hints that another, *better* story is in there, ready to be unlocked. Many are the scoops that emerge unbeckoned from otherwise routine interviews.

Second, don't go directly, quickly or bluntly to the core question. Circle the story you want, probe gently and go at it subtly; wait patiently for it to emerge in its own form. If that doesn't work, then, indeed, go straight in. But hold the really tough questions until late in the interview. Ask them up front and the interview may terminate quickly!

Third, maintain eye contact and *listen*. You're not a stenographer who ducks into a notebook and scribbles furiously throughout the interview. You're a reporter who *thinks* during an interview and takes *selective* notes to catch only crucial facts and quotes.

Fourth (and this takes practice), as you listen, prioritize information in your head. "Ah, that's my lead," you think, and you begin formulating follow-up questions. On really important points, ask the same question two or three different ways to nail down top-priority information.

Fifth, control the interview by jumping in (yes, *interrupting*, particularly if the interviewee drones on). Say, "Excuse me, but what does that mean?" or, "Well, could you answer this ... ?" Media-savvy sources know how to deliver a 15-minute monologue, then abruptly end an interview, which can leave you defeated, exhausted and newsless.

Sixth, be persistent. This is how it works: *We* ask questions, *they* answer them. If they don't, we ask again, and again. If the source says no, write that. If the answer is evasive, write that, too.

Seventh, *always* conclude an interview with, "Is there anything else you can tell me?" You'll be amazed what that unlocks in your pursuit of the human element in sports reporting.

Eighth, be prepared, as you walk toward the door, to hear, "Say, this is off the record, isn't it?" You can say, "No it's *on* the record," and risk losing a source. Or, you can try to save the story *and* the source with something like, "C'mon, there's nothing really damaging here and, anyway, we agreed it was on the record." Your solution comes down to a simple equation: Is the story worth more than the source? Truth is, many reporters stifle their anger and sacrifice the short-term story to preserve the long-term value of the source. *You* have to make the call when it happens to you (as it will).

Key Element #2: What Happened?

Basic, right? Reporting what happened is *so* basic it doesn't need discussing?

Agreed—except that when they ask, "What happened?," true reader-fans want your reporting to probe far beyond the obvious of merely who won, who lost and what the score was.

Your readers want to know what *really* happened, and your reporting must answer:

- What really were the winning (and losing) strategies?
- What were the real turning points in the contest?
- What remarkable individual efforts were behind the outcome and, particularly, how did star athletes perform?
- What other not-so-obvious factors influenced the outcome—weather, injuries, coaching decisions or officiating?

Note how a *Philadelphia Inquirer* reporter, Bob Ford, goes *far* beyond the score in reporting a baseball game:

> CLEVELAND—The Boston Red Sox completed a stunning division series comeback against the Cleveland Indians last night with a 12-8 win that sent the Red Sox into the American League Championship Series against the New York Yankees.
>
> Boston lost the first two games of the best-of-five series before battering Cleveland for 44 runs in the next three games to leave the Indians stunned. After determining they also had no effective pitching and not much hope of outlasting the Indians, the Red Sox went to the bullpen last night and brought in ... the next Cy Young Award winner.
>
> Pedro Martinez, shut down since Game 1 by a strained back muscle, got well against the Indians after entering a tied slugfest in the fourth inning. He finished the game, pitching the final six innings without allowing a hit and striking out eight.
>
> The Indians didn't have a Cy Young in their bullpen. They had only the motley collection that helped blow a two-games-to-none series lead.

Note above that writer Ford quickly reports (third and fourth grafs) *the pivotal event*: Boston brings in Martinez, and he holds Cleveland hitless in the final six innings.

And that—pitching—is the dominant theme of Ford's reporting. The answer to, "What happened?" is that Boston won. The answer to what *really* happened comes in Ford's analysis of the pitching strategy that brought about the win.

Martinez is "the slender Dominican" who becomes a "nightmare" for Cleveland, and just a few grafs later, Ford reports the behind-the-scenes pitching story:

That both teams came into the game short on starting pitching and long on potential bullpen trouble was no surprise. Starters Charles Nagy of the Indians and Bret Saberhagen of the Red Sox were working on three days' rest, without much hope of support behind them.

Before the game, Boston manager Jimmy Williams said Martinez, out since pulling a back muscle in Game 1, would be available, but that news was greeted with a certain amount of skepticism.

Desperate times lead to desperate measures, of course, and who could know this game would be calling for desperate measures by the fourth inning?

"We'll deal with that if it comes," Indians manager Mike Hargrove said. "We have to beat the Red Sox no matter who is pitching. If Pedro is pitching, if he's healthy, that's a whole different story. But we still have to beat the Red Sox."

> Bob Ford
> *The Philadelphia Inquirer*[10]

Next, a writer *opens* with the "real what"—how a team won and why another lost (emphasis added):

ANN ARBOR, MICH.—*Hampered by dropped passes and harassed by swarming defenders,* Purdue junior *quarterback Drew Brees had the worst game of his career today* in the one he called his team's biggest. Fourth-ranked Michigan silenced questions about its secondary in a convincing 38-12 victory over the 11th-ranked Boilermakers before 111,468 at Michigan Stadium.

After stifling Wisconsin running back Ron Dayne last week, Michigan's defense has cast serious doubts on an opponent's case for the Heisman Trophy, but for the first time this season, no one is calling the Michigan secondary "suspect" anymore.

"It's as fast a secondary as I've seen at Michigan," said Wolverines' fifth-year senior quarterback Tom Brady, who threw two first-quarter touchdowns. "This defense, when they run some of their dime packages, and [linebackers] Ian Gold and Dhani Jones are in there ... no, I don't want to throw against those guys."

> Rick Freeman
> *The Washington Post*[11]

Note the use of a quote to back up the theme—that Michigan's defense turned the game. Well-selected quotes add great strength to reporting, "What really happened?"

A *Washington Post* reporter finds—and highlights—an *influencing factor*, an injury (emphasis added):

MORGANTOWN, W. VA.—With West Virginia quarterback Marc Bulger *sidelined with a broken finger*, Navy found a ray of hope in its season.

Slotback Dre Brittingham ran for a career-high 124 of Navy's 388 rushing yards, and Tim Shubzda kicked a 29-yard field goal with 2 minutes 53 seconds left to lead Navy to a 31-28 win today over the struggling Mountaineers.

Navy quarterback Brian Broadwater led four touchdown drives of 80 yards, but it was Navy's defense that made the biggest impact.

Facing sophomore quarterback Brad Lewis (17 of 31, 172 yards), who was starting in place of Bulger, the Midshipmen (2-3) allowed a season-low 264 yards and stopped the Mountaineers (1-4) on 7 of 9 third-down conversions. The lowest yardage total by a Navy opponent last season was 383.

> Rich Scherr
> *The Washington Post*[12]

An Associated Press reporter finds an influencing factor that's *overcome* by a star player:

ATLANTA—Chipper Jones was consumed by *personal turmoil* in the off-season.

He admitted having a child out of wedlock and his marriage collapsed, tarnishing his All-American image.

Somehow, Jones managed to put aside those problems once he stepped on the baseball field. This off-season, he might enjoy a more pleasant task: picking up his first Most Valuable Player award.

> Paul Newberry
> The Associated Press[13]

Key Element #3: The Statistical Context

Understand: Reader-fans appreciate your solid reporting, your pearly prose and your insider wisdom.

But they want more—much more.

To the near despair of sports editors, readers want columns—pages, even—of stand-alone statistics and numbers: box scores, line scores, scoring summaries and other statistical esoterica. And it all must be fitted into a newshole not nearly large enough.

Moreover, reader-fans want you to select key elements from the statistical context and weave them into your story, along with the *human element* and the *real-what*, to form a meaningful story.

Get the picture: *The Boston Globe* runs a half column of agate (small type) on a Mets-Diamondbacks baseball game. The box score and scoring summary would take up an entire column of newsprint, at least, if printed in "body" type, a larger type size used for news stories.

Reader-fans easily could spend an hour reading that agate, digesting its meaning and "playing" the game all over again in their minds. And many do just that.

However, the *Globe*'s Shira Springer, who covered the game, must select key statistics and include them in his story, as well. He does this:

> NEW YORK—If any team in the playoffs knows how to provide a dramatic finish, it's the Mets. If any team has taught baseball fans to expect the unexpected, it's the Mets. After all, who would have thought backup catcher Todd Pratt would replace injured star Mike Piazza and hit the series-winning solo home run in the 10th inning? But that's exactly what happened yesterday.
>
> On a 1-0 count in the bottom of the 10th, Pratt sent a blast 414 feet over the center-field fence to give New York a 4-3 victory over the Diamondbacks. Arizona center fielder Steve Finley jumped and reached for the ball. He thought he made the catch and looked in his glove, but then reality set in. A home run was signaled, Pratt slowed into his home run trot, the team streamed onto the field and the Shea Stadium crowd of 56,177 went wild celebrating the Mets' Division Series triumph, 3-1.
>
> Shira Springer
> *The Boston Globe*[14]

Note the statistical context created above by Springer's second graf: Score, attendance, key play and distance of a homer. It's created in open, inviting and readable writing.

Another *Globe* writer ups the ante with even more statistics and *still* writes an engaging, readable story:

> PHILADELPHIA—This was a loss that was four victories in the making.
>
> After Boston College bumbled, stumbled and fumbled its way to a 4-0 record against teams that had a collective 4-14 record, things finally caught up to the Eagles in yesterday's 24-14 Big East loss at Temple before a Veterans Stadium crowd of 15,067.
>
> It is now 45 years since the Eagles won their first five games of a season, as they couldn't handle the lowly Owls (1-5, 1-1). And the Eagles (4-1, 1-1) lost to Temple at the Vet for the second time in three years. The Owls handed BC a 28-21 loss in the debut of Eagles coach Tom O'Brien Sept. 6, 1997.
>
> BC's offense was outgained for the second game in a row—this time, 429 yards to 328—after showing signs of slippage in a 33-22 victory last week over Northeastern, which was throttled yesterday by UMass, 77-0. After taking a 14-0 lead in the second quarter, BC allowed Temple to score 24 unanswered points. Meanwhile, the offense squandered three red zone opportunities when John Matich missed a 35-yard field goal in the first quarter, backup quarterback Brian St. Pierre threw an interception in the end zone in the

second quarter, and Cedric Washington fumbled at the Temple 19 as the Eagles were driving for a fourth-quarter score that would have tied the game at 21.

Michael Vega
The Boston Globe [15]

In any other form of journalism—including business news—I would tell you that writer Vega, in the example above, jammed too many statistics down his readers' throats too fast. I count *30 numbers* in the four grafs.

In most newswriting, it's mandatory—parcel out numbers slowly and carefully and don't choke your readers. But sports readers easily swallow huge quantities of numbers and call for more.

Nevertheless, in reporting the statistical context, pacing the numbers carefully *does* enhance readability. Note in the following example how the numbers are spread carefully throughout three grafs and not jammed into one:

> Several NFL players apparently were victims of a high-roller accused by federal investigators of bilking investors for at least $31 million, the *Austin (Texas) American-Statesman* reported yesterday.
>
> FBI agents believe the players, including three members of the Arizona Cardinals and one Cleveland Browns player, contributed to a $5.5 million investment wired to (John Doe) by Los Angeles sports agent (Fred Smith).
>
> (Doe), 29, was arrested at his $2.2 million Lake Austin, Texas, home last month. The FBI seized the house, two jets worth more than $10 million, a $2 million helicopter and $800,000 in vehicles, plus undisclosed amounts of money in bank accounts.

The Associated Press [16]

And, Be Precise!

Without precision reporting, the statistical context is meaningless. Note how the pros do it:

- Pat Sullivan of the *San Francisco Chronicle* doesn't report that a golfer makes a "challenging" or "difficult" putt. Rather, it is "a 40-foot putt with a 15-foot break for a birdie at No. 3."
- Steve Hummer of the *Atlanta Journal-Constitution* writes that the fairways are trimmed to "exactly 1 3/8 inches in height" for the Masters Golf Tournament at Augusta National.
- Joseph Durso informs *New York Times* readers not that Charismatic had a "good workout" at Churchill Downs but, rather, that the horse "went five furlongs handily in 1:00 2/5 and galloped out six furlongs in 1:14."
- Jack Hodges reports in the *Chattanooga Times* not that a basketball team

had "a lot" of turnovers but, rather, that it "had 30 turnovers—15 against the press in the first half and 15 against the zone in the second."

See the difference?

Key Element #4: The Look-Ahead Angle

For true reader-fans of any sport, the season never ends. There is only a pause before the games begin again. Tonight's game, win or lose, always is followed by tomorrow's.

For these avid readers, your reporting is meaningful only if it contains the "look-ahead angle"—the effect tonight's game will have on tomorrow's and how *this* season affects the *next*.

Such look-ahead reporting takes different directions.

The Situationer

This look-ahead form enables you to report periodically about an event that is even a year or more ahead, as a *Washington Post* reporter does in October 1999 on preparation by the U.S. women's basketball team for the 2000 Olympics:

> Teresa Edwards sprinted ahead of her teammates on the U.S. women's senior national team halfway through a two-hour practice this past week at George Washington University. After beating her teammates up and down the court, she gave them high-fives as they got ready for another drill.
>
> "I just love the game, working on the game, getting better at the game," Edwards said after practice as she sat with ice packs on her knees. "When it comes time to perform ... good things have happened for me."
>
> Edwards, 35, has been a member of the U.S. women's basketball team in four Olympics, winning three gold medals and a bronze. Anticipating an appearance in the 2000 Olympics next fall, she is one of 12 players on the squad that will play against various college and professional women's teams the next few months to get ready for Sydney.
>
> Athelia Knight
> *The Washington Post* [17]

Note two points about the situationer above:

- It's timeless, and whether it's written today, tomorrow or next week is irrelevant. That is, you don't need a specific news break to establish the timing for reporting this type of look-ahead.
- It's written with imagination—cleverness, even—to lift it from the deadly dull, "U.S. women basketball players are working hard to prepare for ... ."

There are no dull stories, only dull reporters.

Here's a situationer that *is* timely:

> Cal's offense faces rock-and-a-hard-place dilemmas.
>
> The Bears need to improve their woeful attack immediately to compete in a there-for-the-taking Pac-10. But with true freshmen starting at quarterback and tailback tonight against Brigham Young, and another true freshman expected to get increased playing time at wide receiver, patience is a must.
>
> Also, offensive coordinator Steve Hagen would love to display all the subtleties of his varied offense, but with two freshmen learning new positions, inexperience at the skill positions and a flagrant shortage of wide receivers—the cornerstone of Hagen's offense—Hagen is forced to limit the playbook.
>
> "Sixty-five percent of this offense is based on a three-wide receiver set," said Hagen.
>
> Jake Curtis
> *San Francisco Chronicle*[18]

Note how the *Chronicle's* Curtis gives insights into a game that will be played tonight: 1) California's position is characterized ("rock-and-a-hard-place dilemmas"), 2) what needs immediate fixing is "their woeful attack" and 3) coach Hagen's game strategy may be limited.

Now, reader-fans, you're primed for tonight's game!

Game-Story Look Aheads

Unlike situationers, the game-story look ahead always keys off a timely development. It uses a specific event—a game, for example, or contest—as a platform for reporting what's likely ahead.

Here is a form frequently used:

> NEW YORK—Undaunted by another devastating injury, inspired by their seemingly hopeless plight, the New York Knicks—or what's left of them—are going to the NBA Finals.
>
> The incredible story of a Knicks team that has overcome wave after wave of adversity took yet another turn Friday night as Larry Johnson, New York's leading scorer in this series, went down in the second quarter with a knee injury.
>
> That didn't stop Allan Houston from having one of the best offensive games of his career, nor did it stop Marcus Camby, Latrell Sprewell and Chris Childs from making several clutch plays as New York defeated the Indiana Pacers 90-82 in Game 6 of the Eastern Conference finals.
>
> New York advanced to its first NBA Finals since 1994, but it may have to go against the San Antonio Spurs without two of their best big men.

Johnson sprained a knee ligament and had to be carried off the court, and Patrick Ewing is already out for the season after tearing his Achilles' tendon in Game 2 of the Indiana series.

Chris Sheridan
The Associated Press [19]

Note that AP's Sheridan assigns top priority to the look-ahead angle—the Knicks are going to the NBA Finals—and that he subordinates to the third graf the fact that they beat the Indiana Pacers 90-82.

Next, a *Philadelphia Inquirer* reporter also subordinates (to his second graf) the outcome of a game and instead, concentrates in his lead on the look-ahead angle. The Cowboys aren't swaggering as in the glorious old days but that's "just around the corner."

IRVING, TEXAS—The swagger wasn't quite there as the Dallas Cowboys went through their paces yesterday, but you could tell that it's just around the corner.

The Arizona Cardinals were definitely accomplices in their own mugging, coughing up the ball five times, but the Cowboys really didn't need the help. They slapped the Cardinals around often in a 35-7 rout.

Mike Bruton
The Philadelphia Inquirer [20]

Key Element #5: Meaningful Quotes

Let's say you're wondering how to report that players got very intense in a game you covered.

You could write it this way: "The team played with great intensity."

Or, you could do as a *Philadelphia Inquirer* reporter does and *let a quote show the intensity*:

Anyone who wondered if Roman Catholic's football team was for real got the answer yesterday when the Cahillites destroyed Cardinal O'Hara, 42-14, in a game that wasn't as close as the score indicated.

"We were out to kill somebody," said junior running back/safety Joe McCourt.

Chris Morkides
The Philadelphia Inquirer [21]

Unquestionably, carefully selected quotes—*meaningful* quotes—lend enormous strength to your reporting. For beginner reporters, two traps await.

First, young writers tend to filter everything in a sports story through their own thinking, in only their own vocabulary. Thus, quotes representing player or coach thinking are not used.

Second is the trap of simply grabbing a quote—any quote—and plugging it into a story, whether or not it has pertinence or meaning. It's the stuff of Hollywood parody: "'Well,' the pitcher said, scratching and spitting, 'I just play them games one at a time.'"

When a good quote presents itself (or, more likely, is developed in smart interviewing), *get out of the way and let it dominate your story.* A Portland *Oregonian* reporter does that:

> ESTACADA—A jubilant coach Greg Lawrence asked his Sherwood team in the post-game celebration Friday night: "How many times have we worked on that punt block?"
>
> The answer was just enough as the Bowmen blocked a punt late in the fourth quarter and recovered it in the end zone to upset fourth-ranked Estacada 21-18 in a Tri-Valley League game.
>
> Tim Sullivan
> *The Oregonian* [22]

Quotes properly selected can provide insight into many sports events. For example, hockey writer Jeff Miller of the *Orange County (Calif.) Register* must report why, contrary to all expectation, the Ducks and Stars don't beat up each other on the ice.

First, Miller sets up the mystery by explaining why a bloody confrontation was expected.

> The Stars were said to be sizzling over last weekend's events, when the Ducks visited Dallas and left behind a broken nose, strained neck, concussion and fractured eye socket. The damage resulted in three Ducks being suspended for 19 games.
>
> Now, while it is true two wrongs don't make a right, they sure do make for grand theater, and everyone figured that's what we'd have here.
>
> There was supposed to be hatred and revenge oozing from this game, staining the ice like a pool of blood. But the gritty edge was gone from the start. ...
>
> Now, the quote that gives one player's explanation:
>
> "I think everyone just wanted to be smart," Ducks winger Teemu Selanne said. "No one wanted to start a war out there. Everyone did what was best for hockey. Everyone did what was right."
>
> Jeff Miller
> *Orange County Register* [23]

Note the expertise added to the following *Boston Globe* story with a third-graf quote.

He has been the missing link for a ballclub that didn't know it needed one. It wasn't like the Indians were a busted chain, not after winning five straight division titles and reaching the World Series twice.

But Robbie Alomar made Cleveland even greater this season. Going into yesterday's Game 3, Sandy's kid brother was looking like the man most likely to get his mates another date with the Yankees in the American League Championship Series.

"There's a tremendous case that should be made for Robbie as the MVP of the league this year," said manager Mike Hargrove. "There are so many ways that he can help your team win. With his glove. With his speed. With his bat. With his knowledge of the game on the field."

John Powers
The Boston Globe[24]

Next, a *USA Today* reporter expertly weaves in meaningful quotes:

The Miami Fusion complained that D.C. United's second goal in Saturday's 2-0 Eastern Conference playoff win was offside.

No way, said Esse Baharmast, the U.S. Soccer Federation's director of officials. He supervises Major League Soccer officials.

"I looked at the video, and he (Jaime Moreno) was a good 2 yards onsides when the ball was released," Baharmast said.

Baharmast said the play could have looked offside because Moreno was ahead of a defender when he received the pass.

"That's not how you judge offsides. It was a correct call," he said, defending the work of referee Tim Weyland.

Barharmast said officials get a lot of flak because players and fans assume the official is wrong. "It becomes a self-fulfilling prophecy."

Peter Brewington
USA Today[25]

Question: Do we quote athletes—even those that are semi-literate—exactly as they speak? Or do we clean up their grammar and save them embarrassment? Consider two points:

First, eliminate gross obscenities, of course, and if a quote is unintelligible, don't use quote marks. Paraphrase. (A cardinal rule: If it's in quote marks it's *exactly* what was said.)

Second, leave in the "ain't" and "me and him" that you hear on the field and in the locker room. It's all part of sports.

Key Element #6: The Enterprise Dimension

Enterprise in sports reporting is difficult to define. But you know it when you see it:

- It's Paul Attner of *The Sporting News* going beyond the usual and spending hours in the Green Bay Packers' draft room as team officials pick players they hope will "end the backward slide that has engulfed the franchise." Attner reports in thousands of words a fascinating inside story of big-time football.[26]
- It's Michael Bamberger of *Sports Illustrated* leaving the beaten path and trekking through the hills to Tannersville, Va., where houses have "tin roofs that produce the most peaceful sound—p-tat, p-tat, p-tat, p-tat—in a rainstorm." Bamberger is exploring the childhood roots of Houston Astros pitcher Billy Wagner because to understand how he "can throw a baseball 100 mph, you've got to examine the dynamics of his rural upbringing."[27]
- It's the *Chicago Tribune* assigning an arts critic, Sid Smith, to compare golf to dance. He discovers that a golfer "may move with grace, in a seemingly choreographed arc and ritualistic thrust of his body, like the dancer."[28]
- It's AP's Gary D. Robertson digging behind the obvious story in stock car racing and finding a church-sponsored driver who races a "Methodist Motorsports Evangelism car" and says, "It doesn't matter whether your brakes fail. With God, you're always a winner."[29]

For your readers (and your career), work to develop a sense of the unusual, the offbeat and, above all, the *meaningful* story that lurks below the surface. So much reporting (and not only in sports) is superficial, ordinary and predictable that enterprise reporting stands out vividly.

Enterprise reporting requires a different mindset—and different tools.

Computer-Assisted Reporting

Using computer-assisted reporting (CAR) as a tool and where to travel in cyberspace is far beyond the scope of this book.

But keep these pointers in mind:

- CAR extends your reporter's reach into the libraries of the world, into contact with news sources virtually anywhere and enables you to transcend time barriers and geographic boundaries. Use CAR to give your reporting historical and wider context.
- Don't accept Internet information as proven fact without doing what all reporters must do with any information—double-check it. Misleading information, erroneous "facts" and outright lies float through cyberspace.
- Your problem with CAR is not obtaining enough information; rather, it is winnowing and sifting through the overwhelming flow of facts and figures available. Use the same news values and judgments you use in any reporting as you discard the irrelevant, retain the meaningful and prioritize news elements.

CAR is useful particularly when doing *in-depth reporting*—discovering how things *should* work and comparing that to how they *do* work. (I avoid the term "investigative reporting" because that implies we are undercover police officers, not reporters.) Search for deviations from the norm, the usual and the expectable.

Doing a story on, say, a city's bid to host the Olympics? CAR can lead you to the rules on how bidding should be conducted. It also points you at how cities in the past actually did bid (under the table as well as over it).

Searching for facts on, say, player salaries and salary caps in pro football? CAR will take you to sources that reveal whether your team is inside—or outside—salary parameters set by other teams.

Using CAR techniques you can aspire to the true goal of in-depth reporting—original work that's unique to you and may bring about change.

This type of reporting places extra (and heavy) obligations on you. Rather than simply seeking balancing comment from all sides in, say, a controversy over big-money professionalism in college athletics, you're required to weigh information carefully for veracity and information.

Merely reporting "he said ... she said ... they said," won't do it in this type of reporting. What "he" said is included in your story *if* you verify the information; what "she" said is discarded if you doubt its truthfulness or relevance.

That is, you become much more *judgmental* in discarding or retaining information and in selecting sources as you lead readers toward meaningful but hidden stories beneath the surface.

We'll look, in the next chapter, at how that approach to reporting takes today's sportswriter far off-field in search of news.

Summary

—Of all fundamentals in journalism, strong reporting skills are most important.

—Even sports journalists who cannot roar and soar in their writing can fashion job success if they are strong reporters.

—Key Element #1 in reporting sports is the human angle, the "people story" that lifts your reporting out of statistics-laden, ordinary journalism.

—For capturing the human angle, people skills in interviewing are more important to a reporter than ability to surf cyberspace (although that's a great reporting asset).

—To develop people *sources* you must know, intimately, your sport; study it to gain their confidence.

—Building a reputation for integrity is essential to your success, and it comes only with demonstrating you are a professional who reports accurately and is trustworthy with confidences.

—Only hard work—and lots of it—will lead you to sources who are authoritative and strategically positioned to give you news your readers need.

—Key Element #2 in a sports story is reporting what *really* happened—winning and losing strategies, turning points, performance of stars and influencing factors such as weather, officiating and injuries.

—Key Element #3 is a statistical context, the numbers drawn from box scores, line scores and scoring summaries that permit reader-fans to "play" the game in their minds.

—Key Element #4 is reporting the "look-ahead angle"—how tonight's game sets up tomorrow night's and how this season leads into the next.

—Key Element #5 is *meaningful* quotes that add valuable dimensions to your reporting.

—Key Element #6 is the enterprise dimension that takes readers behind the obvious and highlights the unusual, the offbeat.

—Computer-assisted reporting is a magnificent tool that enables you to transcend time barriers and geographic boundaries, extending your reporter's reach worldwide.

Exercises

1. Read today's *USA Today* sports section (or another designated by your instructor) and analyze, in 350 to 400 words, how sportswriters do (or don't) get Key Element #1—the people angle—into their reporting. Give examples of what you think are strong reporting emphasis on the people angle, as well as weak examples.

2. Discuss, in about 300 words, the challenge of developing a reputation for integrity as a reporter. What specific (not general) reporting techniques and "people skills" would *you* use on the sports beat to convince sources you are a professional reporter who can be trusted to handle information accurately and protect confidences? Do you know of reporters who fail the test of integrity?

3. Read the front page of a sports section designated by your instructor. In about 300 words, discuss whether reporters capture the *real what*. Do they report true turning points in a game? Do they highlight winning (and losing) strategies and individual efforts, particularly by stars? Are influencing factors—officiating, injuries and weather—reported clearly and fully?

4. Obtain and discuss, in about 300 words, an example of a sports story that you think reports properly the statistical context of a game or contest. Discuss how the reporter introduces the key numbers and statistics so essential to understanding a sports story. Are the numbers paced evenly to produce readable writing? Are the numbers the *right* numbers, in your opinion?

5. Obtain and discuss, in about 400 words, a sports story that you think does a good job of reporting the *look-ahead angle* and, also, displaying an *enterprise dimension* that lifts the story out of the ordinary. Discuss the reporting techniques apparently used in fashioning the story.

Recommended Reading

Sources for help in computer-assisted reporting:
Computer-Assisted Reporting & Research (CARR-L)
  CARR-L@ulkyvm.louisville.edu
Investigative Reports & Editors (IRE-L)
  IRE-L@lists.missouri.edu
Society of Professional Journalists (SPJ-L)
  SPJ-L@psuvm.psu.edu
Computer-Assisted Reporting (NICAR-L)
  NICAR-L@lists.missouri.edu

Christopher Callahan, assistant dean at the University of Maryland's College of Journalism, is a recognized expert on Internet reporting. He is at ccallahan@jmail.umd.edu

Also helpful:

John Ullman, *Investigative Reporting* (New York: St. Martin's Press, 1995); Lauren Kessler and Duncan McDonald, *The Search* (Belmont, Calif.: Wadsworth, Inc., 1992); Donald L. Shaw, Maxwell McCombs and Gerry Keir, *Advanced Reporting*, 2nd ed. (Prospect Heights, Ill.: Waveland Press, 1997); Carl Hausman, *The Decision-Making Process in Journalism* (Chicago: Nelson-Hall Inc., 1991).

Notes

1. "Serena Williams Breaks Through, Captures Open," Sept. 12, 1999, p. D-1.
2. "Capitalizing A's," Sept. 9, 1999, p. D-1.
3. "Battered Young Tries to Stay Upbeat," Sept. 21, 1999, p. B-1.
4. "Pro Basketball," Sept. 13, 1999, p. 56.
5. "Inside Move: Casey Gets Nod to Coach Nets," June 26, 1999, p. D-1.
6. "Rangers Keeping Leetch," May 21, 1999, p. 35.
7. Dispatch for morning papers, May 10, 1999.
8. "Lions' Sanders Says He's Down, But Watch Out for a Reverse," July 30, 1999, p. D-3.
9. Op. cit.
10. "Super Saver," Oct. 12, 1999, p. C-1.
11. "Michigan, in a Breeze," Oct. 3, 1999, p. D-9.
12. "Midshipmen Topple Mountaineers, Oct. 3, 1999, p. D-1.
13. "A Run at MVP," Oct. 3, 1999, p. D-1.
14. "Just Another Amazin' Win for Mets," Oct. 10, 1999, p. D-2.

15. "Not Wise to Owls," Oct. 10, 1999, p. C-1.
16. Dispatch for morning papers, Oct. 9, 1999.
17. "Edwards Already Good as Gold," Oct. 3, 1999, p. D04.
18. "Cal Keeps Faith in Freshmen," Oct. 9, 1999, p. E-8.
19. Dispatch for morning papers, June 12, 1999.
20. "Sanders Helps Cowboys Rip Cards," Oct. 4, 1999, p. E-8.
21. "Roman Trounces O'Hara, 42-14," Oct. 12, 1999, p. C-7.
22. "Blocked Punt Sends Bowmen to Victory, 4-0 Start," Oct. 3, 1999, p. D-9.
23. Dispatch for Sunday papers, Oct. 10, 1999.
24. "Alomar in the Family," Oct. 10, 1999, p. D-5.
25. "MLS Defends Referee's Call," Oct. 21, 1999, p. C-17.
26. "Draft Day," April 26, 1999, p. 48.
27. "Astro Physics," Sept. 20, 1999, p. 66.
28. "Golfers Dance to a Completely Different Tune," Aug. 13, 1999, Section 4, p. 6.
29. Dispatch for Sunday newspapers, Aug. 8, 1999.

Reporting the Wider Picture

JUST HOW wide is this *wider picture* of the sports world you'll be reporting?

Item: *The Wall Street Journal*, that bible of the investment world, *leads* Page One with a story on player unrest in the National Basketball League.

Item: The *Economist* of London, strong on Japan's trading practices and banking in Zurich, reports on the soaring popularity of U.S. women's soccer.

Item: *Forbes* magazine, which boasts millionaire business leaders for readers, examines the financial structure of team ownership in the National Football League.

Item: *The New York Times*, panoramic in its concern over the compellingly important social, political and economic issues of the day, *fronts*—above the fold, with a four-column headline and massive photo—the retirement of hockey star Wayne Gretzky.[1]

That is, the wider picture of sports is very wide, indeed, and as a sports reporter you'll be covering a societal phenomenon of many dimensions off court and off field, as well as on, for newspapers, magazines and other media of all types.

In Chapter Four, Reporting the Wider Picture, we'll broaden our look at your role as a reporter. We'll discuss:

- How to find, evaluate and develop those off-court and off-field stories that are so revealing about sports as a societal phenomenon.
- How to develop the precision techniques of reporting in highly technical areas such as sports business and sports medicine.

Three Crucial Areas

In sports reporting, as in all journalism, news is defined in large part as what reader-fans *want* to know but also by what you, as a trained journalist, think they *need* to know.

Casting your reporter's net that wide will take you far from the grunts and groans of the on-field game or the on-court contest. Broadly, three news sectors are crucial:

- The lifestyle and personal lives—yes, *private* lives—of athletes. It's not tawdry voyeurism we're talking about here; rather, it's balanced and fair but probing news coverage of men and women whose personal lives are part of the public persona they voluntarily assume as sports figures (not to say, heroes) in America today.
- The business structure of sports. It's big business indeed, and learning how to report that in meaningful dollars-and-cents terms is essential to your career in sports journalism. So is handling sports-world controversies fought out in court—the *law story* in sports reporting.
- Health, injuries and, unfortunately, drugs. In every sport, you'll find this news pivotal in the performance of individual athletes and teams. And learning to report it with careful fact-finding and precise writing—*as in science news*—is important.

What's "Fair Game" After the Game?

If news is defined as what interests readers, virtually *everything* in an athlete's private, as well as public, life is "fair game" for a reporter.

If, however, you agree that reader curiosity is only one element defining news and your reporter's sense of ethical responsibility is another, then the question of what's "fair game" is more complex.

For that question, many sports reporters have *two* answers.

First, if an athlete's private life is thrust into public view by a *public act*—domestic violence or drug arrest, for example—it's news to be reported. In tomorrow morning's paper. In full detail.

Second, however, if no such single public act focuses the spotlight on an athlete's private life, a more considered approach is taken.

Here is how a sports reporter for the *Atlanta Journal-Constitution* reacted when a star athlete's privacy went public in a hurry:

HOUSTON—On a May night in Gulfport, Miss., a 34-year-old man who should have known better sat cringing in a casino hotel room, his arms filled with drug money, a cop's pistol barrel screwed into his ear, his head spinning, looking across the room at the dealer who gave him up and asking the same question his friends have asked for months.

Why?

That's Jeffrey Denberg reporting on an NBA star who has earned about $7 million playing basketball. Denberg continues:

> This week, Greg "Cadillac" Anderson, dapper as always in a gray suit, sat in a conference room in Houston with Tim Johnson, his attorney, and remembered his desperate words:
>
> "'Why did you do this to me?' That's what I asked him."
>
> Perhaps the better question would have been: Why did Anderson, a 10-year NBA veteran, do this to himself?
>
> The truth is that Anderson, who pleaded guilty on Oct. 20 to participating in a drug deal five months ago, can't come up with one rational explanation for his behavior and can't put the blame on anyone else.
>
> He didn't do it for the money. Anderson never took the $1,000 the dealer offered. He didn't do it for the drugs, either. Anderson never was a hard-drug user.
>
> ... this man who earned about $7 million playing basketball was caught in the web of drug dealers and government agents because he lacked the smarts and the backbone to walk away.
>
> "I could have said I don't want to be affiliated with this," he said Tuesday. "When I knew what they were doing, I could have said no. But I didn't."
>
> Now, Anderson says, he understands the damage was self-inflicted, that he is guilty of negligence and, worst of all, participating in a drug deal. That's why he twists in the wind, awaiting his sentence on Feb. 9 for the crime of possession of cocaine and intent to distribute. He tries to keep his life together—and his relationship with four children who were removed from his home by a wife who is suing for divorce.
>
> Anderson is living, breathing proof that you don't have to be a bad guy to get in trouble.
>
> "No, you sure don't," Anderson said. "I wasn't."
>
> He should have known better.
>
> Jeffrey Denberg
> *Atlanta Journal-Constitution*[2]

Note the wrenching detail, the inclusion of humiliating quotes, the reporter's extension of the story from the star himself into the intimate circle of Anderson's family—his relationship with his wife and four children.

Deeper in the story, Denberg also addresses the impact on Anderson's team, the Atlanta Hawks. ("The organization was shocked. Anderson just didn't fit the profile.")

It is that very public connection with professional sports, of course, that makes Anderson a *public figure* and open to public scrutiny.

Lesson: Good reporters today, unlike many reporters in times bygone, don't cut slack for sports heroes in trouble with the law. There is no special "zone of privacy" when public-figure athletes, many of whom become multimillionaires performing for the public, go down in drug busts or otherwise.

However, let's say you learn unflattering details about the private life of a high-profile sports figure, and no single public act, such as a drug bust, provides the "news peg" for a story. How do you handle that?

Another *Atlanta Journal-Constitution* reporter, Jeff Schultz, faces that question in covering Evander Holyfield, the heavyweight fighter. Schultz spends weeks on the story and, importantly, *holds it until he can interview Holyfield* and thus provide balancing context and background.

Note the reporter's straight-in, no-hold-barred approach: The private conduct of this public figure is of concern and is news for the reader-fan public. Period.

> As he closes in on becoming boxing's undisputed heavyweight champion, Evander Holyfield has come to realize his personal life is in far more need of repair than his professional one. That the enlightenment has arrived belatedly at age 35 is not without cost.
>
> One week after his second wife, Janice, gave birth to the couple's first child, Holyfield confirmed in an interview that he has fathered two children out of wedlock in the last year with previous girlfriends. He now has nine children ... the newborn ... three with his first wife ... five others born out of wedlock to four women.

There's even more intimate detail:

> In the interview on his Milburn estate, Holyfield described Janice as "my best friend" but admitted regretting the couple's union almost immediately after they were wed in October 1996, one month before his first victory over Mike Tyson.

Now, the reporter advises reader-fans how he handled this delicate story *and* why the contrast between the fighter's public persona and private life is news.

> He added, "I'm not perfect. But I have overcome other things in my life, and I will overcome this."
>
> The *Atlanta Journal-Constitution* became aware of some elements in Holyfield's personal life about a week ago, but he declined to discuss them until after his latest victory, Saturday night over Vaughn Bean at the Georgia Dome.
>
> Holyfield, who professes to be a devout Christian and maintains a posi-

tive image worldwide, understands he is subjecting himself to criticism from family and religious concerns. But he said, "I know everything comes out of the dark and into the light sooner or later. It might as well be now. If you don't want nothing [known about your actions], then do nothing."

Jeff Schultz
Atlanta Journal-Constitution[3]

In addition to the story above, the *Journal-Constitution* published an extensive question-and-answer sidebar giving Holyfield opportunity to tell, in his own words, of the conflicting currents in his private life.

Fair coverage? Balanced? Yes. Is such behind-the-scenes coverage *news*? Certainly.

WHAT GETS HIGH PRIORITY?

High news priority should be assigned any "private-life" event in an athlete's life if it likely will affect a team's performance or the wider sports world.

Thus, it's top news when a Houston Rockets basketball star is arrested on suspicion of drunk driving. AP's Michael A. Lutz goes directly to the point. "The player will miss workouts, the team's performance could be affected, and coach Rudy Tomjanovich is quoted as saying, 'I hope it won't be a distraction.'"[4]

Thus, it's news—in all newspapers—when Peter Warrick, star Florida State receiver, pleads guilty to misdemeanor petty theft, misses two football games and takes himself out of contention for the Heisman Trophy.[5]

But, even if there is no special "zone of privacy" around an *active* athlete, can a *retired* athlete step out of the public spotlight and erect barriers against continued coverage?

Opinions differ among journalists, as well as athletes.

For example, after earning fame and fortune in the public spotlight, Joe DiMaggio tried to go private when he put down his New York Yankee bat. Even when seriously ill, near the end of his life, DiMaggio roused himself to complain that he didn't care whether his illness was considered by reporters to be a big story—the hospital shouldn't be releasing details to them.

Ethicist Kenneth W. Goodman of the University of Miami commented, "The daily updates about his health served no public good beyond the satisfaction of curiosity."[6]

Another view came from Robert Lipsyte of *The New York Times*, who looked deeply at Dimaggio's desire for privacy, and, by extension, the broader question of privacy for all athletes—and also examined the role of the press:

> Private to the point of paranoia, DiMaggio took charge of his final illness with the same steely reserve that informed his baseball career, his marriage to Marilyn Monroe, his afterlife as living legend. He was his own curator. He allowed us to believe that his genius, like Albert Einstein's, Greta Garbo's,

Orson Welles', had earned him the right to be left alone except when he wanted attention, to be excused whatever smudges might appear on the shiny image.

We scrabbled to justify his aloofness as dignity (but never shyness or contempt), to find grounds for forgiveness in his coffee-maker commercials, to place him in historical context. He had ridden into our consciousness just as the myths of the frontier West were receding, one of a posse of cowboys in the outfield who became our new manly heroes, lone individuals standing just outside the group, our last defense.

He was the son of an immigrant, but graceful and cool, so all the immigrants' sons who were writing about sports identified with him, and in the words of the old sports editor Stanley Woodward, "Godded him up."

"Godded him up" ... It's the fear of discerning journalists: Does coverage of athletic stars, on field and off, approach beatification of the living? And, is the sudden demand for privacy at career's-end just another public relations ploy?

Again Lipsyte:

> (DiMaggio) didn't embarrass us, perhaps because we never got into all the nooks and crannies of his life. He was just smart enough to know he wasn't smart enough to unspool soundbites and commentary. We saw just enough to be able to make up the rest of him. Always dressed for dinner at the "21" Club, he drifted through the rest of his life with the same outward economy he displayed as he drifted under fly balls. He knew just where they would drop.
>
> Robert Lipsyte
> *The New York Times*[7]

How and *when* we pursue off-field stories makes a difference to many reader-fans.

For example, Jim Gray, an NBC sports reporter, drew heated criticism for 1) pressing Pete Rose for comment on his lifetime ban from organized baseball for betting on games and 2) pressing Rose on a lovely evening—the celebration of the All-Century Team, televised from Atlanta before Game 2 of the 1999 World Series.

The interview was short (less than three minutes) but criticism was widespread. Furman Bisher, a leading sports columnist for the *Atlanta Journal-Constitution*, turned over one of his columns to his stepdaughter, saying she expressed what was on his mind. She wrote:

> Not only did Mr. Gray ruin a wonderful moment for Pete Rose, but he managed to sour something magical for the rest of us, too.
>
> Here, we, the American public, were happily witnessing some of the best parts of our collective history. For a few splendid moments, sports were healthy, clean and innocent. There was no salary bickering or drug allega-

tions, spitting in umpires' faces or choking coaches, no accusations of cavorting with prostitutes. Last night was simply a positive celebration of the good and pure energies that make up the American Dream.

Behind the mostly graying and weathered faces of the Team of the Century, we still saw the shadows of the boyish gleam, the focused intensity and well-earned, youthful cockiness of baseball's greats ... .

Then Jim Gray comes on camera and not only pops the bubble, but tramples it. There's a time and place for everything, and whether you believe Pete Rose is guilty of gambling on baseball or not, bringing it up then wasn't right.

Furman Bisher
The Atlanta Journal-Constitution[8]

Lesson: To us, probing deeply into the tawdry side of sports is strong and necessary journalism; to reader-fans it can be trampling on the "American Dream."

Athletes Are Role Models?

Anyone who has made it through a paragraph or two of anything I've written knows I believe fearless but fair reporting and honest commentary have an essential place in a sports section. With escalating amounts being spent on the great escape that is spectator sports—with so many parents presenting wealthy athletes as role models—fans deserve to know the truth about the teams they patronize and the stars they idolize.

Skip Bayless
Chicago Tribune
"In the Wake of the News," *Chicago Tribune,* Oct. 30, 1999,
Section 3, p. 1.

Reporting the Business of Sports

In reporting sports, both amateur and pro, you'll need the skills of business-beat reporters who prowl the corporate world of high finance and industry.

And, as in business news reporting, you'll find the numbers—the dollars and cents—are stunning.

On the pro side, people who run faster than most or hit balls farther become overnight millionaires in contract negotiations as complex as any in the business world. Team owners plunk down hundreds of millions to buy franchises, then twist taxpayers' arms for hundreds of millions more to build stadiums. One way or another, fans—your readers among them—pay for it all.

On the so-called amateur side, huge amounts of money drive enormous sports programs. The University of Wisconsin at Madison, for example, fields more than 700 athletes on 13 women's and 10 men's teams with a budget predicted to hit $50.4 million in 2004-05. Again, fans and taxpayers pay.[9]

Unquestionably, the money of sports is a high-priority news story in which the public and you, the reporter, as the public's surrogate, have not only a legitimate interest but also *a need to know.*

Understanding the business organization of sports and reporting it in meaningful terms for your reader-fans and all those taxpayers out there is a challenge, indeed.

Some suggestions:

ADJUST YOUR MINDSET AND DON'T PANIC

Yes, I know: You didn't get into sports journalism to report like an accountant or write like a stock analyst.

Indeed, like many journalists, you may have entered journalism because of a bad case of math fright, then gravitated specifically to sports to avoid the numbers in business writing.

But, get used to it. The business of sports must be your business. Covering only games won't do it anymore. You won't truly grasp the dynamics of sports today unless you penetrate the business and organizational structure of the sports world and understand it.

You need to understand the numbers—how to both report and write them—to protect the pocketbook interests of the public, fans and taxpayers alike, which are linked directly to the dollars and cents of sports. Your readers have a legitimate *need to know*, for example, about how much they're going to pay for tickets and how they will be taxed for a new municipal stadium.

Changing your mindset from covering games to also covering the money surrounding games requires you to regard individual athletes and their sports organizations as necessarily open to public scrutiny in financial matters as in any other dimension of sports. Athletes, remember, are public figures who live, and prosper, in the public spotlight; teams live off fan largess and, often, public tax funding.

So, don't panic because your reporter's responsibility extends far beyond the playing field and into the counting house. A careful reporter can cover a quarterback's multimillion-dollar contract negotiation as well as a quarterback draw and a team's salary cap as well as a team's win-loss record.

CHOOSE YOUR NUMBERS CAREFULLY

You don't need an accounting degree to sort through the blizzard of numbers you'll encounter. Use your *reporter training* to discard the irrelevant and incorporate the meaningful numbers in your writing.

As in any form of journalism, first answer the question all readers ask, "What's it going to cost *me*?"

That is, ticket prices are numbers with high priority in sports reporting. So are any numbers with implications for taxpayers or the public at large (those tax-funded stadiums, again, or the huge economic impact of sports on local economies).

Quickly look, also, for the numbers affecting individual players, particularly the stars all fans watch closely. Salary negotiations get high priority because the team loyalty athletes showed in days bygone is virtually absent today. Salaries—hard, cold dollars and cents—determine whether a beloved star stays with the hometown team or departs.

Teams ("franchises" in the lingo of big-time sports) move, too. So, team finances—whether they're making money or losing it—are big news.

REPORT NUMBERS WITH PRECISION

As you know, it'll cost you your job to report, "Quarterback John Jones had a pretty good night, hitting, oh, I'd say about half of his passes, for, I guess, a couple hundred yards, or so."

The same is true with dollars-and-cents stories. *Precision is mandatory.* Note:

> The average price of a ticket to a major league game has increased 9.7 percent, to $14.91 from $13.59.
> The Red Sox, whose Fenway Park is the smallest stadium in the majors, is still the most expensive team to see.
> Boston raised its tickets 16.6 percent to an average of $24.05, according to the Team Marketing Report, which released its annual study yesterday ... .
> Seattle, which moves from the Kingdome to Safeco Field on July 15, had the highest increase, a 27.2 percent rise to $19.01. The Mets raised prices 23.5 percent to an average of $19.98.
> Minnesota again has the least expensive average ticket price, even after a 2.9 percent increase to $8.46.
>
> The Associated Press[10]

Note in the preceding example how AP's pro reports ticket prices down to the last penny. No imprecision there. Two other factors of note:

- Each dollar figure is presented in a percentage, an enormous aid to reader comprehension. Here's what I thought when I read that first graf: "I didn't get a 9.7 percent raise in salary this year." That type of linkage with your readers' lives is how to make figures meaningful for them.
- The structure of this numbers story enables all fans everywhere to compare the ticket prices *they* pay to prices elsewhere. Such *comparatives* are essential in reporting numbers.

TRANSLATE WHAT NUMBERS MEAN

Forbes reports a baseball team's managing partner "spent $119 million last winter to sign six hotshot free agents."

So what? Here, *Forbes* translates "so what":

> The [managing partner] ... is digging himself into a big hole with his baseball franchise, which he and 29 limited partners bought for a record $130 million expansion fee.
>
> Thanks to those high-priced free agents, ... payroll has nearly doubled to $65 million—the third highest in the National League, behind only the New York Mets and the Los Angeles Dodgers. ...
>
> Add on the $20 million cost of operating, and servicing the debt on a spiffy new $355 million ballpark.

Now, the *Forbes* writer gets closer to "so what" for taxpayers:

> Taxpayers put up $240 million of the stadium's cost. But the team had to take out a $115 million loan to cover its portion of the cost.
>
> Including the stadium obligations, the team's total debt is $134 million, the fifth biggest in baseball. With total annual expenses now approaching $100 million, [the managing partner] needs to average 40,000 fans to break even. This year he has been averaging 37,000.
>
> Given the team's winning record, shouldn't fans be breaking down the gates? One reason they aren't is that many of them are still smarting from the way politicians financed the stadium.

Forbes now translates the meaning of all this for fans:

> [The managing partner] announced a 12% ticket price hike last September during Fan Appreciation Weekend. That puts home plate club-house seats at $55.
>
> Mary Summers
> *Forbes* [11]

Another example of effective translation:

Isaiah Rider of the Atlanta Hawks skips a practice and is suspended for one game. That means Rider won't be paid for one of the 82 games the Hawks will play. So?

So, a reporter who knows how to handle numbers translates that into meaningful terms:

> The suspension will cost Rider $65,853.66, equal to 1/82nd of his salary of $5.4 million. With fines, he has lost about $100,000 since joining the team, for the third practice of training camp.
>
> Jeffrey Denberg
> *Atlanta Journal-Constitution* [12]

PUT NUMBERS IN LOOK-AHEAD CONTEXT

Successful business executives study today's numbers and find tomorrow's meaning. That's where profit comes from.

Your readers deserve the same look-ahead context for numbers you report.
Note how Hal Bodley of *USA Today* "sets up" readers with the puzzle: Why
are the Cleveland Indians being sold?

> The Cleveland Indians earned $144.6 million in 1998. They will make
> even more than that when accountants complete this year's report.
> Since early 1995, the Indians have sold out every game at Jacobs Field, a
> major league record. And, yes, they've won five consecutive division titles.
> At a glance, this franchise is profitable and successful. Why then would
> Richard Jacobs sell his gem to Larry Dolan for a record $320 million?

Now, reporter Bodley provides the look-ahead context that answers the question:

> The answer is what's wrong with baseball. Even with the sellouts, Jacobs
> has maximized revenues. The Indians' payroll this season was $68.1 million.
> To continue with a championship-caliber team, the payroll for 2000 will
> jump as much as $10 million.
> Jacobs is certain revenues won't keep pace with escalating salaries when it
> comes time to retain premier players such as power-hitting outfielder
> Manny Ramirez—or lose them via free agency. So, he's selling high.
>
> Hal Bodley
> *USA Today*[13]

Again, you need no accounting degree for this numbers-orientated journalism. *USA Today*'s Bodley does just what you do in analyzing, say, the numbers
on a football team's ground game and their meaning for forthcoming games
and opponents.

In seeking context for numbers keep this in mind:

- *Historical trends* can give your readers much help in understanding numbers. If ticket price increases average 6 percent annually for 10 years, but jump 19 percent this year, significant meaning emerges from the numbers!
- *Deviations from the norm* can be extremely revealing. If, as a *Forbes* reporter discovered, major-league batters on average hit .273, why is Jeff Blauser of the Cubs, who hit .240, paid $4.2 million—particularly when five players earning Major League Baseball's minimum wage of $200,000 had higher averages than Blauser?[14]
- *Compare and characterize* numbers to illuminate their meaning. A $600 million offer is made for the Yankees baseball franchise. Is that much? In these days of mega-deals in business, who knows? *Forbes* does—and characterizes it as a "rich price." Cablevision is behind the offer. It took in $10.51 in ad revenue per subscriber last year. Standing alone, that means nothing. So, the reporter *compares and characterizes*: The $10.51 was

"more than double the figure for Fox Sports New York. Even ESPN, Disney's cable giant, made only $8.78."[15]

FOLLOW THE STARS

Let's face it, star athletes—and what they earn—are news, just as movie stars and business moguls are news. So, find and report the numbers on the stars.

Steve Hershey, golf writer for *USA Today*, like most golf writers, follows Tiger Woods' climb in the winnings column. His lead, highlights the magic number:

> LAKE BUENA VISTA, FLA.—After seven weeks away from the PGA Tour, Tiger Woods is returning rested and positioned to become a $6 million man.
>
> Steve Hershey
> *USA Today*[16]

Hershey covers the race for winnings just as he would cover any contest in sports. Woods is at $4,266,585 in winnings, his nearest competitor at $3,538,706; only two other golfers have a chance of passing Woods, and he "would have to collapse."

In following the stars, don't forget the millions they make in product endorsements and other sidelines. Even autograph-signing is a money-making business these days.

BE IMAGINATIVE IN USING NUMBERS

Conquer your math fright and you'll discover wonderfully imaginative stories can tumble out of those long grey columns of numbers. For example:

Two *Wall Street Journal* writers determine which player is highest paid for each position on National Football League teams. In a major takeout that fronts the newspaper's sports and entertainment Friday section, *The Weekend Journal*, Sam Walker and Jonathan B. Weinback, write:

> Welcome to *Weekend Journal*'s 1999 All-$tar team, where the players might not be the best, but their agents sure are. Just in time for the National Football League regular season, which begins next Sunday, we put our computers and financial experts into motion to determine which player will bank the most money this year at each position. ...
>
> ... The big news is how sharply salaries are rising in pro football, which has generally lagged far behind other pro sports in athlete pay. ... The league's average salary will likely surpass $1 million for the first time this year.

Now, the *Journal* reporters discuss how star salaries are increasing even more rapidly (quarterback Troy Aikman of the Dallas Cowboys is high, with $16 million), and the kicker:

In all, the players on our team will earn $90 million—about twice what they would have banked if we had done the same math four years ago. The bottom line: 1999 is shaping up to be, in the words of Dallas Cowboys owner Jerry Jones, "the greatest time on Earth to be a football player."

Sam Walker and Jonathan B. Weinbach
The Wall Street Journal[17]

Note the *timing and context* in the *Journal* story above. It's published on a Friday, before next Sunday's season opener, and today's top salaries are compared to those of four years ago. The story (in *thousands* of words) discusses star players by name, thus alerting fans to how their heroes are doing. The writers also signal the real meaning behind the numbers. Some teams risk spending themselves into financial trouble in the race to sign superstars.

Who said dollars-and-cents reporting in sports is dull?

BEWARE OF BEING MANIPULATED

It's a truism in business news writing (and should be also in sportswriting): 2 + 2 doesn't always equal 4.

That is, *be careful of numbers.* They may not mean what they appear to mean.

An accounting course or two in college (or later in night school) would be excellent preparation for a career in any sector in journalism, including sports. If nothing else, such instruction will put you at ease with searching numbers for their true meaning.

Seek help with complicated numbers stories. Talk to editors, senior reporters or experts in your newspaper's accounts section (where we journalists are legendary for our lack of basic math skills).

Recall the earlier example of two *Wall Street Journal* reporters who put "our computers and financial experts into motion" on the story about NFL salaries. Seeking help is smart.

Consider carefully the motives of sources who slip you numbers, just as you examine the motives of any news source.

Here's another truism in reporting: Powerful people and organizations attempt to manipulate reporters in their battles over money.

Thus, media commentator Allan Wolper finds major league baseball handing out free-lance assignments to newspaper reporters to write stories that are part of efforts to "blackmail" cities and taxpayer fans into financing new stadiums.[18]

Thus, players and team owners use the press and, by extension, public opinion in their war with each other over money. For example, you can tell contract negotiations are warming up, when this type story, published in the *Chicago Tribune*, appears:

Frank Thomas does not want to jump ship.
Sure, he's frustrated that the White Sox likely will still be rebuilding a

year from now. And, yes, he has been annoyed by manager Jerry Manuel's attempts to have him play first base. But neither is enough to make him want to leave Chicago.

"I'm not going to change my tune," he said. "Anything can happen, but I think I'll be here. After the two years I've had, I don't know if anyone would pick up the contract anyway."

The contract extension Thomas signed in 1997 calls for this provision: If he is traded, the deal is fully guaranteed through 2006 at about $10.3 million a year starting in 2001. If Thomas stays with the Sox, much of the money can be deferred over 10 years.

Teddy Greenstein
Chicago Tribune[19]

LEARN HOW TO REPORT LAW STORIES

Know anything about labor law and how the National Labor Relations Board works?

Baseball writers had to know much about that federal body in 1999 when umpires tried to muscle organized baseball for improved contracts, and a dispute arose.[20]

Baseball writers also found themselves covering a heated labor dispute when players struck in 1994, and the Federal Mediation and Conciliation Service made headlines.[21]

On a single day in 1999, these stories broke: contract litigation between universities and coaches, an athlete's arrest on child-molestation charges, sexual harassment lawsuits and race discrimination lawsuits.[22]

That is, the wide, wide wonderful world of sports reporting sometimes takes you into police stations and courtrooms.

A couple points:

First, the law of business is highly complex and far beyond the scope of this book. But, approach reporting it with the same careful, methodical techniques you take to any complex sports story. Find authoritative sources among lawyers and litigants. Go to the official record or official proceeding for definitive details. Write with fairness, accuracy and balance. And, remember, the law of defamation covers corporations as well as individuals.

Second, questions of ethical fairness frequently arise when sports figures are accused of illegal or immoral conduct.

Because they are public figures, sports notables become news for even minor infractions that might go unreported otherwise.

For athletes, there is danger that pretrial news coverage will prejudice the legal outcome or, at the very least, prejudice public attitudes. Proceed carefully when reporting accusations yet unproven. Your ethical responsibility is to be fair—to the athlete, as well as your reader-fans.

And always (as noted in Chapter Two) check and double-check any story that might inflict financial loss, harm to reputation or emotional distress. Stories take you into the law of defamation if they include accusations of illegal or immoral conduct.

Knees, Tendons and Other Body Parts

It was a dramatic sports moment, and Thomas George caught it beautifully for his *New York Times* readers:

> EAST RUTHERFORD, N.J.—The game was not yet 23 minutes old, the Jet's Super Bowl-dreaming season had not even reached its first halftime, when quarterback Vinny Testaverde went down, on his knees, hunched into a human ball. Howling.
>
> With his left Achilles' tendon ruptured, he had a pain in his head and in his heart that told him it was over for him for the year, right then, right there, on a Jet fumble that bounced around, with Testaverde spinning, twisting, trying to pounce on it. Snap. It was over.
>
> Off the field he went, on a cart, with all the Jets' eyes following him, with the 78,227 fans in Giants Stadium watching as if in a trance. The New England Patriots were mesmerized, too. How could such a thing happen? In the first game? With your starting quarterback? With an All-Pro quarterback? Snap.

In an instant, on field but also off, athletic careers, games, title hopes, personal and team fortunes—all can turn on what happens when the human body is pressed beyond its physical limits.

Reporting that in precise, accurate and authoritative detail is a major responsibility in sports journalism.

Things to remember:

CAPTURE THE WIDER MEANING

Stories such as Testaverde's injury carry great drama, and capturing that is important, of course. So is quickly exploring the *wider meaning* of injuries.

Reporting Testaverde's injury, the *Times'* George moves quickly to the *look-ahead element* so crucial in any sports story:

> The Jets spent the rest of the game wondering one thing: How are we going to recover from this? They asked themselves that daunting question for this game and for the season. For the game, they could not, losing, 30-28, on Adam Vinatieri's 23-yard field goal with three seconds left.
>
> For the season?
>
> "When you lose your quarterback, everybody is going to have to adjust," Jets Coach Bill Parcells said.

> Parcells knows that Testaverde—who, a few hours after the game was scheduled for surgery at Lenox Hill Hospital in Manhattan—faces a grueling recovery.
>
> Thomas George
> *The New York Times* [23]

For the same edition, *Times* writer Dave Anderson explores the *cause* of Testaverde's injury, looking ahead to the ongoing controversy over whether artificial turf is the cause of many injuries in football. Anderson's approach:

> EAST RUTHERFORD, N.J.—Stretched out face down, Vinny Testaverde was pounding the artificial turf with his right fist in frustration. Or maybe in retaliation.
>
> Nobody had to tell the Jets quarterback that the Achilles' tendon in his left heel was ruptured. He knew. In the second quarter of the Jets' opener yesterday, he also knew he was out for the season in which he was supposed to lead the Jets to Super Bowl XXXIV. ...
>
> Even more frustrating, Testaverde knew he hadn't been hit, hadn't even been touched. When he saw Curtis Martin fumble, he tried to pursue the loose ball, but he suddenly collapsed with one of sports' most painful injuries apparently caused by one of sports' most treacherous dangers—artificial turf.
>
> "I don't know," Coach Bill Parcells would say later when asked if the turf had caused Testaverde's injury. "I'd hate to say that."
>
> But just about everybody else on the Jets was talking about the Giants Stadium turf as if it were a killer at large. ...
>
> Nine days earlier, wide receiver Wayne Chrebet broke his left foot when he simply tried to cut on the new artificial turf, which had been installed that week.
>
> Dave Anderson
> *The New York Times* [24]

When quarterback Steve Young of the San Francisco 49ers was sidelined with successive concussions, fans naturally wondered if he would retire. *USA Today*'s Richard Weiner looked ahead wonderfully to the wider meaning:

> Young, 38, is torn. A fourth concussion in three years left him unconscious Sept. 27 at Arizona. Since, Young has sought medical opinions while those close to him have urged him to retire.
>
> Even if Young decides, here's why an official retirement announcement isn't coming soon:
>
> If Young were to retire before June 1, the transaction would represent a $5 million salary-cap hit to the already financially strapped 49ers. ...
>
> But if Young were to wait until after June 1 to retire, the 49ers would be hit with just a $1.2 million cap number for Young next season ...

Young, who in 1997 became the NFL's highest-paid player with a six-year, $45 million extension, would then cost the cap $3.75 million in 2001.

Besides, if Young were to announce his retirement next week, when the 49ers have a bye, he would lose 10/17ths of his $6.25 million salary this year: a total of $3.67 million.

Richard Weiner
USA Today[25]

REPORT IN AUTHORITATIVE DETAIL

In reporting sports injuries—as in writing science news generally—it's crucial that you recount precise details and *quote experts on their meaning*.

Here's precise reporting on surgery performed on Pat Croce, president of the Philadelphia 76ers, who was injured in a motorcycle accident (emphasis added):

UNIONDALE, N.Y.—A two-hour operation on 76ers president Pat Croce was labeled "a success" yesterday, but the next three months will be critical.

According to William Delong, the doctor who performed surgery on Croce's left leg after X-rays on Monday showed no bone growth, two screws were removed from a rod near the fractured area of Croce's leg, and marrow elements from Croce's pelvic area were injected into the injured area. *DeLong, who said* Croce had an 85 percent change of a successful recovery, said the operation marked yet another step toward trying to save Croce's leg.

"The operation was a success," *said DeLong, chief of orthopedic trauma at the Hospital of the University of Pennsylvania.*

Stephen A. Smith
The Philadelphia Inquirer[26]

Note how a *USA Today* writer strengthens an injury story with detail crucial to players (and their parents) *and* pulls in impressive and authoritative sources:

University of Florida women's soccer star Erin Gilhart retired last month, worried that heading balls was damaging her brain.

Gilhart began suffering blurred vision and memory lapses last year. When the symptoms returned after a game vs. UCLA, the All-America defender walked away, ending her career 1½ years early ...

Her decision, while rare, is a sign of the times in world soccer, where evidence is growing that head blows could be causing concussions and diminished mental functioning.

In a two-year study of 57 soccer players ages 11 to 14, David Janda, an orthopedic surgeon and director of the Institute for Preventive Sports Medicine in Ann Arbor, Mich., found nearly half had symptoms of concussion. Those symptoms—blurred or double vision, headaches, ear ringing, nausea—were most common in kids who headed the ball most often.

In September, *The Journal of the American Medical Association* published a report with similar conclusions. Dutch researchers compared the brain functions of 33 adult amateur soccer players with 27 middle-distance runners and swimmers. Most of the tests showed decreased performance in memory and planning among the soccer players.

Peter Brewington
USA Today[27]

A baseball writer for *The Sporting News* helps readers understand the precise nature of an injury to Wilson Alvarez of the Tampa Bay Devil Rays:

The Rays say Alvarez has inflammation in the AC joint—which is at the top corner of the shoulder, where the clavicle and scapula meet—and that the injury does not appear serious. The Rays say this injury is unrelated to and in a different spot than the shoulder pain that forced Alvarez to miss six weeks in the middle of last season.

Marc Topkin
The Sporting News[28]

An AP writer *characterizes* an injury suffered by wide receiver Robert Brooks of the Green Bay Packers (emphasis added):

His problems began on the first play of 1996. He tore his right anterior cruciate ligament, ruptured the patellar tendon and separated a large chunk of cartilage from the bone, *virtually an explosion of the knee.*

Greg Beacham
The Associated Press[29]

A *USA Today* reporter describes an injury in terms any fan can understand:

The American Academy of Neurology defines concussion as "trauma-induced alteration in mental status that may or may not involve loss of consciousness." *Simply, the brain gets shaken. You needn't be out cold.*

Beyond familiar symptoms such as headaches, nausea and loss of memory, there are others.

Seattle linebacker Chad Brown on the emotional effects: "I cry. I have no control over it. I can usually tell how severe my concussion is by how much of my emotions I lose."

Gary Mihoces
USA Today[30]

In summary, three characteristics must mark your reporting of sports injuries (or *any* medical or science news stories):

- Accuracy. It's paramount. Report carefully, with precision, and double-check.
- Quote authoritative sources. They include physicians, not linebacker coaches. And, as illustrated above, the Institute of Preventive Sports Medicine and *The Journal of the American Medical Association*, not locker-room rumor, are appropriate sources.
- Translate all medical terms. Readers may not understand a concussion is a "trauma-induced alteration in mental status" but they *will* understand "the brain gets shaken."

Now, About Drugs ...

Drug stories will enter your sports-reporter life in roughly two forms:

Illicit drugs, unfortunately, frequently are sports-section news, along with stories about rape, drunk driving, spousal abuse and other illegal off-field activities. The full range of human frailties is present in sports, as in all other sectors of society, and when they become illegal, you have a *crime story* with a sports twist.

Crime with a sports twist still is crime—even if sports heroes are involved—and it must be reported with all the frank detail and, importantly, the care given any story that reports illegal or immoral conduct.

That is, do as police reporters do: go to the official record, to authoritative sources, then check and double-check.

Stories about *performance-enhancing drugs* also are in the news frequently. They require very special handling.

First, if used carelessly, the term "taking drugs"—whether the good kind or the bad—carries a connotation of illegality and/or immorality.

Second, the sports world—both amateur and pro—is very unsure about what constitutes proper use of performance-enhancing drugs or stimulants.

For example, an enormous flap erupted in 1998 with reports that home-run king Mark McGwire of the St. Louis Cardinals took a nutritional supplement that supposedly builds muscle and a testosterone-producing stimulant.

Almost lost in the furor was the fact that the testosterone-producing supplement, though banned in some sports, was perfectly legal in baseball.

Somewhat plaintively, McGwire said, "Everybody I know in the game of baseball uses the same stuff I use."[31]

In 1999, a drug story became front-page news when it was revealed bicycle riders in the Tour de France, which *The New York Times* described as "one of Europe's legendary sporting events," were taking banned substances. Blood tests, urine tests and "masking substances" designed to conceal the presence of banned substances in the bloodstream became daily fodder for sportswriters everywhere.[32]

In sum, the "drug" story is filled with nuances and subtleties. Don't throw the word "drug" around loosely. Choose your language very carefully.

Summary

—Reporting the wider picture of sports involves covering societal phenomenon of many dimensions off court and off field, for media of all types.

—One crucial area of off-field sports reporting is the lifestyles and personal lives of athletes, which must be a subject of legitimate news coverage but not tawdry voyeurism.

—A second crucial area is the business structure of sports, where you must learn to report meaningful dollars-and-cents stories.

—The third crucial area involves learning to cover health, injuries and, unfortunately, drugs—all pivotal in the performance of individual athletes and teams.

—In determining what's "fair game" in covering athletes' personal lives always consider the readers' right to know but also your ethical responsibility to do the right thing.

—Unlike some sports reporters in times bygone, good reporters today don't cut special slack for sports heroes in trouble with the law; athletes get no special "zone of privacy."

—Any "private-life" event involving an athlete gets high news priority if it likely will affect a team's performance or the wider sports world.

—In reporting either amateur or pro sports, you'll need the skills of business-beat reporters to cover the business of sports.

—Unquestionably, the money of sports is a high-priority news story in which the public has a legitimate right and need to know.

—Reporting the business of sports requires you to adjust your mindset and realize it's big news and then to avoid panic over handling numbers (not a strong skill for many journalists).

—Discard irrelevant dollars-and-cents numbers and incorporate only the meaningful ones in your story, and report them with precision.

—Always translate the meaning of numbers by comparing and characterizing them. (For example, translating a one-game suspension of a basketball player into what it cost him in lost salary—$65,853.66!)

—When searching for the meaning of numbers look at historical trends (ticket-price increases over the past 10 years, for example) and deviations from the norm. (A baseball player is paid more even though his batting average is below the league norm.)

—Learn to report law stories—the business law of big-time sports, as well as contract negotiations, sexual harassment and race discrimination lawsuits and the arrest of sports figures.

—Injuries and health are big stories on the sports beat because they can change dramatically the fortunes of an athlete or entire team.

—Report injury stories in authoritative detail, being certain to quote experts on their meaning—as you would in any science-news story.

—Use of illicit drugs is a crime story, as is news about rape, drunk driving, spousal abuse and any other illegal off-field activity. And, crime with a sports twist still is crime to be reported with all the frank detail—and care—of any story on illegal or immoral conduct.

—Covering performance-enhancing drugs requires very special handling because the sports world is unsure about what constitutes proper use of stimulants, so don't loosely use "illegal" or "immoral" in such reporting.

Exercises

1. Study four issues of a newspaper designated by your instructor. Identify sports stories in the three crucial areas discussed in Chapter Four: stories on a) the lifestyles and personal lives of athletes, b) the business structure of sports and c) on health, injuries and drugs. In about 350 words, analyze this off-field coverage for its newsworthiness, topicality and importance to reader-fans. Is a well-rounded picture presented of the wider world of sports?

2. In about 300 words, discuss whether you agree that athletes are public figures whose lives—private as well as public—are "fair game" for sports reporters. Do you believe *all* dimensions of the lifestyle of a public-figure athlete should be covered? Why? Should there be a "zone of privacy" around some aspects of athletes' private lives?

3. Identify three campus stories you would write that involve reporting on business aspects of sports at your college. In about 50 to 75 words each, describe your story ideas, which sources you would approach in your reporting and, generally, the thrust of how you would write the stories.

4. This exercise will test your ability to use interview techniques discussed in Chapter Three and your understanding of the importance of sports injuries discussed in Chapter Four. Interview a trainer from one of the teams on your campus or a physician specializing in sports injuries. In 350 to 400 words, write a story on what precautions are taken to protect players from injuries, particularly concussions and knee injuries.

5. Interview the director of intramural athletics at your college. Use the wordage necessary for a story on how much money is budgeted for intramural sports and, particularly, for individual sports within that program. Present your readers with some historical context, such as total spending for each of the three previous years.

Recommended Reading

Highly-skilled coverage of sports business appears regularly in *The Wall Street Journal*, where any aspiring sportswriter can find superb examples of reporting accurately and interpreting meaningfully the intricacies of business and the numbers that drive it. *The New York Times* and *The Washington Post* cover the business of sports with highly-talented writers.

See *Fortune, Business Week* and, particularly, *Forbes* for examples of business writing in magazine style.

Though not focused on sports business, helpful guidance is in Louis M. Kohlmeier Jr., Jon G. Udell and Laird B. Anderson, *Reporting on Business and the Economy* (Englewood Cliff, NJ: Prentice-Hall, 1981).

I devote special sections to business, sports and science reporting in *Introduction to Professional Newswriting,* 2nd ed. (New York: Longman, 1998), *Introduction to Magazine Writing* (New York: Macmillan Publishing Company, 1993) and *Bottom Line Writing* (Ames: Iowa State University Press, 2000).

See also *The Business Journalist*, published by the Society of American Business Editors and Writers Inc. (www.sabew.org).

Notes

1. These stories respectively, were John Helyar, "Power Plays," *The Wall Street Journal*, Aug. 7, 1955, p. 1; "Girl Power Plays," *The Economist*, June 26, 1999, p. 35; Daniel Fisher and Michael K. Ozanian, "Cowboy Capitalism," *Forbes*, Sept. 29, 1999, p. 170; Joe Lapointe, "With a Few Tears and a Final Assist, Gretzky Says Goodby," *The New York Times*, April 19, 1999, p. A-1.

2. "Anderson Blames Self for Woes," Oct. 29, 1998, p. D-1.

3. "Infidelity is Holyfield's Toughest Foe," Sept. 22, 1998, p. F-1.

4. Dispatch for afternoon papers of April 23, 1999.

5. Dispatch for Saturday papers, Oct. 23, 1999.

6. Kenneth W. Goodman, "A DiMaggio Rule on Medical Privacy," *The New York Times*, Dec. 30, 1998, p. A-17.

7. "A Nation Turns Its Eyes to Center Field, One More Time," April 25, 1999, Sports Sunday, p. 31.

8. "One Viewpoint from Afar: Reporting at Its Worst," Oct. 26, 1999, p. F-6.

9. "Athletics," *The Chronicle of Higher Education*, Nov. 12, 1999, p. A-57.

10. Dispatch for morning papers, April 2, 1999.

11. "Bottom of the Ninth, Two Out," Nov. 1, 1999, p. 69.

12. "Rider Earns One-Game Suspension," Nov. 16, 1999, p. F-1.

13. "Indians' Success Comes at a Higher Price," Nov. 5, 1999, p. C-15.

14. Dan Seligman, "The Baseball Enigma," *Forbes*, Nov. 15, 1999, p. 176.

15. Jan Akasie, "Out of His League," *Forbes*, Sept. 20, 1999, p. 54.

16. "Woods Could Become First $6 Million Golfer," Oct. 21, 1999, p. C-7.

17. "All-$tars of '99," Sept. 3, 1999, p. W-1.

18. Allan Wolper, "The Ethics Exchange," *Editor & Publisher*, March 20, 1999, p. 48.

19. "Inside the White Sox," Aug. 12, 1999, Section 4, p. 12.

20. For an example, see Mark Asher, "Umpires Set to Vote on Phillip's Future," *The Washington Post*, Oct. 29, 1999, p. D-4.

21. An example is Murray Chass, "Baseball Takes a Third Strike: No Hope for Talks," Sept. 1, 1994, p. B-15.

22. AP covered all these in dispatches for Saturday papers, Aug. 21, 1999.

23. "For Stunned Jets, First-and-Long," Sept. 13, 1999, p. D-1.

24. "Unnatural-Born Killers: Turf That Stopped the Jets," Sept. 13, 1999, p. D-6.

25. "Money Matters Muddle Young's Decision," Oct. 21, 1999, p. C-1.

26. "Surgeon Sees Success in Operation on Croce," Oct. 13, 1999, p. E-4.

27. "Headers Face Scrutiny in Soccer," Nov. 5, 1999, p. C-3.

28. "Alvarez's Injury Puts Pressure on Bullpen," April 26, 1999, p. 32.

29. AP dispatch for Sunday papers, Aug. 8, 1999.

30. "Dangerous Head Games," Nov. 5, 1999, p. C-1.

31. For a summary, see Mark Fitzgerald, "Furor Follows AP Disclosure on McGwire," *Editor & Publisher*, Aug. 29, 1998, p. 10.

32. An excellent wrap-up in Christopher Clarey and Samuel Abt, "Drug Scandals Dampen Cycling's Top Event," *The New York Times*, July 3, 1999, p. A-1.

PART THREE

Making the Writer's Muse Move

True writing genius is found in sports pages. Some of journalism's best writers hang out there.

To join those writers, you should start—now—developing a distinctively personal and strong writing style. It's long, hard work, but the rewards can be huge. Although strong reporting skills can get you a *job*, adding strong writing ability can get you a *career*.

In Part Three, we will explore techniques you can use to jump-start your search for such a personal style.

What we *won't* do is worship leads like this:

> Outlined against a blue-gray October sky, the Four
> Horsemen rode again. In dramatic lore, they are known as
> Famine, Pestilence, Destruction and Death. These are only
> aliases. Their real names are Struhldreher, Miller, Crowley and

Layden. They formed the crest of the South Bend cyclone before which another fighting Army football team was swept over the precipice yesterday afternoon as 55,000 spectators peered down on the bewildering panorama spread on the green plain below.[1]

Surprised that we're *not* going to linger worshipfully over such writing? After all, that lead—published in 1924—was written by the now-lionized Grantland Rice, and certainly is one of the most-quoted leads in the history of sportswriting.

You also may be surprised at something else we're *not* going to do: practice writing that slips the moorings of reality and pants over sports stars by, for example, assigning them fanciful nicknames such as Sultan of Swat for a baseball player (Babe Ruth), Manassa Mauler for a boxer (Jack Dempsey) and Galloping Ghost for a football player (Red Grange).

Do I suggest sports sacrilege? No, because that lead—and those nicknames—are examples of florid, overwritten prose that is scorned today by our best writers.

Interestingly, even those sports reporters who wrote that way in the 1920s and 1930s knew they were stretching. One colorful (and very clever) writer of that era, Paul Gallico of the *New York Daily News*, acknowledged he was a "Gee-whizzer" who churned out "the most florid and exciting prose."[2] Gallico & Co. were enormously talented writers, but their keyboard excesses led to myth-making in sports, to drawing a picture of games and athletes that, though exciting and colorful, was untrue.

Well, those times are gone, so we'll look at writing styles that are more accurate, styles that have both feet on honest ground—but still are no less open, engaging or readable.

We'll start in Chapter Five, Writing It Straight, by looking at writing styles for basic spot-news stories that go directly and quickly to the point, in minimum language but with maximum impact to *tell the news* simply and clearly.

Then, in Chapter Six, Taking Readers Beyond the Score, we'll study styles that let you spread your writer's wings in analytical and interpretive writing.

5

Writing It Straight

LET ME guess your career goal: sportswriter-analyst at the very least, but renowned (and well-paid) sports columnist-essayist by preference.

So, why don't we just skip this business about writing it straight? Why linger over that old Five-Ws-and-How stuff?

Because:

- We write for *news*papers and other *news* media. Despite our strong move toward writing that's entertaining and analytical, there is need, in every newspaper and in every magazine, for *telling the news* and not just *pontificating* about it.
- Learning to write straightforward hard-news stories is an essential technical step before you spread your wings with analytical and interpretive writing. The basic news story is the foundation of all we do. So, don't try to move your writer's muse too far, too fast. First, learn to report and write straightforward game stories and news breaks.

The Basic Story's Minimum Goals

What's "good" in writing, like what's "good" in any art form, is pretty much up to individual taste. Readers—and writers—sometimes react with astonishing disagreement over how we define news, report it and write it.

Nevertheless, reasonable journalists can agree on minimum requirements for the basic news story. Nothing beats the old trick of sitting back after you've written one and ticking them off: Does your story answer who, what, where, when, why and how?

Here, in its most basic form, is a story that meets all those needs in clear, minimal language:

> OXFORD, MISS.—Keith Carter tied a career-high with 33 points as Mississippi beat No. 21 Arkansas 89-81 Saturday to complete a regular-season sweep of the Razorbacks.
>
> The Rebels (15-7, 5-4 Southeastern Conference), who had to overcome a 10-0 deficit to start the game, have won five of the last six games against Arkansas (15-6, 4-4).
>
> Carter's 3-pointer with 12:02 left put Ole Miss ahead for good, 60-57. That was part of a 16-5 run and ended a two-minute explosion by Carter in which he scored 10 straight points.
>
> Freshman Chris Jeffries had 19 points to lead Arkansas.
>
> The Associated Press[3]

The preceding story can be read and its crucial information absorbed with almost at-a-glance quickness. It was one of scores transmitted by AP one night and published the next morning in newspapers across the nation to give eager basketball fans a sweeping view of court action. (*The Aiken [S.C.] Standard* published this and 10 other similar stories on a single page.)[4]

This type of basic story has these characteristics:

- Crisp and clean language, short and punchy sentences. Note AP's lead is just 24 words; the story's five sentences average 19 words.
- "Where and when" are handled smoothly and quickly: The dateline (so-named even though it contains no date) answers "where?"—Oxford—and "Saturday" answers "when?"
- "What?" is in the score.
- The "why?" of the outcome and "who?" are answered with, "Keith Carter had a career-high with 33 points." ... *Always* get star performance into your story, in a high position. This, along with pivotal plays, injuries or coaching decisions, almost always answers "how" a game was won.
- Minimum "color" is inserted in such basic stories because getting poetic uses wordage that is needed to provide the news fundamentals. The closest AP comes to color in this story is the third-graf mention of a "two-minute explosion."
- Context for the outcome must be provided, no matter how brief or "hard-news" the story. Note how neatly that is done: "career-high" and "regular-season sweep" (first graf), "five of the last six games" (second), plus the bracketed win-loss records (second, again).

This lead about a hockey game highlights *star performance* (emphasis added):

> FAYETTEVILLE, N.C.—*Frankie "The Wall" Ouellette saved all five Fayetteville Force shootout attempts* to lead the Columbus Cottonmouths

to a 4-3 victory at the Crown Coliseum Thursday night.

The Cottonmouths (39-17-6) *got two goals from Rob Sinclair, one goal from Dave Neilson, two assists from Mike Martens* and *one assist each from Jerome Bechard and Grady Manson.*

Ouellette saved 27 of 30 Force shots in regulation to earn his 22nd victory of the season. Ouellette is 12-0-1 in his last 13 starts.

Matt Musgrove
Columbus (Ga.) Ledger-Enquirer[5]

Here's a spot-news lead built around the *turning point* in a game (emphasis added):

BLOOMINGTON, IND.—Candi Crawford's layup with 21 seconds remaining capped No. 17 Purdue's *rally from a 10-point deficit* and the Boilermakers beat Indiana State 69-67 in the Big Four Classic.

The Associated Press[6]

Another *reports the tone* of a game in just five words (emphasis added):

BOSTON—Becky Gottstein had 26 points and Kim Mackie added 17, both career-highs, as No. 24 Boston College *coasted to an 83-70 victory* over Kent on Saturday.

The Associated Press[7]

This lead *serves as a roundup* by combining two games in one story:

EVANS, GA.—George Matthews scored 20 points to lead South Aiken High School to a 70-43 rout of Lakeside (Ga.) High School in boys basketball Saturday night.

In girls action, South Aiken dropped its seventh consecutive game with a 47-39 loss to Lakeside.

In the boys game ... .

The Aiken (S.C.) Standard[8]

The more distant a game, the more background your reader-fan needs. Just how much background to insert is a judgment you must make carefully.

Below, a writer for the *Oneonta (N.Y.) Daily Star* inserts considerable background for a game distant not only in miles but, perhaps, also distant from reader-fan mainstream thinking (emphasis added):

MIDDLEBURY, VT.—Middlebury scored seven goals over a 25-minute span, holding Oneonta State to none during the same time frame, on its way to a 19-6 *men's lacrosse victory* Wednesday in *the first round of the NCAA Division III Tournament.*

The two-time Empire Lacrosse League champion Red Dragons (10-4), *ranked 11th in the country*, took their only lead of the contest at Youngman Field with 5:29 gone in the first period. Brian Dooley scored to give O-State a 2-1 lead, but the Panthers came back with the next seven goals.

Oneonta (N.Y.) Daily Star[9]

Below, an AP correspondent in London stacks background in the first two grafs of a spot-news story written for U.S. readers not intimately familiar with the event (this was published by *The New York Times*):

Paul Scholes scored twice as England beat Scotland, 2-0, yesterday in Glasgow, Scotland, in the *first leg of their playoff for a berth in next summer's European Championship.*

The Manchester United mid-fielder scored in the 18th and 42nd minutes, *giving England a commanding lead in the home-and-away, total-goals series, which finishes Wednesday at Wembley in London.*

The Associated Press[10]

Sometimes, *off*-field events outweigh what happens *on* the field, and when that happens you must use the same spot-news reporting and writing techniques you would use in, well, covering a street brawl:

BALTIMORE—The Cuban batters weren't the only ones hitting hard at Camden Yards.

An anti-Castro demonstrator was body-slammed and punched by a Cuban umpire behind second base in the middle of Monday night's game between a Cuban all-star team and the Baltimore Orioles.

The Associated Press[11]

Lesson: You're a *reporter* first, a *sportswriter* second. So watch for news of all sorts, wherever it breaks.

The Good Ol' Inverted Pyramid

Those bare-bones leads you just read really serve best atop the *inverted pyramid* structure, used for generations by newspapers and still the workhorse for thousands of sports stories published daily.

The fundamental strengths of this structure, and its enduring popularity with editors, flow from this: Writers can write their hearts out, to virtually any length, and cool-headed editors ("cold-hearted" you'll sometimes think) can slash their stories, from the bottom, to fit the limited newshole available and still present readers with essential details, even if in only a single lead graf.

To understand why you'll have to endure such slash-and-publish editing, you must realize AP alone throws *hundreds* of game stories and spot-news stories on editors' desks every night, in just a few hours. Local reporters add dozens more. And most must be squeezed into the sports section.

Below, an AP reporter uses the inverted pyramid for a New York hockey game. The first graf alone can be plugged into a sports page jammed with thousands of words on other sports events. In this case, the story is run at length in a Georgia paper because an Atlanta team is involved. Note how you could trim this story easily from the bottom:

UNIONDALE, N.Y.—Mike Stapleton scored his second goal of the game with just 30.7 seconds left to give the Atlanta Thrashers a 4-3 victory Saturday night over the New York Islanders.

The expansion Thrashers have won only two road games and both have come against the Islanders. Atlanta has as many victories this season at Nassau Coliseum as the Islanders, who now have the fewest points in the NHL with 15.

Stapleton's stunning game-winner came as he carried the puck into the Islanders' zone and beat Felix Potvin with a slap shot high on the stick side.

The Islanders tied it 3-3 in the final period on Mariusz Czerkawski's power-play goal at 10:07. Jamie Heward fed the puck to Czerkawski in the right circle, whose shot deflected into the net for his ninth of the season.

With just over two minutes remaining, Norm Maracle, who stopped 34 shots, kept the game tied when he made a stick save on Czerkawski, who came in on a partial breakaway.

The Islanders were 2-for-3 with the man advantage after not scoring a power-play goal in their previous four games ...

Ira Powel
The Associated Press
(Published in *The Athens (Ga.) Daily New & Banner-Herald*)[12]

Now, the AP's writer goes on for hundreds more words, *chronologically* recounting pivotal plays during the game. The chronology, like the preceding six grafs, *can be trimmed easily from the bottom*.

Note this about the inverted-pyramid structure:

- It requires extremely strong understanding of news values and priorities. You must weave important developments (including the score) into the first graf and no later than the second and third grafs.
- You cannot write a color narrative with intricately linked elements—a descriptive introduction tied, say, to a chronological middle and to a finely tuned, featurish "kicker" at the end. This workhorse structure has to endure slash-and-publish editing from the bottom up and *still* give reader-fans the essentials.
- The inverted pyramid *assumes reader-fans haven't seen the game on TV* and don't know the outcome or details from the Internet or other media. If reader-fans stayed up to watch "Monday Night Football" on ABC, can you attract them Tuesday with a lead that reports simply who won the game? No.
- Like a workhorse pulling a wagon, the inverted-pyramid story sometimes just plods along. It can be dull reading and, because it's used so much, can inflict a dreary sameness on readers.

Writing to Compete Against Television

It's challenging, but possible, to write an interesting game story for reader-fans who already know the outcome. Keep these points in mind:

- The outcome—the score—now is secondary as you assign writing priorities to other news elements of your story.
- Top priority must be given to color details and reporting who or what was responsible for the outcome.
- Coming off television's see-it-now reporting, your reader-fan wants a confirmation of what was seen—an explanation, perhaps, of a key play or coaching decision and, above all, a pleasurable reading revisit to a sporting event that was watched with excitement.

Note below how a *Los Angeles Times* writer focuses superbly on *color descriptive* for a spot-news story written after a Monday night game and published Tuesday morning:

> LAHAINA, HAWAII—The sweat-soaked red-and-gold uniforms and the late gasps for air told as much of the story as the final score.
> There are going to be games in which having only five or six players to count on is not going to be enough, no matter the heart of the effort. USC

found that out Monday, getting worn down and ultimately worn out by fifth-ranked North Carolina, 82-65, in the first round of the 16th Maui Invitational tournament.

> Mike Terry
> *Los Angeles Times* [13]

Another *Los Angeles Times* writer focuses on a *star performer* to lead a spot-news report, for Wednesday morning reading, on a game played and televised Tuesday night:

> DENVER—Marcel Cousineau got by with the help of his friends Tuesday night.
> A lot of help.
> From a lot of friends.
> Cousineau, along on the two-game trip as a goalie insurance policy, was cashed in for the final two periods when Jamie Storr suffered a groin strain stopping a breakaway 17:27 into the Kings' 6-2 win over Colorado at the Pepsi Center.
> The victory broke a two-game losing streak, and the game ended under a dark cloud. Storr was injured when he went down to block a shot by Joe Sakic. He stayed down briefly, rose to play the final 2:33 of the period and then sat in a tunnel alongside the bench, becoming president of the Cousineau fan club.

Now, the *Times* writer inserts game details and background on teammate injuries that put Cousineau, a backup goalie, in position to star in the game.

What's still missing?

It's elaboration of the news peg in the lead—that Cousineau got help from friends. Here is how the *Times* writer handles that:

> Several things worked in Cousineau's favor Tuesday night, including goals by Vladimir Tsyplakov and Rob Blake 52 seconds apart. Cousineau had a 3-1 lead to nurse and had played only 2:28.
> Also, the Kings outshot Colorado, 6-0, in that span. By game's end, the Kings had their largest scoring output of the season.
> "That helped a lot," Cousineau said of the pressure-reducing offensive benevolence. "You get a good feeling right away when you get a lead like that."
> More help came from a King defense that took things personally around the net.

> Jim Hodges
> *Los Angeles Times* [14]

Make it a rule that when you peg a lead on a single element, *always* back up that element with elaboration. And, the higher in the story that you flesh it out, the better, especially in what might be called a "hero lead."

For every hero in sports there's always a goat (or two), and *that* also can be a wonderful peg for a spot-news lead. Note this "*goat lead*":

> FOXBORO, MASS.—Two defensive blunders by the Los Angeles Galaxy were all D.C. United needed today to capture its third title in the four years of Major League Soccer with a 2-0 victory before 44,910 at Foxboro Stadium.
>
> Alex Yannis
> *The New York Times* [15]

Here's another spot-news lead designed to take reader-fans beyond what they already know, the outcome. You judge whether the writer succeeds.

> The Escape Artists, also known as the UCLA women's basketball team, brought their act home to Pauley Pavillion and pumped up the drama on Tuesday night.
>
> So no, if you weren't aware that the Bruins could wiggle out of the tightest of spots, well, they made it two for two in this young season. Fourth-ranked UCLA stayed on the tightrope—barely—as it defeated Texas, 84-77, on overtime.
>
> Lisa Dillman
> *Los Angeles Times* [16]

Do you like that lead above? I have several objections.

- "Escape Artists" takes me back to the Galloping Ghost and Manassa Mauler of the 1930s. The cutesy nickname is too much.
- The writer *tells* me there was drama in the game rather than providing exciting detail that lets me *see* the drama for myself.

In sum, the spot-news lead is alive and well in this era of ubiquitous television coverage. But you must write carefully to make it work for you.

Precedes, Follows and Look-Aheads

Can you solve the following equation?

voracious reader-fan interest + gameless days = pressure on you

Pressure comes from having to develop spot-news stories when there isn't major spot news to report. Teams may play only a couple times or even once a week, but the true reader-fan wants to read about them *seven* days a week. Fortunately, three story forms help you solve the equation:

- *Precedes* are vehicles you can use to inform readers of a forthcoming game or event.
- *Follows* are stories in which you can pick apart, to the delight of reader-fans, the game just past.
- *Look-aheads* enable you to look further with long-range visions for the rest of a season or for next year's season.

The Precede

Does the following lead work?

> MILWAUKEE—Villanova and Mississippi meet tonight in the first round of the NCAA Midwest Regional.

Nah! I wrote that just to show you how dull your writing will be if you peg a story to "meet tonight" angles. The following is how a pro writes precedes.

> MILWAUKEE—It's the age-old question whenever basketball teams are being judged or evaluated: Does the tall team or the quick team have the advantage?
>
> . Villanova and Mississippi will debate that issue tonight on the court at the Bradley Center in the first round of the NCAA Midwest Regional (Channel 3, approximately 10:20).
>
> The Wildcats (21-10), seeded eighth, have the size edge. With 6-foot-10 Mark Allen starting at center and 6-10 freshman Brooks Sales at forward, they have two players with at least four inches on the tallest Rebels starter.
>
> On the other hand, Mississippi (19-12), the ninth seed, plays up front with two 6-6 players, Jason Smith and Marcus Hicks, while going with a three-guard attacked sparked by 6-4 senior Keith Carter, the team's leading scorer. The Rebels do have a 6-8 player, Rahim Lockhart, who comes off the bench.
>
> "If you have a big team, it can be a tremendous advantage," Villanova coach Steve Lappas said after the Wildcats went through a brief workout last night at the Bradley Center. "But their quickness is a tremendous advantage for them. Their two 6-6 kids are quick, high-jumping kids. We'll come out with two big kids who are not as quick and don't jump as high. It will be interesting to see how it plays out at the end."
>
> Joe Juliano
> *The Philadelphia Inquirer*[17]

Note that what could have been a dull story is turned into a winner. How?

- Writer Juliano is a basketball expert and uses his expertise to focus on what is an "age-old question" about the game. To succeed in sportswriting you must know your game.

- Juliano *reports with precision* the size of opposing players, which backs up the tall vs. quick peg in his lead. Report thoroughly, and your story often writes itself.
- The Lappas quote nicely fleshes out the thrust of the story. Search for—and use prominently—strong quotes.

Incidentally, note that the *Inquirer*'s Juliano includes TV channel and time for reader-fans who want to watch the game. You'll compete against television, but don't carry the battle to ridiculous lengths by ignoring it. Your job is to serve reader-fans, and TV listings can be part of that.

Note in the following article how a superb writer takes her Pennsylvania readers on a jaunt through a distant Connecticut town, under "snow-dusted trees," as a precede for tonight's game.

> STORRS, CONN.—The scene is daunting for a visiting team. It sends chills, breeds fear. Everything in this college town seems blue and white and emblazoned with "Go Huskies" in these March Madness days.
>
> The women's basketball players from No. 16-seeded St. Francis of Loretto, Pa., insist the surroundings will not shake them.
>
> Not the University of Connecticut banners hanging from balconies and rooftops, not the pictures of the wolf-like dog that grace the portals of bars and restaurants, not the radio disc jockeys talking of basketball-ticket giveaways.
>
> In this town tucked behind snow-dusted trees and left alone by nearby Hartford and not-so-distant Boston, UConn basketball fans are ebullient and the home-court advantage never higher than when a Huskies team hosts an NCAA tournament game at the mystifying Harry A. Gampel Pavillion.
>
> Visitors are not welcome.
>
> Tonight, the No. 4-ranked UConn women's team (27-4), the No. 1 seed in the Mideast Region, hosts insistently unintimidated St. Francis (18-11), the Northeast Conference champion Red Flash.
>
> Marcia C. Smith
> *The Philadelphia Inquirer* [18]

Does that beat a precede pegged to, "St. Francis plays Union tonight"? You bet.

Here's a precede that focuses on a player injury and its possible meaning for a forthcoming game (emphasis added).

> GREEN BAY—All-pro wide receiver Antonio Freeman hasn't played back to that level of excellence this season, partially because of a lingering groin injury that the Green Bay Packers believe has diminished his speed and quickness.

> Coupled with the concussion that he suffered Sunday on an illegal hel-
> met-to-helmet hit by Detroit safety Mark Carrier, Freeman's physical condi-
> tion *is forcing the coaching staff to take a long look at withholding him from the
> game Monday night against the San Francisco 49ers.*
>
> "We've got to make a decision pretty soon whether we're going to rest
> him, or whether he'll get better with rest or not," offensive coordinator
> Sherman Lewis said Wednesday."
>
> Bob McGinn
> *Milwaukee Journal-Sentinel*[19]

Unless you've lived in or visited "Packer-land," you may not understand how
those sore spots on opposite ends of Antonio Freeman were discussed throughout Wisconsin. Fans there want precedes on *everything* that can influence forthcoming Packer games.

The Follow

Ah! The memory lingers on—forever in sports, it sometimes seems.

So, occasionally look backward for your reader-fans. Walk them over old bat-
tlegrounds, dissect old fights, *analyze the why and how of past outcomes.*

Here's how AP, *for Thursday morning publication*, looks back at a *Sunday*
game and, with new information (an interview), writes a perfect *follow*:

> GREEN BAY (AP)—Packers offensive coordinator Sherman Lewis finally
> found the spark he was looking for in the no-huddle offensive.
>
> The Packers ran four plays against Detroit in the no-huddle before the
> first quarter expired, registering two first downs, including a 53-yard pass
> play from quarterback Brett Favre to running back Dorsey Levens.
>
> The Packers beat the Lions 26-17 last Sunday.
>
> Opening up the second quarter, the Packers went back to the huddle, but
> the drive finished with a field goal.
>
> "I thought it got us kind of going," Lewis said, "We were struggling a lit-
> tle bit. We went three-and-out, three-and-out. I thought that was the time
> for it.
>
> "Just to change the tempo of the game, jumpstart us a little bit and I
> thought it did. We got first downs. That's the way I'd like to use it. I was
> thinking about using later if we needed it."

Note these characteristics of the follow:

- Its news peg is serious study of a game tactic that reader-fans (this being
  "Packer-land") undoubtedly discussed with friends all week. Again: know
  your game, its nuances and its subtleties.
- The follow—*like any sports story*—treats as *news* any major events shown
  on television. A surprise tactic, a key play, an injury, a fistfight at mid-

field—they all need explanation in print coverage if television coverage has left millions of viewers wondering the next day what happened.

- The follow rides on a meaningful interview with an authoritative source—the offensive coordinator who engineered the tactical change. An explanatory quote is used at length. Don't simply talk to yourself, then write. That almost always yields only what we call a "thumb-sucker"—an empty, superficial story written without any original reporting.
- The game's time element, "last Sunday," is subordinated to third-graf position. The new interview with Lewis "freshens" the time element.

Now, as interesting as this follow is, it still looks backward, and we're forward-looking writers for news media that always must answer the question, "What's next?"

Well, AP's writer makes an excellent transition to what's ahead for *next* Sunday:

> But Lewis said he won't be overusing the changeup.
> Wide receiver Antonio Freeman is listed as probable on the injury report with a groin injury, which indicates his chances of playing are good.
> They could be thinking about resting Freeman for a week when he's really needed.
> "We have to kind of see as we go," Lewis said, "We have to make a decision if he'll get better with rest. We're going to need him big-time down the stretch.
> Whatever's best to get him 100 percent we're going to have to do."
> Freeman also suffered a concussion against Detroit last Sunday.
>
> The Associated Press [20]

Here's a follow by George King of *The New York Post* that exudes expertise.

> BOSTON—Consider the moves the Yankees made yesterday as a line change instead of a major shakeup that would lead everybody to believe panic had settled into the Yankees' universe.
> In order to make room for reliever Jeff Nelson's return from the DL after an inflamed right elbow, the Yankees designated lefty reliever Tony Fossas for assignment.
> Knowing that he wouldn't have Ramiro Mendoza for last night's game against the Red Sox at Fenway because Mendoza worked 3 2/3 innings Wednesday, Joe Torre requested another pitcher be available in long relief last night.
> So Todd Erdos was summoned from Columbus (Triple-A) to be on call in case Orlando "El Duque" Hernandez' struggles continued. Right reliever Jay Tessmer was optioned back to Columbus to clear a locker for Erdos.

If you're not an expert on baseball, don't try to write the way George King does. And, if you're not an expert reader-fan, don't try to read him! King *writes for insiders* enthralled with the game. Note his insider language—"DL," for example, which all true fans know means "disabled list."

Like all good *news*paper writers, King has to "kick" his follow ahead to the news. He does this:

> Another move has to be made today to make room for Roger Clemens' return from the DL. That could be Erdos going down or righty reliever Dan Naulty, who is nursing a stiff neck, could be placed on the DL. And of course the Yankees could come to their senses and place third string catcher Mike Figga, the only player in the majors on a roster from Opening Day who hasn't played yet, on waivers.
>
> George King
> *New York Post* [21]

The Look-Ahead

"Yes, but ... what does it all mean?"

That's your reader-fan, inundated by daily journalism's bits and pieces from around the sporting circuit, trying to see the broader picture of what's ahead.

The *look-ahead* is a reporting and writing approach well-suited to gathering those bits and pieces, making them into a coherent whole for reader-fans and directing them ahead to the understanding they seek.

Note: The look-ahead is a *reporter's* device, one *solidly based on spot-news reporting*. It isn't the highly-personalized analytical writing, featuring the perpendicular pronoun "I," created so effectively by many sports columnists (and which we will study in future chapters).

For example, a superb reporter, Jason Diamos of *The New York Times*, sniffs around the New York Rangers hockey team, puts together a pattern of developments and comes up with the following look-ahead:

> Whether it is fair or not, Rangers Coach John Muckler is in dire jeopardy of losing his job, possibly as early as this week.
>
> The Rangers' president and general manager, Neil Smith, would not comment on Muckler's status after the Rangers were embarrassed by the Boston Bruins, 5-2, at Madison Square Garden on Saturday, a loss that left the Rangers 0-5-1 in their last six games at home.
>
> With a league-record $59 million payroll, the Rangers are a major disappointment at 6-10-3 over all.
>
> Smith's refusal to comment was not a surprise. His superiors at the Garden ordered him not to discuss anyone's job status after he talked candidly about Muckler's situation in Chicago the previous weekend.

Even if Smith had decided it is time for a drastic change, such a move would take time given the management structure of the Garden and its owner, Cablevision.

Jason Diamos
The New York Times [22]

In subsequent grafs, Diamos lays out some of the bits and pieces that went into his look-ahead: Only one player has spoken in defense of the coach, tension between the coach and club president increased in recent weeks with team losses, the club is doing so badly that it's either fire the players or fire the coach—"So it looks as if Muckler ... is set to take the fall."

Here's a look-ahead published on a Monday that's built around recent time elements—a meeting the previous Friday and an interview on Sunday:

Having seen their investment suffer a late-season implosion for the second straight year, the people who own the Phillies have decided it's time to get serious about improving their ball club.

They're going to spend some money.

In their quarterly meeting Friday, the team's investors informed general manager Ed Wase that he will have more financial freedom to improve the team this winter.

"I'm not telling you I have $65 or $70 million to work with," Wade said yesterday. "There are limitations. But the limitations aren't as dramatic."

"The partners are in agreement about improving the club. The baseball decisions we make to improve it will not necessarily be encumbered by numbers. I've been given significant leeway to make improvements."

Wade, who is presiding over a team that is blessed with offense but short on pitching, said he will have the freedom to pursue significant free agents this winter.

Jim Salisbury
The Philadelphia Inquirer [23]

There, reader-fans, is something to look ahead to—a winter of watching your team woo high-priced free agents.

Below, Dave Sheinin of <i>The Washington Post</i> surveys not the outcome of a meeting yesterday and not an interview the day before. Rather, he looks at a team's performance over three-quarters of a season and takes a futuristic look ahead:

CLEVELAND—With the Baltimore Orioles' trying season nearly three-quarters over and the focus having shifted to the future, fundamental questions hang over this veteran-heavy team. As Frank Wren prepares for his first full off-season as their general manager, he is ushering in a major organizational shift in the way the Orioles build their team.

Traditionally, the Orioles put together their team based on available free agents.

"Those days are over, absolutely over," Wren said. "I don't want to be part of an organization that builds that way. This has been a summer where, with our draft and what we have now in our farm system, we won't have to be a major player" in free agency. Wren, however, noted that the team may still shop the free agent markets in some way.

In recent weeks, Wren has been spending more time with the team's minor league teams, charting progress of prospects, listening to managers and coaches, assessing where the organization stands.

"This year and next year, to a certain extent, are both transitional years," he said. "We feel like we have the first group of young players in place who can be part of helping our club going forward."

While he would not discuss individual players, Wren is committed to making the Orioles younger and faster next season.

Dave Sheinin
Washington Post [24]

Here's a *game story* published on a Monday that has a strong look-ahead spin:

SALT LAKE CITY—The two-time kings of the Western Conference are alive and well and heading into the second round of the NBA playoffs.

The Kings aren't. Sacramento's odds-defying bid to oust the Utah Jazz died Sunday in a heart-stopping 99-92 overtime loss in Game 5. The Kings fell off their high-wire act in the final 59.9 seconds of regulation when Vlade Divac missed two potential game-winning shots in the paint with Karl Malone draped all over him.

Malone added 20 points and 12 rebounds to his game-winning defensive work against Divac, and Shandon Anderson scored six of his 16 points in OT. Utah hosts Portland on Tuesday in Game 1 of the best-of-seven second-round series.

Greg Boeck
USA Today [25]

The look-ahead, then, has these characteristics:

- Strong reporting that gives reader-fans clues on the shape of the even distant future but stops short of outright predictions (which are better reserved for opinion writing by columnists).
- Writing that lays out, for reader-fans to see, the bits and pieces that are the evidence supporting the story's general conclusion (coach-president tension, for example, and player discontent, picked up in interviews, are evidence that a coach's job is in jeopardy).
- Time elements that can be specific and recent (such as an interview yesterday) or nonspecific (such as when a reporter collects bits and pieces over days or weeks, then writes without a peg to any one event).

Beyond the Basics

Now you can handle comfortably the straightforward basic story: the who-won-and-why structure.

What's next?

For you, it should be *constant* effort to expand your spot-news writing skills beyond the basics, into multiple-element leads and keyboard tricks of the trade that enliven your writing.

For your readers, what's next, if you succeed, will be their association of your byline with writing that's expansive, enjoyable and more informative.

Multiple-Element Leads

Your key aim with this structure should be to compress more drama, color and detail into your first several grafs *but not to lose control of writing flow or reading ease.*

Recall an earlier example of a 24-word AP lead, then look at this one:

> BOSTON—The New York Yankee-Boston Red Sox rivalry, relatively dormant for some 20 years, erupted into a ninth-inning volcano of flying debris and angry words Sunday night, marring the Yankees's 9-2 victory in Game 4 of the American League championship series in Fenway Park.
>
> A crowd of 33,586, flushed with the frustration of two controversial calls that didn't go their way and the inevitability of the Yankees taking a commanding 3-1 lead in the best-of-seven series, littered the field with plastic water bottles and other trash after Nomar Garciapara was called out on a close play at first.
>
> <div align="center">Mike DiGiovanna
<i>Los Angeles Times</i>[26]</div>

Read that lead once again—this time aloud, which is an *excellent* way to let your ear tell you if writing flow is maintained. Note those *45 words* in the first graf hold together beautifully.

The following is a multiple-element lead that concentrates on development *in a game*:

> Tim Duncan scored 31 points, grabbed 15 rebounds and scared the Spurs when he hit teammate David Robinson in the head as San Antonio cruised to a 121-98 victory over the Celtics on Wednesday night in Boston.
>
> There was little doubt the defending NBA champions would win their third consecutive game after building a 33-20 lead after the first quarter. But near the end of the second, Duncan, following up his own miss, inadvertently hit Robinson on the top of the head.
>
> The Spurs' stunned center crumpled to the court, first holding his head,

then his right shoulder. He lay under his own basket for more than two minutes as many of his teammates surrounded him.

Robinson went to the locker room with 1:21 left in the half and San Antonio leading 60-39. But he returned to play the first eight minutes of the third quarter before sitting out the rest of the game and finishing with 10 points and nine rebounds in 26 minutes.

The Associated Press [27]

Now, a multiple-element lead that carries the story *beyond the game itself*:

Texas Tech coach Spike Dykes, who made a career out of upsetting rivals Texas and Texas A&M on the way to becoming the Red Raiders' winningest coach, announced his retirement after Saturday's 38-28 win over visiting Oklahoma (6-4, 4-3).

The announcement came after a week of rumors that Tech was seeking a new coach.

"There really wasn't any pressure put on me. This is something that I've been thinking about for a long time," said Dykes, 61.

Texas Tech went 6-5 and was 82-67-1 under Dykes, who joined the school in 1984. The Red Raiders have recently gained notoriety for playing spoiler to Texas A&M, beating the Aggies this season, 21-19 while they were ranked No. 5.

The Associated Press [28]

Characteristics of the multiple-element lead:

- Its strength is that it widens your readers' view, enticing them with color and details far beyond the humdrum recital of who won and who lost.
- Its weakness is that unless you write very carefully, you can drown your readers in meandering sentences and meaningless detail that leave them breathless and perplexed. Read your writing aloud; your ear will tell you when you are straying too far.
- The second and subsequent grafs must be written carefully to elaborate on the multiple points made in your lead graf. Note above how DiGiovanna of the *Los Angeles Times* quickly explains ("littered the field") his lead's mention of angry fans; note how AP maintains the thread of Robinson's head injury through his recovery and return to the game; note how the Texas Tech coach's retirement is backed up immediately with a quote from him.

Tricks of the Writing Trade

Yes, a basic, straightforward writing style should be your first goal. But your challenge extends far beyond that.

Think of this: Research shows that readers spend 26 to 28 minutes on average reading a newspaper. That's less than half an hour for *everything in our pages*.

So, how can you catch readers before they skip away to world news, state news, local news, business news and the comics?

With imaginative writing.

The You Lead

Here's something else research tells us: Readers view us as distant, cold, arrogant and removed from them and their daily lives.

Getting close to readers and *warming up to them* is one purpose of the "you lead." Note how a writer brings reader-fans into the game and into analysis of what's happening:

> ORCHARD PARK, N.Y.—You remember the drill from last year.
>
> First, the score: The Eagles lost to the Buffalo Bills, 26-0, yesterday.
>
> Next, the litany of embarrassing facts: The Eagles are 0-3 for the first time since—well, since last season. They haven't won a road game during Bill Clinton's second term, having gone 0-17-1 on the road since December 1996. They are approaching the NFL record of 23 straight road losses. They have scored exactly eight points in the 11 quarters since they took a 21-0 first-quarter lead over Arizona in their season opener. The offense has scored two field goals, the defense one safety, in 165 minutes of football. The Eagles have been shut out four times in their last 19 games.
>
> "I'm getting tired of standing before you with the same thing over and over," coach Andy Reid told reporters. "I've got to find a way to change this."
>
> Phil Sheridan
The Philadelphia Inquirer[29]

Another *Inquirer* writer brings readers into a chatty conversation, *as if across the kitchen table*:

> You had to see it to believe it.
>
> In the fourth quarter of his team's 24-14 victory over Boston College on Saturday at Veterans Stadium, Temple defensive back Kevin Harvey intercepted a pass and juked, slithered and spun his way down the left side of the field for an apparent 59-yard touchdown.
>
> The crowd went wild, and though the scintillating run was negated by a personal foul penalty on Temple, it was another indication of the emergence of Kevin Harvey.
>
> After two injury-plagued, and frustrating seasons trying to make it as a quarterback on the Division I college level, Harvey has become the all-

around threat that he was billed to be after a spectacular career at Paulsboro (N.J.) High.

> Kevin Tatum
> *The Philadelphia Inquirer*[30]

A *USA Today* writer challenges readers to solve a problem:

> You do the arithmetic. The tottering Pacific 10 Conference has all of two teams with winning records at the moment—Arizona and Stanford—and five bowl berths to fill by season's end.
> Understandably, officials with the tied-in Aloha and Oahu bowls in Hawaii are beginning to cast their eyes for alternatives.

> Steve Wieberg
> *USA Today*[31]

The Question Lead

Like the "you lead," this structure reaches out and takes your reader by the hand:

> Savior? Protector? Scapegoat?
> Which label will be placed around Hideki Irabu's thick neck at the end of September?
> Will his right arm, equipped with high-octane fastballs and nasty forkballs, be the force behind the Yankees chasing down the Orioles in the AL East?
> Can Irabu add just enough to a deep pitching rotation to ward off all AL wild-card challengers and put the Yankees in the playoffs for the third straight season?
> Or will he be a colossal waste of $12.8 million of George Steinbrenner's money and be blamed for a miserable second half?
> Tonight, at what is expected to be a packed Yankee Stadium, the answers begin to take shape.

> George King
> *New York Post*[32]

An AP writer involves readers with a question widely discussed at the time:

> AUSTIN, TEXAS—Texas was not supposed to be this good this fast.
> After a surprising 9-3 record last season, the Longhorns were expected to step backward. Ricky Williams was gone, the nation's best recruiting class was still too young and the sophomore quarterback Major Applewhite—who looks so small on television—could not really have been that good, could he?

One year later, the 9-2 Longhorns have risen to No. 6 in both polls, tied for sixth in the Times ranking and a place in the Big 12 title game in Coach Mack Brown's second season.

The Associated Press [33]

A *USA Today* writer asks a question baseball fans were asking:

What paucity of pitching? Some good ones have emerged from unusual places in the National League.

Entering this season, righthanders Paul Byrd, Russ Ortiz and Kent Bottenfield were aiming no higher than managing to win a spot, any spot, in their club rotation. They have done much more.

Byrd, 28, joined his fourth organization when the Philadelphia Phillies claimed him on waivers from Atlanta last August. Since then, he's 10-4, including his win Sunday.

Ortiz ... .

Bottenfield ... .

Rod Beaton
USA Today [34]

Note: When using the question lead, always *answer* the question high in your story.

Write in Conversational Tones

When appropriate (and sometimes it isn't), you can touch readers with a conversational—even slangy—tone.

Masters at this are among writers for the New York City tabloids, the *Daily News* and the *Post*. A *Post* writer "talks" with his street-smart readers (emphasis added):

BOSTON—Chuck Knoblauch stood behind the batting cage fitting his frigid bat with a weighted donut as he prepared to step in and find a stroke *that has vanished faster than a mob informant.*

"It's coming," Knoblauch said *as he walked toward the cage for his hacks.*

George King
New York Post [35]

A *Daily News* writer raps with the crowd about a prep game:

This kind of win, the kids from Prospect Heights hope, *is a rep-maker.*

The Cardinals rallied from a 13-point, fourth-quarter deficit yesterday to knock off city power Lincoln, 66-64, in the Gobbler/Snowflake Classic at Adelphi Academy.

Sherman Windley sank two free throws with :10 left to seal the victory.

"Now maybe we can get some recognition," said PH's Michael Thomas, who led the Cards with 21 points.

Anthony McCarron
New York Daily News [36]

One danger in stretching for a conversational tone is that you can lapse into slang that is inappropriate for a newspaper. What do you think about featuring so prominently the quote in the following lead?

PHILADELPHIA—Jason Isringhausen didn't have any answers. "If I did," he said, "the problem would be fixed and I wouldn't be going through this crap."

Anthony L. Gargano
New York Post [37]

Yes, I know. That's the way they talk in the lockerroom. But ...

The Quote Lead

Punchy quotes enormously strengthen your writing—if they truly are punchy (and relevant) and if you choose them with care.

A *Washington Post* writer adds nicely to her story through selective use of a partial quote in the first graf, followed by a full quote in the third:

Saying it was "time to let go," Washington Redskins linebacker Ken Harvey announced his retirement yesterday, drawing accolades from coaches and teammates for his ferocity on the field and benevolence off it.

Harvey, 34, reached his decision Wednesday morning, roughly halfway through training camp, as he prepared for what would have been his 12th season in the NFL and his sixth as a Redskin.

"All my life I've wanted to give 100 percent," Harvey said. "I said in the beginning that if I couldn't, then it would be time to go. This was the one time I couldn't. As much as I wanted to mentally, the body wasn't as good as I wanted it to be."

Liz Clarke
Washington Post [38]

Could you paraphrase a coach's feelings better than the coach expresses them himself in the second graf of the following AP story?

MILWAUKEE—Milwaukee coach George Karl sure didn't sound like the winning coach.

"I'm concerned and I'm disappointed and I'm angry," Karl said after his
Bucks survived a second-half scare from the lowly Chicago Bulls to win
102-95 and snap a two-game losing streak.

The Associated Press [39]

The Chronological Structure

When you're guaranteed sufficient newshole and don't have to risk slash-
and-publish editing, you can inject drama into your writing with chronological
coverage of key plays or key moments in a game.

For example, the *Chicago Tribune* grants its writers huge newshole for coverage of athletics at Northwestern University in suburban Evanston. Thus protected from bottom-up editing, a *Tribune* writer leads readers, at a run, down
the basketball court for a key play:

> Mateen Cleaves had missed 7 of 9 shots Friday afternoon and 37 of 44
> in the United Center over the last two seasons.
> But as Michigan State's star guard dribbled into the heart of the
> Northwestern defense with the score tied and the clock running down, the
> Spartans' Antonio Smith had only one thought: Put it up, Mateen.
> "I don't care if he goes 1 for 20," Smith said. "If we're down at the end of
> the game and we need a bucket, I'm going to give him the ball and get out
> of the way."
> And that's what the Spartans did this time. Cleaves steamed into the
> lane—painted green, fittingly enough—and tossed a prayer over
> Northwestern center Evan Eschmeyer.
> When the ball slipped through the net, second-ranked Michigan State
> had survived Northwestern 61-59 in the quarterfinals of the Big Ten tourna-
> ment. The Spartans advance to face Wisconsin, the only conference team to
> tame it this year, in Saturday's first semi-final.

Andrew Bagnato
Chicago Tribune [40]

Colon and Dash Leads

For a change, a colon lead works nicely occasionally:

> The education of New Orleans Saints running back Ricky Williams con-
> tinues. The latest lesson: dirty play.

Mike Freeman
The New York Times [41]

> Allen Iverson's eyes filled with tears Tuesday as he announced the news:
> The highest-scoring hand in the National Basketball Association is broken.

Iverson, the league's scoring leader, will miss three to six weeks with a broken thumb on his shooting hand.

The Associated Press[42]

Virginia Tech fans: Don't make those reservations to New Orleans just yet.

The No. 2 Hokies (10-0), who finish the regular season Friday against Boston College, received a jolt Monday from the newest Bowl Championship Series rankings.

Tony Barnhart
The Atlanta Journal-Constitution[43]

A dash lead can single out for emphasis a key point:

GRAND BLANC, MICH.—He's been at it now for nine or 10 years, groping that golden ring on the PGA Tour merry-go-round—coming close, never giving up.

Knight Ridder Newspapers[44]

As the Giants prepared this past week to face Brad Johnson, the highly rated Washington Redskins quarterback whose passing destroyed them two months ago, defensive end Michael Strahan heard the suggestion—on radio talk shows and elsewhere—that the Giants had squandered their chance to obtain Johnson last winter because they were unwilling to trade Strahan.

This did not sit well with Strahan, the Giants' two-time Pro Bowler.

Bill Pennington
The New York Times[45]

The Cleveland Browns become the first NFL team to open training camp when they welcome their rookies Wednesday, but they're already league leaders in one category—free-agents signings.

Larry Weisman
USA Today[46]

Other Things You Can Do

You can get *imagery* into your writing:

Patrick Ewing is as stubborn as a grass stain on white linen. As he marched defiantly down a set of stairs leading from the practice floor to a locker room last week, he shook his head "no" like a toddler to every question floating in his wake.

Selena Roberts
The New York Times[47]

Stop reading (if you can) after the first-graf imagery of this one:

> MIAMI—The sequence was rim, glass, ecstasy.
>
> In a matter of seconds and two beautiful bounces, Allan Houston sent a jolt of electricity into the Knicks' season and Jeff Van Gundy's career.
>
> "It sent chills up my spine," said Charlie Ward. "We got the good roll today."
>
> The eulogy for the 1999 Knicks and their head coach will not be delivered this morning. Today, the Knicks are headed to the second round and Pat Riley is out of the playoffs. Does it get any better than that?
>
> Houston, the son of a coach, hit a pullup jumper in traffic with eight-tenths of a second remaining as the broken down and wounded Knicks shocked Miami, 78-77, in Game 5 on Sunday for the second straight year.
>
> Frank Isola
> *New York Daily News* [48]

This lead drew readers deep into a story (which, unfortunately, we don't have room to reproduce here):

> PHOENIX—It was a game with a message, delivered by a weeping coach, dancing players and red-eyed fans who hugged late into the desert afternoon.
>
> Bill Plaschke
> *Los Angeles Times* [49]

Note how a *Boston Globe* writer plays nicely with words:

> NEW YORK—In the final hours before Evander Holyfield stepped into the ring with Lennox Lewis last night, *the weightiest subject under discussion in Madison Square Garden was the respective tonnage of two champions.*
>
> On Thursday, Holyfield weighed in at 215 pounds, the exact weight he carried in his first fight with Mike Tyson, while Lewis tipped the same rusty scale Muhammad Ali and Joe Frazier used in 1971 at a svelte 246 pounds, having earlier claimed he might weigh as much as 260.
>
> Ron Borges
> *The Boston Globe* [50]

Sometimes, just two words do it all:

> Continuing his *birdie binge*, David Toms maintained his distance from an elite field by posting a tournament-record 29 points for the second-round lead Friday in the Sprint International in Castle Rock, Colo.
>
> The Associated Press [51]

Or, even, a single word can add spice:

> Stefan Koubek seemed the least surprised, so perhaps only he could explain it. Needing just 56 minutes, the Austrian left-hander became the first qualifier and lowest-ranked player ever to win the AT&T Challenge when he *thumped* fifth-seeded Sebastien Grosjean 6-1, 6-2 Sunday in the final at Atlanta Athletic Club.
>
> Todd Holcomb
> *The Atlanta Journal-Constitution*[52]

Don't you wish *you* had written the following lead?

> Public floggings may be illegal, but Lindsay Davenport inflicted one on top-ranked Martina Hingis yesterday at Madison Square Garden. Davenport wielded her racket like a weapon in a shockingly one-sided 6-4, 6-2 victory in the final of the Chase Championships, and Hingis, who usually thinks her way out of intimidating situations, never came close to escaping this one.
>
> Robin Finn
> *The New York Times*[53]

Things Not to Do

Don't jam too much into a lead. Read this one aloud—and listen to yourself choking for air:

> LAUSANNE, SWITZERLAND—At the conclusion of an unprecedented two-day session called to address the worst corruption scandal in Olympic history, International Olympic Committee President Juan Antonio Samaranch today declared the organization successful in enacting promised reform and ensured he would control further change by installing himself as the head of a new committee created to examine the structure and operation of the 105-year-old body.
>
> Amy Shipley
> *The Washington Post*[54]

Don't get corny:

> Jamir Miller sees a time when the Cleveland Browns will be winners instead of winless. The Browns looked at Miller and saw the linebacker they want to anchor their defense.
>
> *Chicago Tribune News Service*[55]

("*Sees*"-"*saw*," get it?)

Don't stretch so far you grasp an awful cliche:

> WHITEFISH, MONT.—Olympic sprinters might consider themselves the world's fastest humans, but they *can't hold a candle* to Whitefish speed skier Jay Sandelin.
>
> Mark Goldstein
> The Associated Press [56]

Don't highlight the irrelevant:

> MIAMI—Jamal Mashburn *scored 22 points on his 27th birthday*, and P.J. Brown added 18 as the Miami Heat snapped Sacramento's eight-game winning streak, 99-88 Monday night.
>
> The Associated Press [57]

> SANTA CLARA, CALIF.—*Two tattooed sophomores* ushered the University of Portland out of the West Coast Conference women's basketball tournament Friday night.
>
> Ken Wheeler
> *Portland Sunday Oregonian* [58]

Don't compare a horse-racing scenario to a book (particularly if you never explain the comparison, as this author didn't).

> BALTIMORE—The post-Preakness scenario is like a chapter from a Stephen King novel for both Arthur Hancock and Elliott Walden—the two men most closely linked to the talented but frustrated colt Menifee.
>
> Matt Graves
> *Albany (N.Y.) Times Union* [59]

Don't forget that *forever* is a very long time:

> WASHINGTON—Two plays will forever be etched in the memories of the players and the crowd of 40,119 in today's international match between the United States and Argentina at Robert F. Kennedy Stadium. The first was a penalty-kick save by Kasey Keller of the United States and the other was Joe-Max Moore's goal that gave the Americans a 1-0 triumph.
>
> Alex Yannis
> *The New York Times* [60]

Don't forget to think again when you're inclined to feature Ross Perot in a sports lead:

> BALTIMORE—Before batting in the ninth inning today, Luis Sojo turned to teammates on the Yankees' bench and predicted he would hit a home

run, which is like Ross Perot guaranteeing he is going to be elected president or Larry Johnson promising he is going to utter something noncontroversial. Sojo had not hit a home run in nearly two years.

Buster Olney
The New York Times[61]

Don't think a bus trip is news:

The Southern Arkansas University women basketball team will travel to Searcy Thursday night to play Harding University in hopes of ending a three-game losing streak.

Steven Herrington
The Bray, Southern Arkansas University[62]

Summary

—The basic spot-news story that goes directly to the point and tells the news clearly is the foundation of all good sportswriting.

—Nothing beats leaning back after you've finished a story and asking yourself if you've answered who, what, when, why, where and how.

—The basic Five-Ws-and-How story is characterized by crisp language and short, punchy sentences.

—Minimum "color" is included in this basic spot-news story because color uses wordage needed to provide details of the news.

—The spot-news story should highlight star performance, pivotal plays, injuries or coaching decisions that explain the "why" and "how" of the out-come.

—The inverted-pyramid story structure endures because it enables editors, always short of a newshole and time, to trim stories quickly from the bottom without eliminating truly crucial information.

—In writing to compete against television, remember that the outcome—the score—is secondary because your readers already know that.

—Reader-fans who have seen a contest on television need from you the color details and reporting on who or what was responsible for the outcome.

—Above all, reader-fans who have seen a televised game need from you a pleasurable reading revisit to the event.

—*Precedes* are stories you can use to inform readers of a forthcoming game or event.

—*Follows* enable you to pick apart, to the delight of reader-fans, a game just past.

—*Look-aheads* are designed to give fans a long-range vision of the rest of the season or of next year's season.

—Once you've conquered the basics of the straightforward spot-news story, you should work to expand your writing skills into multi-element leads.

—The key to multi-element leads is compressing more drama, color and detail into your first several grafs but not losing control of reading ease.

—The "you lead" addresses the reader directly and is a wonderful device for warming up your writing.

—The question lead takes your readers by the hand and involves them in your story.

—Write in conversational tones—even slang, sometimes—but don't overdo this effort to get close to readers.

—The quote lead enormously strengthens your writing if you select truly punchy and relevant quotes.

—If you're guaranteed sufficient newshole, and thus protected against bottom-up editing, you can relate details chronologically, which puts readers on the field or on the court.

—You can achieve emphasis—like this—if you use dashes; sometimes this is effective, too: the colon.

—Strive to get imagery into your writing but don't stretch too far by using cliches or corny irrelevancies.

Exercises

1. Study the sports section of today's *USA Today* (or another newspaper designated by your instructor) and select four stories you think meet the fundamental goals of a basic spot-news story. Clip these stories and attach them to your analysis (in about 300 words) of how well the stories provide readers with clear, engaging, Five-Ws-and-How information. Are *all* those basic elements in the stories? Is the writing open and engaging?

2. Select four AP stories published in a nearby metropolitan daily (or another newspaper designated by your instructor) and analyze, in about 350 words, the sentence structure and language of each. Are sentences short and clear? What is the average word count for each lead? Is the language crisp and clean? Punchy?

3. Analyze leads from a nearby metropolitan paper (or another that your instructor designates) that are pegged to a) a star's performance, b) a turning point in a game, and c) an injury or coaching tactic. Analyze each in 50 to 75 words. Did the writers accomplish their apparent objectives? In your opinion, did the writers select the proper peg? How would you have written each differently, if at all?

4. Select two "precedes" from a nearby metropolitan sports section (or another designated by your instructor) and, in about 150 words each, analyze whether the writers selected news pegs and writing approaches likely to satisfy discerning reader-fans. Are the news pegs sufficiently newsworthy to hold read-

er interest? Is the writing open, engaging? Would you have written those stories differently? If so, how?

5. Cover a campus (or local community) sports event selected by your instructor. Write one lead and subsequent 150 words as if the outcome was *not* known to your readers. That is, write in straightforward, spot-news style, stressing the Five Ws and How. Write the *same* story a second time, again in about 150 words but as if your readers had seen it on television. That is, write a multiple-element lead for the second version and try for a look-ahead angle that reports the event within the context of the team's next game or the outcome of the season.

Recommended Reading

Two sources are particularly helpful for aspiring writers trying to develop their strengths in basic spot-news stories. The sources are The Associated Press and *USA Today*, whose writers are adept at packaging maximum information in minimum wordages, yet writing with readable and engaging openness. Virtually every daily newspaper's sports section carries many AP spot-news game stories, each written so editors can publish them as one-graf briefs or in hundreds of words. Careful study of AP style can be very helpful. *USA Today's* sports section probably is the most tightly edited of all. Study how its writers, showing their knowledge of sports, pick crucial information and write with a highly developed sense of news priorities.

Notes

1. For this lead and a wider discussion of sportswriting in this earlier era, see Robert Manning, "Good Sports," *Columbia Journalism Review*, January/February 1994, p. 52.

2. Ibid.

3. Dispatch for morning papers, Jan. 31, 1999.

4. The Jan. 31, 1999 edition, p. B-1, et seq.

5. "Cottonmouths Cut Cats' Division Lead With Victory Over Force," March 19, 1999, p. B-1.

6. Dispatch for morning papers, Dec. 5, 1999.

7. Dispatch for morning papers, Dec. 5, 1999.

8. "Matthews Paces S.A. Boys in Rout of Lakeside," Jan. 31, 1999, p. B-1.

9. "O-State Lacrosse Loses in NCAAs," May 13, 1999, p. 13.

10. Dispatch for morning papers, Nov. 14, 1999, published that day in *The New York Times*, p. 41.

11. Dispatch for morning papers, May 4, 1999.

12. Dispatch for Sunday papers, Dec. 5, 1999, published that day in the *Daily News & Banner-Herald*, p. C-7.

13. "Trojans Fade Out into Maui Sunset," Nov. 23, 1999, p. D-1.

14. "Couisneau Minds Net for Storr," Nov. 24, 1999, p. D-1.

15. "It's No Contest in M.L.S. As United Takes 3rd Title," Nov. 22, 1999, p. D-3.

16. "Bruins Prove Very Elusive Again," Nov. 24, 1999, p. D-4.

17. "Villanova's First-Round Foe Is Smaller but Much Quicker," March 12, 1999, p. D-10.

18. "St. Francis Women Looking For a Win in the Huskies' Den," March 12, 1999, p. D-12.

19. "Groin Pains: Injury Has Slowed Freeman," Nov. 25, 1999, p. C-1.

20. Dispatch for morning papers, Nov. 25, 1999.

21. "Yankees Reactivate Nelson," May 21, 1999, p. 110.

22. "Rangers Downfall Endangers Muckler," Nov. 15, 1999, p. D-4.

23. "Phillies Vow to Spend More Money to Attract Talent," Sept. 27, 1999, p. D-1.

24. "Orioles' Season Raises Questions," Aug. 13, 1999, p. D-1.

25. "Jazz Finally Drive Out Kings," May 17, 1999, p. C-1.

26. "Amazin' Night for New York," Oct. 18, 1999, p. D-1.

27. Dispatch for morning papers, Nov. 25, 1999.

28. Dispatch for Sunday papers, Nov. 21, 1999.

29. "Birds Lay Another Goose Egg," Sept. 27, 1999, p. D-1.

30. "Harvey Starting to Prosper as a Temple Defensive Back," Oct. 13, 1999, p. E-8.

31. "Pac-10's Losing Season Has Hawaii out Looking for Bowlers," Oct. 22, 1999, p. C-17.

32. "Stadium Is House," July 10, 1997, p. 86.

33. Dispatch for Sunday papers, Nov. 21, 1999.

34. "NL Pitching Produces Plenty of Surprises," May 17, 1999, p. C-3.

35. "Chuck Primed for Breakout," May 21, 1999, p. 110.

36. "Prospects High for Heights," Dec. 15, 1997, p. 72.

37. "Izzy: It's No Fun on the Losing End," July 4, 1996, p. 64.

38. "Redskins' Harvey Decides to Retire," Aug. 13, 1999, p. D-1.

39. Dispatch for morning papers, Nov. 25, 1999, p. B-1.

40. "Cleaves' Forgettable Day Ends Memorably," March 7, 1999, Section 3, p. 6.

41. "Williams Retaliates Against Dirty Tactics," Nov. 21, 1999, p. 42.

42. Dispatch for morning papers, Nov. 24, 1999, p. C-3.

43. "Margin Closes in BCS," Nov. 23, 1999, p. B-1.

44. Dispatch for Saturday papers, Aug. 8, 1998, p. B-3.

45. "Defense Looks for Atonement as Giants Play the Redskins," Nov. 21, 1999, p. 37.

46. "New Browns Ready to Get Busy at Camp," July 20, 1999, p. C-1.

47. "With Ailing Ewing, the Spirit is Willing," May 30, 1999, Section 8, p. 1.

48. Dispatch for morning papers, May 17, 1999.

49. "Two for the Show," March 21, 1999, p. D-1.

50. "Weight Disparity a Heavy Topic for Holyfield, Lewis," March 14, 1999, p. E-10.

51. Dispatch for Saturday papers, Aug. 21, 1999.

52. "Koubek's up to the Challenge," May 3, 1999, p. D-1.

53. "Hingis Is No. 1, But Davenport Has Her Number," Nov. 22, 1999, p. D-1.

54. "IOC Head Proclaims Meetings A Success," March 19, 1999, p. D-1.

55. "Browns Reward LB Miller," Oct. 30, 1999, Section 3, p. 5.

56. Dispatch for Sunday papers, March 28, 1999.

57. Dispatch for afternoon papers, Nov. 30, 1999.

58. "It's Final for the Pilots, But Not the WCC Final," Feb. 28, 1999, p. C-4.

59. "Scenario Favoring Menifee?" May 17, 1999, p. D-1.

60. "At Long Last, Some Brilliance Displayed Inside the Beltway," June 14, 1999, p. D-4.

61. "Sign of Success: Jeter Sits Out, But Sojo Homers," June 28, 1999, p. D-1.

62. "Riderettes Pounded on Boards, in Games," Dec. 10, 1999, p. 11.

6

Taking Readers Beyond the Score

So, YOU'VE conquered the basic spot-news story concept that's so essential to your first mission as a journalist: communicating *news*, simply and clearly.

What's next?

If you seek that sportswriter *career* we've been discussing (and not just a *job*), you now must spread your writer's wings into analytical and interpretive writing that takes readers well beyond the score, beyond who won.

Analytical writing strongly founded in sports expertise is a trademark of some of our very best writers, those whose bylines attract a crowd, every time, whatever the subject.

It's those bylines that readers seek when struggling with sports complexities, when they're trying to figure out what *really* happened, and what it *really* means.

We still are dealing in Chapter Six with *reporting* for *news* pages. Yes, our subject is writing that moves well beyond ritualistic and objective recital of the Five Ws and How. *But,* it is writing that stops short of subjective opinion writing (which we'll cover in later chapters on column writing).

The line we're treading between objective and subjective writing is more blurred in sports than in any other form of journalism because over decades, newspaper-writing guidelines developed with dramatic differences.

Reporters on "cityside," who wrote for hard-news front pages, were required by generations of tough city editors to keep their opinions out of their copy. Straightforward, objective reporting became the goal in general news.

In sports, described jokingly by even sportswriters as the "toy department," those rigorous standards were not applied to reporting on games and the people who play them. Sports reporters, consequently, generally were freed to develop their own writing styles, which on many newspapers became warm, inviting and conversational. And today, even in covering spot news, many sportswriters inject their own expertise into their analytical reporting.

Nevertheless, analytical writing that is still as objective as possible is the strength of many of the nation's best sports sections. We turn now to a few hints you can use as guidelines for expanding into it. (These are guidelines *only*, because you must strive for a unique, highly personalized style of your own.)

Winning Combo: Writing Flair Plus Analytical Expertise

Here is an example of how you can score with a careful combination of writing flair and analytical expertise:

> NEW YORK—Day turned to night, gray turned to rain and the sweet thought of champagne suddenly turned sour for the Atlanta Braves.
>
> The longest game in postseason history, a war of attrition, lasted almost six hours Sunday, but it may last a lifetime for a rookie pitcher named Kevin McGlinchy.
>
> Unable to hold a 3-2 lead in the 15th inning of a historic game, he will be forced to carry the burden of a 4-3 loss to the New York Mets, who are back from the grave again, heading to Atlanta for a Game 6 Tuesday night and trailing in the National League's best-of-seven championship series only 3-2.

Note above these characteristics:

- The lead is neatly crafted with imagery obviously drawn from the writer's wider experience in literature. Spend your life reading nothing but box scores and your writing will read like a box score! Good writers read great writers—wherever they are found.
- The second graf sketches the wider context ("longest game") and, impor-

tantly, focuses on an individual performance (in this case a "goat," the losing pitcher).

- The third graf is the "housekeeping" graf, where important statistics are
  stored. Note that who won, who lost and the score are subordinated to
  the color of the lead and the pitcher angle of the second graf. This game
  was widely televised, and who won no longer is top-priority news.

Now, two grafs of analytical reporting (emphasis added):

> For the Braves, attempting to underscore their reputation as the Team of
> the Decade, *it should never have come down to McGlinchy, to a sixth pitcher.*
> *They could have buried the resilient Mets in Game 4 on Saturday and*
> *should have buried them Sunday.*

But, this is a *news* story, so the writer introduces an *authoritative source*:

> The telling line wasn't McGlinchy's. The telling line was delivered by bat-
> ting coach Don Baylor after the Braves struck out 19 times and left the
> same number of runners on base.
>
> "Terrible," Baylor said. "That's the worst approach I've seen from our hit-
> ters all year. We had another clinching game and lost our focus.
>
> "At one point, Orel Hershiser [the second of nine Met pitchers] threw 18
> pitches, 17 of them were balls, and I think we swung at all of them.
>
> "I mean, you come down to the last part of the game and wonder why
> you get beat? Just drive in a run instead of swinging for the fences. Suddenly
> everybody is pressing and wants to be a hero."

Now, the writer turns to those numbers so beloved by baseball fans:

> The Braves left 11 runners on base in a five-inning stretch starting in the
> fourth inning.
>
> In 33 innings of three games at Shea Stadium, they scored only six runs
> and won only on the basis of an unearned run Friday night, 1-0.
>
> Chipper Jones, who again heard a crowd of 55,723 chant his given name
> of Larry in derisive fashion, awakened Sunday with three hits, but the
> Braves are batting .211 for the series with Brian Jordan, Ryan Klesko,
> Gerald Williams and Andruw Jones all below the Mendoza line of .200, and
> Bret Boone only slightly above at .222.

In just that fashion, the writer "walks" reader-fans through the game, highlighting key plays, inserting more comments from the batting coach. But how
about the goat, the losing pitcher? He, too, gets his say:

> The 23-year-old McGlinchy had appeared in 23 games with the Braves
> this year, recording a 7-3 record with a 2.82 earned-run average, but in the

15th inning of his first post-season appearance, with the remnants of the Shea crowd up and screaming, with the rain falling and his spikes clogged by mud, with the Braves needing only three outs, he couldn't locate the plate.

"I knew I was the last guy standing," he said. "I knew it was up to me. It was as pressure-filled as it gets, and as loud as it gets, but I don't feel that was the issue. I was going after guys, but I just couldn't command my fastball. It was cutting a lot, running out of the strike zone. I was getting behind, and you can't do that at this level."

Ross Newhan
Los Angeles Times[1]

Note that Newhan limits his personal analysis to what actually are journalistically sound, objective *observations*—the "should" and "could" of the fourth graf. *The truly analytical and interpretive dimension of this reporting is created by appropriate arrangement of facts, timely insertion of telling statistics and extensive quotes from authoritative sources.*

That is, don't do "thumb suckers" for news pages—don't pass off as *news* only your analysis, only your interpretation.

Here's a superb combination of clever writing and (second graf) brief analysis that highlights a star performance:

ITHACA, N.Y.—For nearly 59 minutes yesterday, Harvard's defense gave highly-touted Cornell quarterback Ricky Rahne all he could handle.

Unfortunately for the Crimson, football games last 60 minutes, *and Rahne, in the waning seconds, proved he's every bit as good as advertised.*

Rahne took Cornell 58 yards in six plays with no timeouts, culminating the march with an 18-yard scoring strike to Keith Ferguson with just 26 seconds to play, to lift the undefeated Ivy League leaders (4-0) to a pulsating 24-23 win at Schoellkopf Field.

John Vellante
The Boston Globe[2]

Below, a *Philadelphia Inquirer* writer lays on heavily critical interpretation— *or*, is it, as he writes, a "fact" supported by evidence?

EAST RUTHERFORD, N.J.—Give the Eagles at least this much: They keep finding new and unforgettable ways to get to the same place.

They lost to the New York Giants, 16-15, yesterday at the Meadowlands. It was their 19th consecutive road game without a victory. They have gone 15 quarters without scoring a touchdown on offense. Their record is 0-4 under Andy Reid, 3-17 in the last two seasons, and 3-20 since their last two-game winning streak, which came back in November 1997.

"It's been kind of mind-boggling the last four weeks," quarterback Doug Pederson said.

The fact is, the Eagles are in the midst of one of the most profoundly wretched stretches of football in their generally sorry history.

When you lose so much for so long, you're bound to do things no one has seen before. The Eagles mined new ore in this one. They scored a touch-down on defense and a safety on offense and still lost. They intercepted three passes and recovered a New York fumble and still lost. They lined up against a Giants offense quarterbacked by Kent Graham and Kerry Collins and still lost.

Phil Sheridan
The Philadelphia Inquirer[3]

It's worth emphasizing: The very best analytical writing for news pages actually is a shrewd arrangement of supporting evidence by clever writers who keep their own opinions to a minimum.

Next, a *Forbes* reporter reaches a grave conclusion—the Women's National Basketball Association is in trouble:

When the National Basketball Association started its professional women's league (WNBA) three years ago, it was a classic brand extension. Create a new market of young women viewers while keeping basketball's name in the public eye year-round—women play in the summer when men are off.

The WNBA is still alive—no small accomplishment for a new sports league—but as a brand extension, it looks like a venture that's got the potential to foul out.

Now supporting evidence:

The WNBA is ... owned by the NBA. Its 16 teams are ... in the same cities as NBA teams and play in the same arenas. But despite the marketing muscle of the NBA, which has thrown millions behind the young league and helped secure vital broadcast contracts from NBC, ESPN and Lifetime, response to WNBA games has been lackluster.

Average attendance in the 1999 season was only 10,207 per WNBA game. ... That's a worse showing than the Arena Football League, which averages 11,000 per game, and represents a decline of 6% from the WNBA's 1998 average.

Nielsen ratings for NBC broadcasts of WNBA games have also slipped from 2 million households reached in 1997—the WNBA's inaugural season—to 1.5 million in 1999. In television terms, this rates popularity of the WNBA on a par with drag racing and not far above pro bowling. On cable, the WNBA fared even worse. Former WNBA sponsor Lee jeans recently declined to renew its three-year con-tract. Sponsors Adidas and Reebok have told the WNBA they may not renew.

Carleen Hawn
Forbes[4]

Mike Freeman of *The New York Times* has supporting evidence so strong that he says his analysis is the "truth" (emphasis added):

> Tim Couch was anointed as top pick in the National Football League draft months ago. The title did not come with a crown, but it should have come with body armor. That is because Couch is now taking more shots than he ever did as a quarterback for the University of Kentucky.
>
> Couch is learning the harsh reality of being rated the top player: every move he makes is scrutinized and every pass he throws in workouts is dissected.
>
> *The truth is* that Couch has made some rookie mistakes in his dealings with National Football League teams and with choosing agents. Those decisions have hurt him, and that has opened the door for the Oregon quarterback Akili Smith to become the first choice of the Cleveland Browns in the draft April 17.

Freeman now explains his second-graf use of "harsh reality":

> It may be harsh, even cruel, to hold a college player to almost unreachable standards. These days NFL teams are so picky, at times so oversaturated with information that if Superman declared himself eligible for the draft some team would find a weakness. Yet the microscopic inspection is understandable, especially in the case of the Browns. This pick may be important to their franchise's history, and one scout for the Browns, who did not want to be identified, said that the closer they look at Couch the more nervous they get.
>
> So it cannot be ruled out that the Browns will pass on Couch.
>
> Mike Freeman
The New York Times[5]

Lesson: In analytical writing, you must not only assemble strong evidence to support your conclusion you also must *let your readers see it.*

Frank Litsky of *The New York Times* does just that:

> HEMPSTEAD, N.Y.—The Jets' secondary is a mess—not its playing, which was effective enough Sunday against the Miami Dolphins—but its health.
>
> Steve Atwater, the free safety, missed two starts because of a strained hamstring, and his availability Sunday against the Dallas Cowboys (7-6) will be limited at best. Ray Mickens, the nickel back, has the same injury and the same prognosis. Otis Smith, a starting cornerback, has missed the entire season because of a shoulder injury, and Kevin Williams, who plays cornerback and safety, had his season ended by a life-threatening virus.
>
> Frank Litsky
The New York Times[6]

When the *Waukesha (Wis.) Freeman* named its High School Offensive Player of the Year, staff writer Steve Zimmerman analyzed—in expert detail—the winner's running style:

> BROOKFIELD—It wasn't blinding speed that left defenders trailing Adam Ciborowski.
>
> It wasn't brute force, either.
>
> What made the Brookfield Central High School senior so tough to stop was his patient and stubborn running style.
>
> Ciborowski gained more than 2,000 yards rushing this season and has been named Offensive Player of the Year by *The Freeman*.
>
> By outsmarting the opposition and often cutting back against waves of tacklers, Ciborowski was able to slither through defenses and turn basic 4- and 5-yard pickups into double-figure gains and immediate first downs.
>
> What separated the 6-foot, 200-pound Ciborowski from many runners was his poise when play got hectic. Instead of forcing his way through tight openings, he waited an extra second or two for sustained blocks to take hold.
>
> Most of his yardage came after initial contact and a quick change of direction.

Now, writer Zimmerman goes to an authoritative source for backup evidence:

> "He's such a natural runner," Central coach Rick Synold said. "We have a few plays that are designed to cut back, but many times he cuts back on his own."
>
> Steve Zimmerman
> *Waukesha (Wis.) Freeman*[7]

Again: Know your game! Zimmerman knows his.

So does Larry Whiteside, who covers baseball for the *Boston Globe*. His analytical writing *exudes* expertise.

> MINNEAPOLIS—One bad pitch is usually all it takes to ruin the best effort of Red Sox knuckleballer Tim Wakefield. He made a dandy last night, and the Minnesota Twins made him pay for it.
>
> Wakefield tried to sneak a fastball past Torii Hunter, and the rookie catcher responded with a grand slam in the fourth inning that erased a 1-0 deficit and sent the Minnesota Twins toward a 6-1 lead through seven innings. The 400-foot drive was Hunter's third homer of the season and his first major league slam.
>
> Larry Whiteside
> *The Boston Globe*[8]

Analysis and interpretation sometimes take just a sentence or two—a few words, even.

Thus Bloomberg News quotes Kansas State's football coach as saying things are coming together for his team in the race for a post-season bowl. The news service adds, "That might not be true, though"—and lays out evidence why not.[9]

Selena Roberts of *The New York Times* finds the New York Knicks "looking dreadfully uninspired" in a 94-88 loss to the Heat.[10]

David Leon Moore of *USA Today* analyzes race driver Arie Luyendyk's winning style—"discipline, experience, guts."[11]

The *Boston Globe*'s Nick Cafardo watches the New England Patriots lose 20-14 to the Redskins, and reports, "This was a stinker."[12]

It's unimaginable that the *Globe*'s Washington correspondent would report in a news dispatch that the U.S. secretary of state had pulled off a "stinker," or that the *New York Times*' White House correspondent would report in a news story that the president was "dreadfully uninspired."

Yet those analytical observations and that language—along with every other example you've seen so far in this chapter—were drawn from sports *news stories*.

Note: The very considerable analytical liberties you are granted as a sportswriter are accompanied by correspondingly great responsibility to get it right, to be accurate and to be fair.

Sometimes, if analytical writing *stretches into prediction*, editors will "slug" it, "Analysis." *Boston Globe* editors did that on a dispatch from Will McDonough, who covered the same Patriot game that Nick Cafardo termed a "stinker." McDonough's dispatch:

> ANALYSIS
> Foxborough—How about fifth place?
> That's what the Patriots will be looking at this year if their varsity players continue to perform like they did last night here against the Washington Redskins.
> Management and players weren't happy when almost every preseason football publication picked the Patriots to finish fourth in the AFC East behind New York, Miami and Buffalo. But in the 20 minutes or so when the Patriots offensive and defensive first units were on the field, the Redskins made them look bad. Not that the Redskins had to work that hard to do it. The Patriots did a lot to help them out.
>
> Will McDonough
> *The Boston Globe*[13]

Capture the Key Moments

We journalists are very lucky. We are paid to go places our readers cannot go, talk to people they never will meet and bring back explanations for mysteries they do not understand.

As you expand your reporting and writing to take readers beyond the score and through those mysteries, your mission revolves, crucially, around analyzing *key moments*—key plays, pivotal decisions, turning points.

Note how Bill Pennington of *The New York Times* does that for his readers in superb analytical writing:

> PHILADELPHIA—Football games are won in focal moments, sequences almost stolen from the game's routine—the stab of hand on ball, a bull-rush to block a kick, a deflected pass that leads to a catch-and-run and touchdown.
>
> The Giants had three such moments today against the Eagles. The first was game saving, the next game tying and the last game winning.
>
> With the Giants trailing by two touchdowns, their season teetering between advancing prosperity or a dreary descent to mediocrity, their defense turned three playmaking moments into a stunning, and perhaps meaningful, victory.
>
> The last act was Giants defensive end Michael Strahan—head back, legs churning to carry his 285 pounds and a pound of pigskin—running 44 yards with an overtime interception return for a touchdown, giving the Giants a 23-17 victory over the Eagles and salvaging a season at its midpoint.

Pennington inserts here his housekeeping graf. (Giants are on a three-game winning streak, have a 5-3 record "that positions them firmly in the chase for a playoff berth.") Now comes the explanation of the three moments Pennington used as a peg in his lead:

> A bizarre game, fitting for the historically quirky nature of the Giants-Eagles series, revolved around three plays during the final half-hour at Veterans Stadium.
>
> First, Giants defensive tackle Christian Peter blocked a Philadelphia field-goal attempt that would have put the Eagles ahead by 10 points with six and a half minutes to play. About four minutes later, Peter's colleague at tackle, Keith Hamilton, knocked the ball from the hands of Eagles running back Duce Staley on the Philadelphia 5-yard line. The fumble, recovered by the Giants, produced a late touchdown that tied the game at the end of the fourth quarter.
>
> And finally, once again it was Peter, fighting his way through a block, who deflected a pass by Eagles quarterback Doug Pederson high into the air roughly four minutes into the overtime period.
>
> Bill Pennington
The New York Times[14]

AP's Steven Wine puts a key moment into freeze-frame, letting readers linger deliciously on a bouncing ball:

> MIAMI—The ball was out of Allan Houston's hands, and so was the

Knicks' fate. He had fired a running 14-foot jumper, and the ball hovered above the rim as the final seconds ticked away.

"It seemed like two minutes," Houston said.

Miami Arena turned quiet for the first time all day as a sellout crowd, the Heat and the Knicks held their breath. The shot bounced off the front of the rim, kissed off the backboard and finally fell softly through the net.

Knicks 78, Heat 77.

The last bounce, last shot and last game went New York's way Sunday. Thanks to Houston's basket with 0.8 second left, the Knicks won the first-round series, 3-2.

Steven Wine
The Associated Press [15]

Even fans who watched the game, in the stadium or on television, wanted to go back over this one:

Just three more yards. The way Tennessee Coach Phil Fulmer saw it Saturday night, three yards stood between the Volunteers and their chance to continue their quest to repeat as national champions, their chance to break a 28-year drought on Florida's home field and their chance to hold on to their No. 2 ranking.

The three yards never came. Playing on fourth down at the Gators' 42-yard line, workhorse running back Jamal Lewis tried to rush behind his left tackle, but got nowhere. With two minutes remaining, Florida took possession and ran out the clock to claim a 23-21 victory. Fulmer never got the chance to get his team in field goal position, leaving many of the Volunteers' hopes for this season sitting on the field, deposited somewhere in the middle of those three yards.

Rachel Alexander
Washington Post [16]

Note above how AP's Wine and the *Post*'s Alexander weave in necessary context—scores, series record and national rankings. These are *news leads* built around key moments that report who won but also how and why, the goal of analytical and interpretive writing.

How many baseball fans would like to have a moment in the Atlanta Braves dugout, talking shop with manager Bobby Cox? All of them would, probably. So, the *Boston Globe*'s Allen Lessels takes his reader-fans there:

ATLANTA—Bobby Cox, all baseball, sits in the Atlanta Braves dugout talking shop.

He tells how one of his mentors, 80-year-old Ralph Houk, called and then stopped down to see him and the Braves this summer.

"He formed a lasting impression on me on the way to treat people," Cox said. "He had a natural way of doing it. He really cared about you, even if you were not an integral part of the team."

Cox, who last night led his team in Game 1 of the World Series talked of the Atlanta way of winning in the '90s.

"We just push hard, as hard as we can," he said. "There's no magic to that. We have good players who want to win. We're paid to win and we want to put on a good show every night."

Now, the essential look-ahead:

Maybe this is the year Cox breaks away from the pack and gets the recognition those around the Braves figure is overdue him as the best manager in baseball. Or at least one of the best.

Allen Lessels
The Boston Globe[17]

In the following, *The New York Times'* Bill Pennington crafts for the *interior* of his story a beautiful inside look at another place reader-fans never go. First, there are two grafs of "set up":

EAST RUTHERFORD, N.J.—It has been 33 years, and 502 games, since a Giants team has given up so many points. No opposing team in Giants Stadium has ever scored as much.

It was, somehow, an upset that the Washington Redskins defeated the Giants by 50-21 today. And upset was what the Giants were in their locker room afterward.

Now, the key moment:

Silence is expected in any losing locker room. Embarrassment, however, is disquieting.

Players slammed equipment in their lockers as others stomped in circles around the cavernous room. Everyone squirmed as the Giants Coach Jim Fassel entered the room to address his charges.

His face red, his eyes glaring around the room, he was expected by many of players to deliver a screaming tirade.

"That was a disgrace," Fassel said with a snarl, but without the yelling they had anticipated. "Don't ever, ever let that happen again."

The coach made it plain that there was going to be a penalty paid for such a performance, promising a tough week ahead as he spread blame to every corner of the room. But the talk didn't last long.

Fassel, his players said, looked stunned.

Who wasn't?

Bill Pennington
The New York Times[18]

Note how the *Times'* Pennington avoids the amateurish mistake of *telling* you coach Fassel was angry; rather, he describes Fassel—"face red, his eyes glaring"—and *lets you see* the coach was angry.

Extraordinary power of observation—the mark of a great reporter—shines through Tim Layden's capture of a key moment for *Sport Illustrated*:

> He lay sprawled on the track in twilight, his chest rapidly rising and falling like a sleeping infant's. On the infield grass a clock illuminated 43.18 in yellow, along with the simple message NEW W.R. Michael Johnson stared at a darkening Spanish sky and at a full moon above the Seville Olympic Stadium, and then he ended a decade's pursuit of the 400-meter record and three years of injury and frustration with one crooked smile.
>
> Tim Layden
> *Sports Illustrated* [19]

That's how to take readers places they cannot go!

Now, how did Melvin Mora of the Mets get off third base so quickly to steal home and win one for the Mets? Jack Curry of *The New York Times* explains with incredible analytical insight into the esoterica of baseball:

> Melvin Mora inched slowly off third base yesterday and stared closely at Brad Clontz's right hand, searching for small clues. Mora was a teammate of Clontz's on the Mets' Class AAA Norfolk team last year, so he was poised when he saw Clontz, now a Pittsburgh reliever, gripping the ball with two fingers pressed close together.
>
> That meant Clontz was throwing a slider that was supposed to dive down to Mike Piazza. That meant the pitch could bounce. Sure, it seemed improbable, but anything and everything now seems probable with the chaotic and wonderful Mets. Anything and everything happened.
>
> Clontz's sidearm slider started a few inches outside and kept drifting outside until it buzzed by catcher Joe Oliver and rolled to the backstop and up on the screen. Piazza stepped back from home plate like a commuter watching the wrong bus pass. That bus was Mora, who barreled home with the winning run in a 2-1 victory over the Pirates, ending a game that had been tense and then became uplifting for the Mets.
>
> Jack Curry
> *The New York Times* [20]

Again, the best analytical writing *takes readers into the game*, providing the color and details they can use for their own interpretation.

Maintain Your Writing Momentum

When writing longer analytical pieces, you cannot simply stack a couple of interesting facts and observations atop your story and then indiscriminately plug in all that follows. Do that and your readers will depart quickly for more interesting pastures.

You can "juice" your writing—maintain its momentum—along the way with three devices.

The Pull-Ahead Quote

You pull readers ahead by inserting meaningful quotes throughout longer articles. *Everybody* reads quotes.

Deep in a story of several thousand words, a *Chicago Tribune* writer inserts a quote that explains why high school players in Flint, Mich., an economically depressed city, so desperately want to make it as basketball players.

> "I have 17-, 18-year-old kids crying in front of me when I've cut them," Flint Northwestern coach Grover Kirkland said. "Kids have told me many, many times, 'This is the only way I can get to college.'"
>
> Rick Morrissey
> *Chicago Tribune* [21]

Owner George Steinbrenner of the New York Yankees is interfering (again) in how interim manager Don Zimmer runs the team. Steinbrenner announces he "hopes" Hideki Irabu will start against the Los Angeles Dodgers. Deep in its story, the AP inserts quotes that let readers analyze for themselves the tension thus created:

> When asked if what Steinbrenner said was a slap at his authority, Zimmer replied, "We'll find out. I'm ready for anything and don't give a damn about it, either. I'm the manager, I try to do what's right for the ball-club. My mind is not going to be changed by anybody."
>
> If given an ultimatum that Irabu is to pitch Wednesday, Zimmer, said, "Would I resign? It won't be resigning if something happens. I'd quit. I'm not saying I'm quitting, but ain't nobody going to tell me one thing and double-talk me on something else. He's fired a lot better people than me."
>
> The Associated Press [22]

The Meaningful Characterization

For all but the most knowledgeable reader-fans, you must be certain a sport's complexities aren't too deep for easy comprehension, *even if you understand them.*

Joseph Durso of *The New York Times* writes with notable expertise about horse racing:

> The great John Henry ran five times as a claimer early on, then raced

until he was 9 years old, won 39 of his 83 starts and earned $6.5 million. At one time, you could have claimed him for $20,000.

Stymie ran 12 times as a claimer for as little as $1,500, then ran in the money 90 times in 131 starts. Seabiscuit, who started his career with a 17-race losing streak, ran four times in claiming races in 1935 on both coasts, then won 33 times.

Now, that's a little deep for me. You, too? That's why Durso adds this:

They were to racing what Don Mattingly, drafted in the 19th round by the Yankees, was to baseball, and what Terrell Davis, drafted in the sixth round by the Denver Broncos, was to pro football: overlooked but marked for greatness.

Joseph Durso
The New York Times [23]

Now, a characterization—and a question for you: Why does a *New York Times* sportswriter bother in the following to explain a trap play? Don't football fans know what that is?

Motley was an inside blaster who had the speed to go outside. He made most of his yardage on trap plays, on which a defensive lineman was allowed to penetrate the line of scrimmage, then was trapped, allowing Motley to run through the vacated area.

Frank Litsky
The New York Times [24]

Frank Litsky explained the trap play because he wrote the above for Marion Motley's obituary, which was published in the *Times' general news section* and thus encountered by *non*-fan readers who didn't know football. Lesson: Judge carefully how much background characterization is required, by determining *who will be your likely audience.*

Jere Longman writes several thousand words on soccer player Mia Hamm, and because the article starts on Page One of *The New York Times* where non-fan readers will see it, Longman creates a picture of Hamm that all soccer fans have seen already:

Although Hamm is reticent off the field, her style of play is dynamically suited to spreading the sport to a wider audience. A fiercer countenance emerges, cheeks hollow and jaw clenched in exertion, her ponytail fanning out behind as she sprints 40 yards to finish a fast break or carves a defender with a deft two-step and makes an inexorable charge toward the goal.

The passion of her game is most evident in the celebrative convulsion when she scores, the tendons in her neck flared, her mouth an open scream, her arms cocked at the elbow and fists closed as if she has just lifted some enormous weight.

She has a dancer's feet, a felon's heart.

Jere Longman
The New York Times [25]

"Dancer's feet, a felon's heart." Wish you had written that? (Me, too.)

The Wink-And-Nudge Insight

Ever wink at friends and maybe nudge them to signal, "Hey, this is a joke" or "Don't take this too seriously"? You can create enormous warmth in your writing with a wink and a nudge that invites readers into an inner circle of understanding, a sort of camaraderie shared by pals.

Jeffrey Scott of *The Atlanta Journal-Constitution* wins me over with this:

> Standing in the doorway of wrestler Bill Goldberg's dressing room at the Bi-Lo Center in Greenville, S.C., is a blockish piece of human granite with what appears to be a bowling ball for a head and tattoos for hair.
>
> "We're good friends," says Goldberg, motioning at his arch-foe in pro-wrestling, 6-foot-3-inch, 325-pound Bam Bam Bigelow.

Now, the wink and nudge (emphasis added):

> Bigelow doesn't speak of friendship, however. *Spotting a reporter, he falls into character, and points at Goldberg: I'm going to get you!" he growls.*
>
> An hour and twenty minutes later, Goldberg—the biggest phenom to hit professional wrestling since pay-per-view—dispatches Bam Bam in trademark fashion.
>
> He spears Bam with his shaved head, then picks him up by his legs and drives him headfirst into the mat with his signature "finishing move," the "Jackhammer."

Jeffrey Scott
The Atlanta Journal-Constitution [26]

There is on-field fighting between members of the New York Giants football team during training camp. Deep in his story, a writer sets up his readers:

> Linebacker Jessie Armstead, who was in the center of one fight and spent the rest of practice taunting his offensive teammates, interpreted the day's events.
>
> "We ain't no choirboys," Armstead said. "It's football not volleyball. I don't mean no harm, but I don't love nobody on the other side of the ball. It's my time to hunt."

Now, the wink and nudge (emphasis added):

> The fighting also didn't seem to bother Coach Jim Fassel, who a year ago threatened his players with punishment for fighting in practice. But today, Fassel was unruffled, even making jokes about it.
> "Hey, I knew we'd eventually get it stopped," he said, *pausing to add*: "By tomorrow."
>
> Bill Pennington
The New York Times[27]

Create New Insights From Roundups

As in assembling bits and pieces of a puzzle, you can create a wider and more meaningful picture for your readers by writing analytical roundups.

Thousands of sport-news bits and pieces surface daily in newsrooms as staff writers and news service reporters cover their beats. Alone, each bit or piece may mean little; combined in roundups they can tell readers important stories that lie behind the score and beyond who won.

For example, *USA Today*'s Richard Winer analyzes bits and pieces floating in from the NFL and detects a trend:

> As the NFL continues its wacky ways nearly halfway through the season, a related trend remains in full swing: Teams keep changing quarterbacks in an alarming fashion.

Winer swings immediately into four grafs of backup.

> — Only 10 of the 31 teams have not been forced to switch quarterbacks because of injury or poor play.
> — Making first starts for their respective teams Sunday: Jeff George (Minnesota) and Damon Huard (Miami) as the Dolphins' Dan Marino (neck) and Vikings' Randall Cunningham (demotion) are the latest big-name passers to sit.
> — Four NFC teams (Washington, Dallas, Green Bay and Carolina) have had the same quarterback all year.
> — In the AFC, the six-team Central Division has made at least one quarterback switch.

Now, the "why" of this trend:

> 49ers general manager Bill Walsh, who is without Steve Young (concussion), cites more four-receiver sets leaving passers unprotected, artificial turf and officials possibly not catching all the dangerous hits.

"There are a lot of calls that are being made," Walsh says, "but they are missing a lot."

Richard Winer
USA Today[28]

Sam Smith of the *Chicago Tribune*, in a roundup headlined, "NBA Report," walks readers around the league (and note his chatty tone that puts him one-on-one with individual readers):

Most NBA teams have played about 15 games, so it's time to reshape the roster, right? That's the dilemma facing teams this week with Thursday's trading deadline looming.

Most general managers are saying they don't expect anything major to occur because they've barely had a chance to look at their own teams. Yet the names of All-Stars David Robinson, Eddie Jones, Terrell Brandon, Glen Rice and Jayson Williams have come up.

Now, quickly, to an authoritative source:

"When you're not doing well, people assume you're going to make all these trades and all kind of stuff," San Antonio coach/General Manager Gregg Popovich said, addressing a Robinson-for-Portland's Rasheed Wallace rumor. "We're not interested in anything like that. Never have been, never will be. I say it every year. I'll say it again. Hopefully, people will listen."

Sam Smith
Chicago Tribune[29]

Most such bits and pieces arrive on AP's sports-reporting network, the world's largest, or from other newspapers whose copy you can access through their own news services or Web sites. Using these resources properly adds enormous strength to your writing.

Here's how Anthony Dasher, assistant sports editor of the *Athens (Ga.) Banner-Herald and Daily News*, used those resources effectively in a roundup focused on two former football players at the University of Georgia in Athens:

On the day Matt Stinchcomb realized his financial freedom by signing a five-year deal with the Oakland Raiders worth $7.2 million, former Georgia teammate Champ Bailey and representative Jack Reale are finding out how exasperating these types of big-money negotiations can be.

According to the Associated Press, Bailey and Reale are asking the Washington Redskins for a four-year contract worth about $3.2 million per season. But, as is often the case, the ownership in D.C. isn't quite as forthcoming, having countered with a five-year deal worth about $1.9 million per season. However, the Washington Post reported Friday that the two sides were making progress. If a deal isn't reached soon, Bailey won't be in attendance Sunday when Redskin rookies are due to report to the team's training camp in Frostburg, Md.

Anthony Dasher
Athens (Ga.) Banner-Herald and Daily News[30]

Two points:

- Major *local* stories can be hidden in those bits and pieces from afar; look them over carefully when they arrive.
- Always credit AP or other newspapers in such roundups. Crediting sources is professionally courteous and, for readers, a mark of your credibility.

Speaking of bits and pieces, just check your own reporter's notebook after covering a major game. You'll have more information by far than you could (or should) pack into your main story. So, use those bits to good advantage in sidebar roundups, as does Rachel Bachman of the *Portland Sunday Oregonian* in covering an NBA game between the Trail Blazers and the Charlotte Hornets.

First, Bachman writes a principal story of about 750 words.

Second, Bachman rounds up bits and pieces in a sidebar titled, "At a Glance." Its components:

- *Why the Blazers lost*: Said Blazer guard Greg Anthony: "We took them for granted."
- *Top performance*: Isaiah Rider had 27 points. ...
- *Trends, milestones*: The Hornets' .750 field goal shooting in the first quarter was the best against the Blazers in a quarter this season. ...
- *Injuries*: The Hornets were missing what would be a decent lineup: starters Glen Rich (elbow surgery) ...
- *Noteworthy*: (An assortment of even more bits and pieces from the game.)

Third, Bachman's notebook yields even more: A sidebar roundup ("Game Talk") quoting players and coaches from both teams, a quarter-by-quarter roundup of key plays and scoring, plus, of course, the box score and other statistics.[31]

Not even by watching at courtside could the average fan collect and analyze the information so knowledgeably presented in Bachman's main lead and sidebar roundups.

Profiles: A Sports Analyst's Best Friend

No writing structure is better-suited than the profile for luring readers far beyond the score and into deeper analysis of sports. Two reasons:

First, of course, people are what sports is all about, and to understand sports, reader-fans must understand people.

Second, people, put simply, are interesting—fun to write about, fun to read about.

Thus, the *personality profile*, because it can be so entertaining to read, is an excellent vehicle for explaining the whys and hows of sports and for performing both of your journalistic missions—informing *and* entertaining.

Because we're *journalists*, the profile is best used not to simply illuminate a single personality but, rather, to shine light in hidden corners of a wider story.

Thus, *USA Today's* Skip Wood focuses on one man to tell a larger story about NASCAR race car owners:

> There's Richard Childress, or if you will, "R.C."
> And there's all the rest.
> Rick Hendrick, Jack Roush, Joe Gibbs and even Robert Yates all deserve respect as NASCAR car owners who have raised the standard by which Winston Cup success is measured. Childress, however, commands an unmatched respect that stems from his 30-year NASCAR background and personality as much as his six championships with driver Dale Earnhardt.

But what's the *news* here? It's this:

> Yet he has slipped behind the aforementioned owners the last several years and is burning to return to the fray.

Now, something *physical* about the man himself:

> Laid back and humble with eyes that sparkle with intensity, Childress spent the better part of 10 years as an independent—and winless—driver. He finally handed the wheel to Earnhardt and began to craft the early model of a modern-day team.

But this profile is designed to do more than merely picture a man. So, Wood quickly moves to the *judgment of peers*:

> Says NASCAR chief Bill France: "Richard's been one of my good friends, really, one of my heroes, for many, many years. I like to look at where he is now, because he and his wife (Judy) boot-strapped that race team right up to where it is now. I mean, some of those other teams got started with left-over factory equipment and kind of had it all just handed to them on a plate, but Richard had to grow his."
> Adds 50-year car owner Junie Donlavey: "Richard came from the old school. He understands what it's like to not have much money to work

with. But he was smart enough to set up his corporation in a way that he went right to the top."

Skip Wood
USA Today[32]

USA Today's profile now broadens for brief looks at other NASCAR team owners, and then returns to a conversation with Childress about his management style and racing philosophy. *Readers who began reading about a man ended up reading about a sports industry.*

With moving sensitivity, Joe Drape of *The New York Times* profiles a jockey to illuminate a darker side of horse racing. First, this set-up:

> Chris Antley, riding afternoon and night at two tracks, once won nine races in a single day. In 1991, he guided Strike the Gold to victory in the Kentucky Derby. And he was a savvy enough player of the stock market that he turned the $6 million he had earned riding racehorses into a fortune big enough to insure that he would not have to work again.

Now, with a harsh jerk of the writer's reins, Drape pulls his readers the other way.

> But none of that mattered 17 months ago. Antley, 32, was back in an alcohol and drug rehabilitation clinic.
>
> Worse, his body was as wrecked as his psyche, crumpled from years of trying to shrink himself into a saddle fitted for a 117-pounder. There had been too many mornings of throwing up his day's one meal, ingesting laxatives, wilting in a sauna.

Drape now recounts the jockey's struggle in a recovery clinic, how he was "directionless and overwhelmed by self-doubt." And now the *news peg*:

> But two weeks ago, only months removed from his most despairing moments, Antley rode a 31-1 long shot named Charismatic to his second Kentucky Derby crown. This time he wept right there in the winner's circle.
>
> "I had dug deep into the depths of my soul and faced down some monsters," Antley said later.

With that poignant (and, for me, irresistible) intro, the *Times'* Drape pulls readers toward the wider story:

> Antley is far from the first jockey to inhabit the dark world of substance abuse. In fact, in today's Preakness, Antley will race against two Hall of Fame jockeys ... who have battled alcohol and drug problems.

Now, a sense of balance—jockeys aren't alone in having addiction problems—and tightly written background that, importantly, cites official statistics on abuse among jockeys:

> Of course, every tale of addiction is shaped by its own particulars, and there is no evidence to suggest race riding is disproportionately rife with substance abuse. But for jockeys, the struggles with addiction are often very public and frequently driven by aspects of their unforgiving work.
>
> Addiction afflicts young riders who suddenly make big money in a grueling year-round sport. It hits jockeys who are forced to be obsessive about their weight, men often struggling with lifelong concerns about being undersized. It grows out of a need to numb oneself after another day of courting catastrophic injury. And it can be a costly consequence for jockeys working in an industry with a reputation for hard living.
>
> In the past five years, state racing commissions around the country have investigated and taken action against at least 160 jockeys for alcohol or drug abuse. There are roughly 900 licensed jockeys in the United States, although not all of them are active at any given time.
>
> Joe Drape
> *The New York Times*[33]

Mark Wiedmer of the *Chattanooga Times and Free Press* profiles key Southeastern Conference football players not to illuminate a sports industry (as in the NASCAR profile) or a problem (as in jockey addiction) but, rather, to draw a complete picture of star athletes. Thus Wiedmer focuses intently on physical traits—and a quote—designed to help readers "see" that picture:

> University of Florida junior wide receiver Travis Taylor wears braces on his teeth, a constant reminder that he is still a young man, under 21 and thus unable to buy a beer—not that he necessarily would.
>
> Taylor also wears a wedding ring on his left hand, a constant reminder that he is both a husband and a father, and thus much deeper into manhood than most of his teammates.
>
> "They put everything in perspective," says Taylor of wife Rashida and 9-month-old daughter Tionna. "No matter how bad a day I have at school or practice, when I come home, everything's fine again. They're always happy to see me."
>
> Mark Wiedmer
> *Chattanooga Times and Free Press*[34]

After that personalized intro, Wiedmer broadens the profile to include the player's performance statistics and his importance to the Florida team. But it is the man, not the team and not the game of football, that is the thrust of this profile.

Above all, the profile gives you opportunity to *write* your way into the sports pages—and readers' hearts. Note this colorful, engaging writing:

> It's a life of mid-size cars, mid-level hotels and drive-thru dinners just off the interstate. Your best friends are talk radio and the *USA Today* box scores. Your worst enemies are a full bladder and a sign that reads "Next Service Area 56 Miles." You work a territory, usually three or four states, and you have to be prepared for all of nature's elements. You learn quickly never to leave home without long johns, a rain slicker and sunscreen.
>
> The life of an area scout for a major league baseball team is a lonely one. High school game one day. College game the next. Juco game. American Legion game. Babe Ruth game. Pull up your folding lawn chair, point your radar gun, click your stop watch. Hundreds of games. Thousands of players.
>
> Then it happens. As quickly as a coach can spank a fungo across a choppy infield in Flint, Mich., you remember why you got into this business. The ball takes a high bounce, then a low one. It begins to roll, then pops up again like bacon grease off a frying pan. A tall, reed-thin shortstop somehow calms the ball. He glides in, reaches forward to glove it, makes the transfer and then fires a smooth, firm throw to first. You are left breathless. The kid is a high school sophomore.
>
> "I see an electric body," Yankees scout Dick Groch recalls. "Thin, but with lithe, sinewy muscle. Classic infielder's body type. Fluid and graceful."
>
> At this moment, the scout gathers himself. Time to find out more about this boy, beginning with the basics.
>
> Jeff Bradley
> *ESPN Magazine*[35]

Incidentally, that profile above is *not* about a baseball scout. Rather, it's about the player he discovered, shortstop Derek Jeter of the New York Yankees.

The successful profile, then, has these characteristics:

- An individual is your writer's vehicle for deeper exploration of an issue or industry but, also, on occasion is the entire focus.
- A news peg—a game just won, a race yet to be run—adds topicality to the profile.
- The detail and amount of your physical description of the individual varies with your mission; drawing a complete "picture" is secondary if you're illuminating an issue or industry but primary if the profile focuses on the individual.
- Honesty, not adoration is a hallmark. Unabashed praise is unworthy of good journalism; portray your subject's weak points as well as the strong.

Summary

—After you've conquered the basic spot-news story, move your writing into the analytical and interpretive dimension.

—Objective writing still is a requirement when analytical stories are destined for *news* pages.

—Strong analytical writing is characterized by writing flair, inclusion of a wider context and statistical background, plus quotes from authoritative sources.

—The best analytical writing is built on journalistically sound, objective observations, rather than mere personal interpretation by the writer.

—In analytical writing, you must not only assemble strong evidence to support your conclusion; you also must let your readers see that evidence.

—The very considerable analytical liberties granted sportswriters, as contrasted with writers in other departments, carry correspondingly great responsibility to get it right, to be accurate and to be fair.

—Capturing key moments—a key play, pivotal decision, a turning point—can take your readers beyond the score and toward understanding the complexities of sports.

—Take your readers to places they otherwise never would visit—a dugout for a talk with a coach or a locker room to see a team in victory or defeat.

—In writing longer analytical pieces, you must maintain your writing momentum by inserting quotes that pull readers ahead or characterizing a sport complexity in terms they understand.

—Roundups written from bits and pieces received via the AP or other newspapers can help you create a wider and more meaningful picture for your readers.

—Search news service reports for nuggets from afar that can be turned into important local stories or laced together to show a trend.

—Profiles let you use a personality as a vehicle for luring readers beyond the score and into deeper understanding of sports.

—The best personality profiles are those that are not used to simply illuminate a single personality but, rather, shine light in hidden corners of a wider story.

Exercises

1. Examine spot-news sports coverage in today's *The New York Times* (or another newspaper designated by your instructor) for examples of writing that combines writing flair and analytical expertise. In about 400 words, describe a) language that displays analytical expertise and b) whether the writers have produced coverage that is objective and balanced as well as analytical. If you find *subjective* writing, comment on whether it is appropriate for news pages.

2. Cover a sports event designated by your instructor and write an *analytical*

spot-news story that contains appropriate arrangement of facts, timely insertion of telling statistics and extensive quotes from authoritative sources. Use as your guide examples from the first section of Chapter Six, "Winning Combo: Writing Flair Plus Analytical Expertise." Use the wordage required to cover the event appropriately.

3. Cover a sports event designated by your instructor and structure your article to focus on key moments, including key plays, pivotal decisions and turning points, as discussed in Chapter Six. If possible, take your readers where they otherwise could not go—into a locker room or dugout. Use the wordage necessary for this assignment.

4. Write a personality profile with minimal focus on the individual and, rather, use this story structure as a vehicle to take readers into deeper understanding of a campus sport. You might profile a coach, for example, with the wider mission of explaining training methods or game strategies. Use the wordage appropriate for this assignment.

5. Write a personality profile that concentrates on describing a campus sports figure—a coach, player or trainer, for example. In this profile, your mission is to describe the individual as a personality rather than focus on an issue or event behind the personality. Be certain you "draw" a word picture of how the personality looks, walks and talks. Use wordage appropriate for this assignment.

Recommended Reading

Writing for *American Journalism Review* (January/February 2000, p. 16), free-lancer Bo Smolka summarized valuable reading found on Internet sites:

espn.go.com carries the NFL's GameDay Live real-time presentation, with detailed analysis of plays and statistics. Some National Basketball Association coverage also is available.

www.cnnsi.com combines strengths of Cable News Network and *Sports Illustrated* in offering real-time play-by-play and statistics.

www.finalfour.net offers NCAA Division I men's and women's basketball tournaments.

www.totalbaseball.com provides baseball statistics from Total Sports Inc., a sports information company.

www.pgatour.com offers golf coverage and statistics.

www.sportsline.com provides real-time NBA coverage and statistics (including shot charts). NFL football and the World Series are covered.

www.broadcast.com offers radio broadcasts of more than 100 university and college football games, along with audio of horse racing and other sports.

www.nascar.com is a source on stock car racing.

Notes

1. "Braves Have a Lot of Wannabe Heroes," Oct. 18, 1999, p. D-13.
2. "Crimson Heartbroken," Oct. 10, 1999, p. C-14.
3. "No Map, No Clue," Oct. 4, 1999, p. E-1.
4. "A Dud of Their Own," Nov. 29, 1999, p. 80.
5. "Couch Learns Hard Facts of Being the Top Prospect," April 4, 1999, p. 23.
6. "Health Issues in Secondary Worry Jets Against Dallas," Dec. 15, 1999, p. D-3.
7. "Ciborowski Excelled With Savvy Style," Nov. 25, 1999, p. B-1.
8. "Twins Leading Red Sox in Eighth," April 27, 1999, p. E-1.
9. Dispatch for Sunday papers, Nov. 14, 1999.
10. "Knicks-Heat Rematch Has a Different Conclusion," Nov. 15, 1999, p. D-1.
11. "Luyendyk Fends Off Ray to Come Away With Indy Pole Spot," May 24, 1999, p. C-13.
12. "A Twisted Debut," Aug. 14, 1999, p. G-1.
13. "This Showing Proves Critics to Be Right," Aug. 14, 1999, p. G-1.
14. "Freeze Frame: 3 Plays Define The Giants' Strange Victory," Nov. 1, 1999, p. D-6.
15. Dispatch for morning papers, May 17, 1999.
16. "Volunteers Sink in Swamp," Sept. 20, 1999, p. D-3.
17. "Braves Pull For Cox," Oct. 24, 1999, p. D-16.
18. "Giants Big Balloon Goes Pffft! in Loss of Eye-Popping Size," Sept. 20, 1999, p. D-1.
19. "Back on Track," Sept. 6, 1999, p. 47.
20. "Mora Used His Memory and His Eyes to Seal Victory," Oct. 4, 1999, p. D-2.
21. "Flint Takes Pride in Spartans' Bedrock," March 27, 1999, Section 3, p. A-1.
22. Dispatch for Sunday papers, April 4, 1999.
23. "From a Claimer to Acclaimed: The Saga of Charismatic," May 28, 1999, p. D-1.
24. "Marion Motley, Bruising Back for Stories Browns, Dies at 79," June 28, 1999, p. B-7.
25. "Show Time for Reluctant Soccer Superstar," June 11, 1999, p. A-1.
26. "Goldberg," March 23, 1999, p. E-1.
27. "The Giants Train and Come Out Fighting," Aug. 3, 1999, p. D-4.
28. "NFL Quarterbacks Are Passing the Baton," Oct. 22, 1999, p. C-1.
29. "Time Is Now for Spurs to Part With Robinson," March 7, 1999, Section 3, p. 9.
30. "Finances the Key for Former Dogs," July 24, 1999, p. D-1.
31. These stories are packages under "Locker Room Is Buzzing Again," Feb. 28, 1999, p. C-7.
32. "Veteran Childress Still Has Drive," Oct. 21, 1999, p. C-15.
33. "An Addict With One Weapon: Hope," May 15, 1999, p. D-1.
34. "Florida's Taylor Ready," Aug. 16, 1999, p. C-1.
35. "2 Hot," May 3, 1999, p. 83.

PART FOUR

Covering the Majors

Check out "job board" at The Associated Press Sports Editors' Web site (apse.dallasnews.com) and you'll see two types of job listings.[1]

One is for jobs some newspaper sports editors offer generalists—a "sportswriter" or "staff writer."

The other is for reporters with specific job skills—"golf writer," "hockey writer," "baseball writer" and so forth.

Some sports editors hire well-trained generalists presumed able to take the same basic reporting and writing skills to any sport, any assignment. But many others seek specialists finely tuned to subtleties and nuances of individual sports.

Whatever the editors' initial hiring practices, they will require you to recognize and adapt to differences that do exist between individual sports.

For example, if you're covering football, you'll face a relatively limited game schedule and thus will spend more time writing the precedes and follows we discussed in Chapter Five and the analytical pieces covered in Chapter Six.

Basketball, with its longer and tighter game schedule, and baseball, with an even longer and even tighter schedule, have different coverage rhythms. Baseball, particularly, requires a different, more spot-news and game-story approach because you're virtually covering back-to-back games all season.

So, yes, all the reporting and writing fundamentals you've studied so far in this book truly are applicable to any assignment in journalism. But, it's equally true that as in all journalism, the day of the specialist reporter is here in sports.

Therefore, we turn in Part Four to three specialist chapters on covering the major sports—football, in Chapter Seven; baseball, in Chapter Eight; and basketball, in Chapter Nine. (Yes, I know, for you, hockey may be "major," and golf or tennis or fishing may be important, too. But we'll turn to them later in the book.)

7

Covering Football:
A Case Study

IT'S A SULTRY September evening in Atlanta. In the Georgia Dome, 69,555 football fans settle down to watch Atlanta Falcons vs. Minnesota Vikings.[2]

The kickoff. The Falcons receive deep in their end zone and run the ball out to the 19-yard line.

Now, first play from scrimmage—and high above the field, in the press box, Mark Schlabach, National Football League writer for the *Atlanta Journal-Constitution*, scribbles this in his reporter's notebook:

1-10 A19 32 3 mid. (57 blitz) (52 T)

Translation:

It is first down and 10 yards to go, on Atlanta's 19-yard line. No. 32 for the Falcons, Jamal Anderson, carries the ball for three yards, up the middle. No. 57 for the Vikings, linebacker Dwayne Rudd, blitzes, and No. 52, Ed McDaniel, makes the tackle.[3]

Two more Atlanta tries fail, and the Falcons punt. Minnesota takes over, makes a first down but a second series of plays ends with a punt.

Schlabach now notes this:

Atlanta (10:02)

Translation: Atlanta again has the ball; 10:02 minutes remain in the quarter.

Atlanta makes a first down, and Atlanta fans begin to hope—then a *turning point*:

3-11 A38 57 sacked 12 blind 12 fumble (58 rec.) (32 bad block)

Translation:

It's third down, 11 yards to go. Atlanta has the ball on its own 38-yard line. Minnesota's Rudd, No. 57, penetrates the Falcon offense and sacks No. 12, Atlanta quarterback Chris Chandler, who fumbles the ball. Minnesota linebacker McDaniel, No. 58, recovers. The villain? No. 32, Atlanta's Jamal Anderson, guilty of a "bad block."

And so it goes throughout the game: Schlabach, the reporter, noting down every play, especially every turning point, in elaborate (if encoded) detail so Schlabach, the writer, can turn to his keyboard the instant the final whistle is blown.

How the Pros Do It

This case study illustrates how highly professional football writers handle game assignments, and how their editors package a wide variety of stories and statistics to give reader-fans a complete picture of what happens on the field.

When that final whistle blew, the *Journal-Constitution*'s Schlabach turned to his writing assignment: A long sidebar examining turning points and Falcon mistakes. The following is what he wrote hurriedly, under intense deadline pressure, for the next morning's *Journal-Constitution* (under the headline, "Mistake = Loss"):

> In their last 20 games, including three playoff contests in last season's improbable flight to the Super Bowl, the Falcons have lost three games. Not surprisingly, Atlanta has committed more turnovers than its opponent in all of those defeats.
>
> In Sunday's loss to the Minnesota Vikings, the Falcons lost three fumbles, committed two costly pass-interference penalties and missed two field goals, including one that could have tied the game with 3:38 left.

Note those two grafs are straightforward, factual statements. Now, a quote from an authoritative source that *supports the story's news peg, mistakes.*

> "It was definitely a team loss, because we contributed in every phase of our football team," Atlanta coach Dan Reeves said. "We missed the field goals and special teams had a fumbled kickoff, which gave them excellent field position. We didn't get the job done there.
>
> "Offensively, we had two turnovers that led to us not scoring and giving them a chance [to score]. We had four penalties for first downs, and they were all big penalties that set up touchdowns for them."

Schlabach elaborates on the mistake peg and, for the first time, inserts personalized and subjective language (emphasis added).

> Overall, it was not a mistake-free performance that was a trademark of last season's 14-2 squad.
> A closer look at *Atlanta's comedy of errors*, which led to the Falcons losing at home for the first time in 12 games:

That colon frees Schlabach to move into compartmentalized "dash matter"—three story segments set off by dashes. This is what he writes:

> — Turnovers: Quarterback Chris Chandler set the tone early in Atlanta's second series. On third-and-11 at the Falcons' 38, Chandler was sacked from his blind side by linebacker Dwayne Rudd, who was barely touched by running back Jamal Anderson's block. Chandler fumbled and linebacker Ed McDaniel recovered at the Atlanta 29. ...
> On Atlanta's next possession, the Falcons moved the ball to their 40, where Chandler hit wideout Ronnie Harris for 15 yards. But Vikings safety Orlando Thomas stripped Harris of the ball and recovered at the Minnesota 42.
> That led to the Vikings' first touchdown—Randall Cunningham's 2-yard pass to Cris Carter—and a 7-0 lead.

For his reader-fans (including the *thousands* who watched on television), Schlabach examines other Falcon mistakes—a kickoff returner runs right out of the end zone, although his blockers go left; another fumble sets up a Viking score.

Now, the second and third segments of dash matter backing up the lead's peg on fumbles, penalties and missed field goals (*Always* back up your leads!):

> — Penalties: Atlanta was flagged four times for 84 yards, including two pass-interference infractions that led to both Minnesota touchdowns.
> — Missed field goals: Morten Andersen, one of the most effective kickers in league history and owner of seven NFL records, had hit 14 consecutive field goals from 30-39 yards. His last miss from that distance was a 30-yarder as time expired in a 19-17 loss at Jacksonville in 1996, which put the Jaguars into the playoffs. On Sunday, he missed from 35 and 39 yards.
>
> Mark Schlabach
> *Atlanta Journal-Constitution*[4]

Note these characteristics of the Schlabach performance:

Football expertise. Though only 27 when he covered the game, Schlabach was well-versed in football and its subtleties. Before joining the *Journal-Constitution*, he wrote sports for two years (concentrating on football) and served as sports editor for one year for his campus daily, *Red & Black*, at the University of

Georgia. During that time, he was campus sports stringer for the *Journal-Constitution*, the *Los Angeles Times*, *Austin (Texas) American*, *Dallas Morning News* and (now-defunct) *Houston Post*.

"I've always read a lot about football," Schlabach says, "particularly coaches' biographies and what George Allen (a former coach) wrote about the game."[5]

Detailed reporting. In most press boxes, particularly for college games, team officials quickly make game statistics available. But only by keeping his own detailed play-by-play could Schlabach achieve deep understanding of the game and, most crucially, turn so quickly to his keyboard and meet his deadline, writing and filing without second thought or any rewriting or polishing.

Develop your own reporter's shorthand and ensure it catches—and highlights for your quick reference—key plays, turning points, mistakes, injuries and penalty calls. Reporting them must buttress any meaningful account of a game.

Conceptual story structure. Although Schlabach, of course, took notes chronologically, *he didn't write a chronological account.* Rather, he built his story around a concept—"Mistake = Loss"—and segmented treatment of turnovers, penalties and missed field goals.

Chronological treatment of a key series of plays or even a single incident as it unfolds can add internal strength to a story. But seldom will you succeed by merely writing a wrap-up first graf or two—a summary lead—then lazily slipping into a play-by-play chronology. Readers seek not a play-by-play walk through a game but, rather, an organized and coherent writing structure built around concepts, such as those highlighted by Schlabach.

In fact, *none* of the *Journal-Constitution*'s extensive coverage of that Falcons-Vikings game takes traditional, chronological approach to who won and why. Let's look closely at the wider structure of the *Journal-Constitution*'s coverage for clues on how you can approach *any* assignment you might receive when you and your sports department colleagues team up for a "takeout" on a major football game.

Wider Coverage Strategy

First hint on how to cover football in a football-crazy town: Take each game seriously!

For the Falcons-Vikings game, actually a routine 1999 season-opener, the *Journal-Constitution* set aside *five pages* of a special 10-page section titled, "NFL Monday." In no other journalism—general news, business, science, lifestyle—would a story of that caliber receive so much valuable newshole and costly staff time.

Second hint: Reader-fans assign news value to almost everything that happens before, during and after the game. Here's how the *Journal-Constitution* served that voracious reader-fan demand:

The special-section's front page was dominated by a huge photo of a Vikings player scoring a touchdown and a *single* staff-written story, all under the banner headline, "KO'd in Rematch."

Matt Winkeljohn wrote that Page One story and it, like Schlabach's Page 4 sidebar, takes a conceptual rather than who-won-and-why approach. *But* note how Winkeljohn weaves into his story the *spot-news essentials*—key play, score, attendance and wider context (particularly the meaning for coach Dan Reeves):

> Spotted through binoculars, the sight of Dan Reeves Sunday evening might have been alarming. The Falcons coach had every right to be steamed.
>
> Morten Andersen's 39-yard field goal try sailing wide left with 3:38 left in the game triggered his barking, but a laundry list of foibles made Reeves a time bomb waiting to go off.
>
> Bad enough that his team lost 17-14 to the Vikings in front of 69,555 while making virtually all the mistakes it had avoided on the way to the Super Bowl last season. Add the status of quarterback Chris Chandler, whose strained right hamstring could keep him out of the next game, Monday night in Dallas, and it was Reeves' worst day at the office since Nov. 9, 1997, when Tampa Bay prevailed 31-10 in the Georgia Dome. The Falcons' streak of 11 regular-season victories in a row at home came to an end.

By reserving the score to his third graf, Winkeljohn assumes his readers know the outcome and that they seek from his writing *deeper meaning*. Winkeljohn turns, in his third graf, to a look-ahead angle—the quarterback's injury and its implications for the rest of the Falcon's season.

> "When I hurt it in practice [in the pre-season], I was able to straighten it," Chandler said of the hamstring injury. "This time, it was hard to straighten my leg out. But we have eight days until the game.
>
> "From a selfish standpoint, it has been 11 years since I have played on Monday Night Football. I want to play. From a team standpoint, I know we have a lot better chance when I'm out there."

Now, Winkeljohn elaborates on his lead's news peg—Falcon mistakes—and inserts, briefly, historical context:

> Last year, the Falcons led the NFL in turnover ratio. Sunday, they had three fumbles and forced no Minnesota turnovers. Atlanta helped the Vikings to at least 10 of their points after first-half fumbles by Chandler and kick returner Tim Dwight.
>
> Penalties gave the Vikings 55 of the 58 yards on the first score, including a questionable 52-yard interference call against cornerback Ray Buchanan, who was defending Randy Moss.

Finally, two colorful quotes *carefully selected to elaborate on the "mistakes" news peg*:

"I couldn't believe they called me on that one," Buchanan said. "Here I am 5-10, and Moss is 6-10 [actually 6-4], and they say they're not going to call that [incidental contact] this year, and they call it on the poodle."

The Vikings led 17-0 at the half. Atlanta tried to recover, but unlike the 1998 NFC Championship Game, Andersen missed after the Vikings' Gary Anderson left the door open with a late miss.

"I never brought a cape," said Andersen, who also missed a 35-yarder in the first half. "I'm not Superman."

Matt Winkeljohn
The Atlanta Journal-Constitution[6]

If *you* one day draw Winklejohn's assignment on a football takeout, remember these characteristics of his Page One story:

- It is designed as a short (just 386 words) and snappy summary of principal points that are discussed in much fuller accounts on inside pages. (Each element in Winklejohn's "mistakes" news peg, particularly the Falcons' bad place-kicking, is listed in an accompanying front-page "teaser" box. Reader-fans are directed to Schlabach's sidebar with, "Mistake-free performances of 1998 weren't reflected in Falcons' opener, E-4.")
- The story sets, briefly, the historical context, with third-graf reference to the coach's "worst day" and the sixth-graf's, "Last year ... ."
- The story has strong look-ahead angles: the quarterback's injury, the outlook for the next game and, by implication, because of the first-graf focus on him, the coach's future (*always* a big story in NFL coverage).

Inside, *Journal-Constitution* editors devote Page 2 to highlights and statistics of other NFL games, then, on Page 3, begin highly detailed coverage of the Falcons-Vikings game.

First up is columnist Mark Bradley (under the slug, "Viewpoints"). His angle:

This undoes nothing. This refutes nothing. The Falcons weren't flukes last season and aren't now. Those who seek to cite Sunday's game as ultimate proof of Minnesota's superiority ... . Well, here's what Jamal Anderson has to say to you:

"I'm tired of proving ourselves. If you believe in us, fine. If not, forget you. I'm tired of this, 'Are you worth it?'"

Mark Bradley
The Atlanta Journal-Constitution[7]

Columnist Bradley thus takes the coverage far ahead, into whether the game's outcome signals the Falcons' future. He also turns quickly (in his fifth graf) to the coach's role, commenting, "If this game did anything, it served to re-prove the Dan Reeves Method."

Huge display (40 column inches) of Schlabach's sidebar and an accompanying photo dominate Page 4, but on this page, *Journal-Constitution* editors begin the "nitty-gritty" coverage loved by reader-fans:

"Game Breakdown"

This includes scoring by quarter and, in 80 to 100 words each, recaps key plays, scoring and play-by-play descriptive (such as, in the second-quarter recap, "Working against the Vikings' 'prevent defense,' Chandler moved the Falcons into Minnesota territory in two plays").

"Drives"

Drawing from play-by-play notations, editors represent statistically the possessions and drives by each team, for each half. On the printed page it looks like this:

Play Summary

TEAM	START TIME	START YD	PLAYS	YDS	TOT TIME	RESULT
Falcons	15:00	F19	3	8	1:47	Punt
Vikings	13:13	V24	6	40	3:05	Punt

Translation of the first line above:

The Falcons took the first possession (with, of course, 15 minutes left in the first quarter) on the Falcons' 19-yard line. In three plays, they gained eight yards and controlled the ball for 1:47 minutes. Then they punted.

"Key Stats"

This records for each team total downs, rushing yards and passing yards.

"Beyond the Box Score"

In its entirety:
What: Randall Cunningham (Vikings' quarterback)
When: 13:02, second quarter
The Play: On second-and-goal from the Falcons 2, Cunningham fired a bullet to receiver Cris Carter, who ran a slant pattern to beat Ray Buchanan for the game's first score.

"Highlight Reel"

Also in its entirety:
Who: Leroy Hoard (of the Vikings)
When: Fourth quarter, 1:52
The Play: If the Falcons' chances were not already shot, they were when Hoard zipped through the middle for 34 yards to the Falcons' 20. It was the first down the Vikings needed to keep the clock moving.

"Falcons Opponents"

Finally (for this page), a box listing the outcome of *every* game played the previous day by teams the hometown Falcons will meet for the rest of the season.

Note these characteristics of the "stats" published on Page 4 and examined above:

- Discerning reader-fans virtually can replay the game in their heads. Complete play-by-play must await television's rerun of the game, of course. But key plays and highlights—all can be "seen" in the *Journal-Constitution* stats.

- The stats are constructed *from reporters' notebooks* (underscoring, again, your responsibility to pay attention, up there in the press box).

- The stats report *tactic* (pass or run), *time* (when the play developed) and *result* (whether the pass was completed; what yardage was picked up in the run).

- The stats give fans the nitty-gritty they want *but*, importantly, are designed to eliminate the need for writers to include all that detail in their accounts. *Writers thus are freed for analytical writing that, in the Page One story and inside sidebars, takes readers far beyond what they saw on television.*

Continuing their panoramic coverage, *Journal-Constitution* editors devote Page 5 to a column and two game stories. All focus on Falcon failures in place-kicking.

First, senior columnist Furman Bisher, in the "off-lead"—or upper left corner of the page:

> As exhilarating, as emotionally wrenching as The Other One was, this one wasn't. As inspiringly heroic as Morten Andersen was in The Other One, this time he let the air out of the Dome. It must be depressing to have one single obligation to your team, and to fail, and to realize that you must wait another week to try again. Such is the life of the man who lives by his

foot in professional football, thus the lives of Morten Andersen and Gary Anderson, one a Dane, the other a South African.

Anderson and Andersen have kicked more field goals than any other players in the history of the National Football League. In The Other Game, when the Atlanta Falcons reached the pinnacle of their existence in the NFC Championship Game in Minneapolis, Andersen the Great Dane was the hero, Anderson the South African was the loser. He had to live a year with his failure. At least Andersen has only to live with it until next week, when he takes his show with the Falcons to Dallas.

Furman Bisher
Senior Sports Columnist
The Atlanta Journal-Constitution[8]

The page lead (upper-right position) goes to staff writer Curtis Bunn:

Two of the most prolific kickers of their era met on the artificial turf of the Georgia Dome and had a long chat before the Falcons and the Minnesota Vikings played their NFC Championship Game rematch. One would suspect they would kick around the nuances and intricacies of a gut-wrenching and often-thankless job. But not Atlanta's Morten Andersen and the Vikings' Gary Anderson.

"We talked about fly fishing," Andersen said.

If only the conversation was so light *after* the Vikings edged the Falcons in a game that Andersen and Anderson had a significant foot in—just like in Minnesota last January.

Curtis Bunn
The Atlanta Journal-Constitution[9]

The third Page 5 article, though focusing initially on kicking, takes a wider view by discussing key plays and quoting Minnesota players.

A Gary Anderson missed field goal. Two, in fact. An Atlanta team that trailed early, then cut the lead to three points.

Just as the echoes from last January's NFC Championship Game overtime loss to the Falcons started getting louder, the Vikings ended the similarities in the most definitive way possible: They won the game.

"We said, 'We can't let the same thing happen that happened last year,'" said Minnesota linebacker Ed McDaniel, who sustained a knee injury in January's matchup. "We tried to put last year behind us. We knew we just had to keep doing what we were doing, because what we were doing was working.

Karen Rosen
The Atlanta Journal-Constitution[10]

Finally, on Page 5, more stats: a box (headlined, "Kicking Problems").

Kicking Problems

Kicker	Qtr.	Time	Distance	Reason
G. Anderson	1st	1:40 left	26 yards	Blocked
M. Andersen	2nd	6:22 left	36 yards	Wide right
Etc. . . .				

You noted, of course, a weakness in coverage we've studied so far: redundancy. Too many staffers writing with essentially the same news peg, focusing on the same element (field-goal kicking).

Well, get used to it. Before a game, editors find it impossible to precisely delineate reporting and writing territorial boundaries (although smart editors *always* try in pregame staff meetings). And, after the game, all staffers write furiously to meet cruel deadlines, and editors cannot order up neatly differentiated stories.

Anyway, redundancy in a sense demonstrates journalistic validity—all *Journal-Constitution* writers interpreted the game, and reasons for the outcome, the same way!

The final (and fifth) page devoted to the Falcons-Vikings game is dominated by analytical writing by Winkeljohn and Schlabach, plus game stats.

Under the slug, "Analysis," Winkeljohn writes:

> The Vikings beat the Falcons on Sunday because they dominated the middle of the field, got three turnovers to none and the worst penalties of the game went against Atlanta at terrible times.
> That pretty much sums it up.
>
> Matt Winkeljohn
> *The Atlanta Journal-Constitution*[11]

Point by point, Winkeljohn comments on the principal elements of his lead—the Vikings' time of possession was more than six minutes over the Falcons', cornerback Ray Buchanan was penalized 52 yards for pass interference.

Schlabach gets even more pointed, under the heading, "Report Card." Schlabach grades the Falcons' "D" for offense ("Once again, Jamal Anderson was shut down by Minnesota. ..."), "C+" for passing game (quarterback Chandler completed 17 of 30 passes for 258 yards and one touchdown). Schlabach's best grade: "B" for defense against Minnesota's running game ("Until Leroy Hoard burst for a 34-yard run with less than two minutes remaining, the Falcons' front seven held the Vikings running game in check.")

Note these characteristics of the news-page analyses by Winkeljohn and Schlabach:

- Both slide across the boundary between objective newswriting and subjective commentary, which, again, is permitted in sportswriting to a degree unacceptable in other news sectors (imagine the *Journal-Constitution*'s White House reporter writing a "report card" on a president's success in, say, economic policy).
- Both writers, however, are strongly experienced professionals, *and they produce, for readers to see, the evidence on which their analyses are based.* It's OK to be judgmental in sportswriting; just be certain your reporting backs up your interpretation.

If you're an aspiring football writer, study—carefully—the *Journal-Constitution*'s final offering of stats. They cover *the key elements of a football game that must be represented in your writing*, whether spot-news or analytical. These categories are crucial:

Game Stats

	MINN	ATL
First downs	19	22
Rushing	6	3
Passing	9	16
Penalty	4	3
Net rushing yards	115	81
Rushing attempts	32	23
Yards average	3.6	3.5
Net passing yards	184	278
Attempted	33	31
Completed	22	18
Had intercepted	0	0
Total net yards	299	359
Offensive plays	65	56
Yards per play	4.6	6.4
Fumbles-lost	0 - 0	3 - 3
Penalties-yards	9 - 81	4 - 84
Interceptions	0 - 0	0 - 0
Punts-yards	3 - 121	2 - 88
Average	40.3	44.0
Punt returns-yards	1 - 1	0 - 0
Kickoff returns-yards	3 - 94	3 - 67
Possession time	33:14	26:46
Third-down conversions	17 - 09	11 - 05
Sacked-yds. lost	0 - 0	2 - 12

Another crucial statistical base for your reporting is in the individual performances by key players in six categories: rushing, passing, receiving, punt returns, interceptions and tackles.

Here is how the *Journal-Constitution* reports the Falcons' rushing stats:

Rushing

	GAME				SEASON			
	ATT	YDS	AVG	TD	ATT	YDS	AVG	TD
J. Anderson	16	50	3.1	0	16	50	3.1	0
Hanspard	3	9	3.0	0	3	9	3.0	0
Christian	1	1	1.0	1	1	1	1.0	1
Chandler	3	21	7.0	0	3	21	7.0	0
Totals	23	81	3.5	1	23	81	3.5	1

And, this is what reader-fans want to know from passing stats ("C-A" translates, of course, as "Completed-Attempts"):

Passing

	GAME				SEASON			
	C-A	YDS	I	TD	C-A	YDS	I	TD
Chandler	17-30	184	0	1	17-30	184	0	1
Graziani	1-1	32	0	0	1-1	32	0	0
Totals	18-31	216	0	1	18-31	216	0	1

Your writing also must draw from the stats above for references to key players.

Case Study Lessons

The *Journal-Constitution* case study illustrates principally these factors you should consider when covering football:

- As illustrated by the newshole and staff resources assigned to this single game by the *Journal-Constitution*, editors regard football coverage as a major reader attraction. Winning assignment to your newspaper's coverage team will put you in the journalistic front line.
- As in all of journalism, detailed and strong reporting must be your core strength in covering football. Although you seldom will write play-by-play chronologies, you must observe closely—and understand—each play

if your writing is to reflect overall professionalism and journalistic integrity.

- The long columns of statistics your paper publishes will relieve you of the need to stuff your writing with figures. Avoid writing news stories that read like accountants' reports. *But* draw factual substance for your writing from these stats: key plays, star player performance, turning points, mistakes, injuries and penalty calls.
- Analysis and subjective commentary is acceptable in even spot-news coverage of football, as in most sportswriting. *But,* your analysis must be supported by solid reporting—factual evidence—your readers can see.
- Each story must be placed in context, evaluating the game against a team's history or season performance, for example, and *always* must include a look-ahead element. There always is another game, another season.

And, it is to another game that we turn in the next chapter.

Summary

—Because each sport has its own rhythm and subtleties, the era of specialist reporters has arrived, although many editors hire writers who can take the same basic journalistic skills to any assignment.

—In football writing, as in any journalism, reporters develop their own shorthand for keeping track of play-by-play action and the statistics that must buttress any well-written story.

—You'll need years of experience and serious study of the sport if you want to report football for a major publication.

—Like most newspapers, *The Atlanta Journal-Constitution* presents readers with panoramic coverage of football and this requires huge newshole and major staff assignments.

—Although you must note each play chronologically, you seldom will succeed by writing a simple wrap-up summary lead, then lazily slipping into chronological recitation of what happened in a game.

—As illustrated by a case study in this chapter, Mark Schlabach of the *Journal-Constitution* successfully covered an Atlanta Falcons-Minnesota Vikings game by building his story around a conceptual structure that focused on "Mistakes=Loss."

—Your newspaper probably will publish long columns of game statistics, relieving you of the need to overload your story with figures.

—Rather than focus on too many stats, peg your writing to key plays, star performers, turnovers, injuries, penalty calls and other pivotal factors.

—In football reporting, as in any sportswriting, you're often permitted to include analysis and subjective commentary, *but* your writing must show readers the evidence you have for your interpretation.

Exercises

1. Examine coverage of a football game in a newspaper designated by your instructor. In 350 to 400 words, analyze the reporting and writing. Is the coverage truly panoramic? Does it achieve balance between spot-news reporting, analysis and statistical backup? As a reader, do you have firm understanding of turning points, key plays, star performances and other influences on the outcome?

2. Your instructor will give you statistics on a football game *but none of the stories written about the game*. Drawing solely from the statistics, write a spot-news story on the outcome. Search the stats for the pivotal factors discussed in Chapter Seven—rushing, passing, penalties, fumbles, interceptions, punt returns and so forth. In about 300 words, write a story that enables your readers to "see" the game.

3. Construct a reporter's "shorthand" for keeping track of play-by-play action in a football game. Use Mark Schlabach's system, discussed in Chapter Seven, as a model. Write this with particular emphasis on how you can arrange your "shorthand" to single out key plays and turning points in a game. Your mission in Exercise 3 is to begin developing reporter's techniques you can use in a sportswriting career.

4. If the season is appropriate, cover a football game at any level—prep, college or professional. Write *two* articles: a spot-news main lead to serve as the principal story for the front page of a newspaper's sports section and a sidebar analysis that grades both teams' performances, as Mark Schlabach graded the Falcons and Vikings in Chapter Seven.

5. In about 300 words, describe how newspaper accounts of football games should be structured to carry readers beyond what they see in watching the games on television. As a football writer, what will *you* seek from a game that will carry your readers' understanding beyond what they have seen? How will subjective commentary and analysis fit into your reporting and writing? What limits will you place on the insertion of your personal viewpoints into the copy you write?

Recommended Reading

You'll need access, of course, to *Total Football II: The Official Encyclopedia of the National Football League (Total Football, 2nd ed.)* It's a huge (1,664 pages) compilation of stats, play diagrams, essays on the sport and the esoterica of the locker room and huddle.

Also see the annual *Official National Football League Record & Fact Book* and *The Sports Encyclopedia: Pro Football: The Modern Era 1974-1998.*

For a quick view of other books available on football, go to *www.amazon.com*. It lists 2,561!

Notes

1. Job offerings also are available in *Editor & Publisher*, a newspaper weekly trade publication, and other industry magazines.

2. This game was played on Sept. 12, 1999, and *The Atlanta Journal-Constitution* coverage discussed in this chapter is drawn from "NFL Monday," a 10-page section published Sept. 13, 1999.

3. Mark Schlabach graciously provided this material and other football insights in a series of interviews in 1999-2000. In the spirit of journalistic openness, let me add that he is a former student of mine.

4. "Mistakes = Loss," Sept. 13, 1999, p. E-4.

5. Interview with author, Jan. 5, 2000.

6. "Chandler Injured As Falcons' Comeback Falls Short," Sept. 13, 1999, p. E-1.

7. "No Handwringing; It's Just One Loss," Sept. 13, 1999, p. E-3.

8. "Anderson-Andersen's Reversal of Fortunes," Sept. 13, 1999, p. E-5.

9. "Tough Day for Kickers," Sept. 13, 1999, p. E-5.

10. "Eerie Repeat," Sept. 13, 1999, p. E-5.

11. "Errors Stall Falcons," Sept. 13, 1999, p. E-6.

8

Covering Baseball

NEW NEWS, old news, non-news, rumors of news.

If you cover major league baseball, you'll write it all.

If you're a sports editor, you'll publish it all—in huge amounts and with gobs of statistics and details.

If you're a fan, you'll read it, whether in the heat of summer or the cold of winter, and demand more.

In sports journalism—nay, perhaps *all* of journalism—there's nothing quite like baseball in what we cover and how. The teams are many, the off-season active, the playing season long and the reader-fans insatiable in their demands.

Consequently, we turn in Chapter Eight to learning to write about baseball, of course, but also learning to *hold an ongoing conversation with readers about it*.

Talking with readers is what baseball writers do in major papers across the country. Much of their writing truly is unusual. For example, football writing frequently swings widely in tone, spiking with a weekly high that sometimes is near frenzy over relatively few games on fall weekends, then quickly subsides emotionally.

Baseball coverage purrs along steadily each day in the off-season, then builds slowly during spring training to a more leisurely momentum during the playing season. And throughout it all, the best writers chat with readers day after day, experts to experts, and assume all along that fans have deep understanding and love of the game.

You can see why baseball coverage has its own pace: Whereas a pro football team plays 16 regular-season games, in major league baseball, 30 teams (16 in the National League, 14 in the American League) play 162 regular-season games each. That totals 4,860 baseball games, and it's too much to expect each to provide high sports drama. And, importantly, it's too much to expect you to deliver unique reporting angles or highly-charged writing for each game.

The writing we'll study in Chapter Eight is perhaps *more even in tone* than some on other sports we've studied in this book. For certain, much baseball writing is extremely technical—sometimes almost esoteric—in its examination of the sport's complexities.

We'll look primarily at covering professional baseball. Prep and college baseball is covered by some newspapers, but not in the depth normally accorded football and basketball. Many large papers pay only passing attention to baseball at those levels.

But if you aspire to cover baseball at the community level, be confident that the reporting and writing lessons ahead are fully applicable to any baseball writing at any level.

Off-Season: The Conversation Begins

It's *December*, surely the season for some football and lots of basketball, but *USA Today's baseball* reporters are sending in important intelligence (some of it in code) from around the circuit. Examples (decoding added):

American League
NEW YORK: Yankees are close to being set, but then you never know. RHP (right-handed pitcher) Hideki Irabu on block (offered for a trade) to make room for LHP (left-handed pitcher) in rotation (schedule for pitchers to start games).
TAMPA BAY: Needs a 3B (third baseman), and maybe it will be Rockies' (Colorado Rockies of National League) Vinny Castilla. RHP Rolando Arrojo is available.

National League
ARIZONA: Signed RHP Russ Springer to free-agent contract (under which players can negotiate their own deals) but still shopping for more relief help (pitchers who come into a game when starting pitchers tire or "lose their stuff").
PITTSBURGH: Needs RH (right-handed) power reliever and third baseman. ... [1]

And on it goes, for *every* team, as one of the nation's most complete sports sections labors through the winter to cover a game played by "the boys of summer."

As spring blooms in the South, fans' interest quickens. It's spring-training time, and all newspapers broaden their coverage. *The Los Angeles Times* certainly does, even if *news* from training camp is, shall we say, scarce. The following was the *lead* story one March day in a *Times* feature titled, "Spring Training: Daily Report."

> *Dodgers*
> Brown Flush With Anger
>
> Pitcher Kevin Brown destroyed a toilet with a baseball bat in the Dodgertown clubhouse Saturday because he was angry about being scalded while taking a shower.
> The water temperature in the shower became hotter when someone flushed the toilet, inciting the all-star right-hander to smash it after grabbing a nearby bat. ...
> Several people familiar with the water situation at Dodgertown said the problem is nothing new. For many years, players have been scalded while taking showers when toilets are flushed in the clubhouse.
> Manager Davey Johnson lived vicariously through Brown.
> "He did something I'd like to do many times when I was in the shower and someone flushed the toilet," Johnson said. "Sometimes it's better to get that [frustration] out. No one was hurt by it. You can repair a toilet."
>
> *The Los Angeles Times*[2]

Things are more serious at training camp in Clearwater, Fla., where the Philadelphia Phillies had a momentary fright. The *Philadelphia Inquirer* is there to cover it in detail, even though the fright seems, well, a bit overdone:

> CLEARWATER, FLA.—Phillies third baseman Scott Rolen will have an X-ray taken on his right foot today to determine whether he suffered any damage when he fouled a ball off the foot in yesterday's exhibition game against the Detroit Tigers.
> Rolen sustained the blow in the first inning, but it seemed rather innocuous at the time because he continued to play. Four innings later, Rolen informed manager Terry Francona that the foot was bothering him and Francona quickly removed his young star from the game. ...
> Rolen seemed confident that there is nothing wrong with his foot.
> "My diagnosis is I'm a big wimp," he said with a smile. "It was bothering me a little, that's why I came out."
> Francona said trainer Jeff Cooper ordered the X-ray as a precaution. Francona agreed with Cooper's thinking.
> "He's a good player," Francona said of Rolen. "We're kind of crazy not to send him (for an X-ray). For Scotty to say something, it must be bothering him."

If there is any team that knows how dangerous a foul ball off the foot can be, it's the Phillies. Two years ago, in his first at-bat as a Phillie, Danny Tartabull broke his foot with a foul ball and was lost for the season.

Jim Salisbury
The Philadelphia Inquirer[3]

Every newspaper, whatever its journalistic character, gets into the swing (so to speak) during spring training. *The New York Times*, best known perhaps for coverage of Afghanistan and other nonsports stories, *fronts* this on A-1:

Jason Grimsley, a relief pitcher in his first season with the Yankees, was among those who flocked to see the movie "Mission: Impossible" in 1996, and as he watched Tom Cruise and an accomplice crawl through an air duct to steal secret information, memories of Grimsley's own impossible mission came back to him.

Grimsley didn't steal government secrets, but he was at the center of a heist that is part of baseball lore for its audacity and ingenuity. For the first time, Grimsley acknowledged last week that it was he who crawled through the innards of Chicago's Comiskey Park into the umpires' dressing room on July 15, 1994, to exchange an illegally corked bat of his Cleveland Indians teammate Albert Belle for one that was cork-free.

"That was one of the biggest adrenaline rushes I've ever experienced," Grimsley said in telling a tale known to others but never addressed by himself.

Buster Olney
The New York Times[4]

Jumping the story inside, the *Times* explains, in hundreds of words and an elaborate artist's rendition of the "crime" scene, that Belle faced suspension for the bat, illegal because hollowing it out, then filling it with cork "makes the head of the bat lighter, increasing the speed of the swing."

Are you trying to get a grip on the journalistic thrust and writing tone of the examples above? Well, think of chatting with your best friend about a topic that absorbs both of you, and you'll understand what those baseball writers are doing.

First, those writers are *talking* baseball in truly conversational tones with *their friends*, those reader-fans hungry for baseball talk, whatever the time of year. For true fans—and there are millions—anytime is baseball time.

Second, standard definitions of what's "news" are suspended as we *vacuum* the baseball circuit for even low-grade tidbits, just as good friends often chat about inconsequentials when a favorite hobby is the topic. (Ever hear two trout fishermen talking? Or antique collectors?)

Third, however, serious baseball intelligence is in those tidbits. It matters a great deal whether the Yankees trade Hideki Irabu. Is a pitcher "losing it" if he busts up a toilet? Will the Phillies' star third baseman indeed be ready for the season's start?

Season Starts: The Game Story

For readers and writers alike, things turn really serious when the season opens.

For many readers, coverage isn't complete unless it includes details on all games, everywhere.

For writers, the challenge is to write *hundreds* of game stories in detail and depth, yet maintain—day after day—writing vigor and freshness.

In coverage that sprawls over many pages, major newspapers generally take two approaches: staff-written coverage of the hometown or home-state team and Associated Press dispatches on distant games.

How AP Experts Do It

Covering *every* game, *every* day, AP writers learn to prioritize news carefully, placing truly important developments high in stories that frequently are trimmed to three or four grafs by newspaper editors who have too much sports news for too little newshole (a task copy desk wags liken to putting six gallons of water into a five-gallon jug).

On one day, for example, editors of the *Schenectady (N.Y.) Sunday Gazette* devote an entire page to National League action alone. They jam in two full columns of league stats, a large baseball photo and *eight* AP game stories plus box scores.

The upstate New York paper leads its page with a northeastern team popular in New York state:

> PHILADELPHIA—Edgardo Alfonzo had an eventful sixth inning Saturday night, driving in the tiebreaking run for the Mets and then getting erased on a triple play in New York's 9-7 win over the Philadelphia Phillies.
>
> Alfonzo went 2-for-3 with three RBI as New York fought back from six runs down to win their third straight game after losing six of seven.
>
> Phillies reliever Ken Ryan (1-2) walked Roger Cedeno to lead off the sixth. Cedeno stole second and scored on Alfonzo's single to center.
>
> After John Olerud walked, Mike Piazza lined to shortstop Alex Arias as the runners were moving. Arias flipped to second baseman Kevin Jordan for the second out, and Jordan then tagged Olerud to complete the Phillies' second triple play in the last two years.
>
> The Associated Press[5]

Those four grafs, plus a box score (which we'll discuss later), are *all* that readers get. Note these characteristics of the writing:

- The writer doesn't assume readers saw the game on television. The lead is written to quickly communicate who won, the score and who was a key player.

- There is no featurish twist on this lead. The writer intends to inform, not amuse; to communicate essential facts, not sketch a color picture.
- The writer sorts through nine innings of action and focuses the lead on the key player, Edgardo Alfonzo, who "had an eventful sixth inning."
- The writer *assumes reader expertise in baseball*, using technical terms without translation: triple play (three outs in one play); Alfonzo went 2-for-3 (hit twice in three at-bats) and had three RBIs (batted in three runs) and so forth. This assumption of reader expertise isn't permitted in other forms of journalism, such as business news or science writing, where translation of technical terms is mandatory.
- Quickly, in minimum wordage, the AP's writer sketches the wider context: New York won their third straight after losing six of seven games; the Phillies completed their second triple play in two years.
- Overall, the writing is clean, open, direct and communicates simply (but don't misunderstand—writing simply isn't simple).

The seven other game stories on the page are presented in standard format: Score in an overline (mini-headline) and three to five grafs of copy, plus box score. Examples in their entirety:

Cubs 5, Braves 1

CHICAGO—Henry Rodriguez hit a two-run homer, backing Steve Trachsel's six-hit pitching, and Greg Maddux's woes continued as Chicago beat Atlanta.

The victory stretched the Cubs' regular-season winning streak against the Braves to seven games. Atlanta has dropped its last three.

After starting the season 4-0 for the first time in his career, Maddux (4-3) is in an uncharacteristic slump. He was tagged for three runs in the first inning, and gave up a total of five runs a career-high 14 hits in seven innings.

The Associated Press[6]

Diamondbacks 9, Rockies 2

PHOENIX—Randy Johnson returned to form with a three-hitter, and Luis Gonzalez extended his hitting streak to 27 games as Arizona beat Colorado.

Gonzalez, who has hit safely in 31 of 32 games this season, matched John Flaherty for the third-longest streak in the NL this decade. Flaherty hit safely in 27 straight games for the San Diego Padres in 1996.

Johnson (4-1), who allowed six runs on a career-worst 13 hits against Montreal in his last start, allowed only Neifi Perez's homer to lead off the game, and singles to Henry Blanco and Derrick Gibson.

The Associated Press[7]

Note above how the AP's writers, responding to varying newspaper needs nationwide, employ expert reporting skills to find *the* crucial play and *the* key player and write in direct, engaging language whose meaning can be absorbed virtually at a glance.

Indeed, AP writers learn to compress minimum essentials into a one-graf lead that, with the overline score, can be used in columns of "briefs" by editors facing newshole shortages. This is how *Sunday Gazette* stories look when cut to a single graf each:

Brewers 7, Marlins 2

MILWAUKEE—Steve Woodard pitched a four-hitter, and David Nilsson, Geoff Jenkins and Ron Belliard homered as Milwaukee beat Florida.

The Associated Press [8]

Pirates 17, Expos 6

PITTSBURGH—Freddy Garcia and Brian Giles hit three-run homers, and Montreal tied a team-record with six errors as Pittsburgh beat the Expos.

The Associated Press [9]

Learning to write in such minimalist language that drives directly and sharply to the news focus is essential to your development as a writer. As your experience broadens, you can spread your writer's wings. But remember that in journalism, *informing* readers accurately and quickly is your first goal.

Nevertheless, notice above how a terrible *sameness* can settle over baseball writing, how the daily grind of covering so many games can trap you into *formula writing*—using the same story structures game after game and simply plugging in, each day, a new crucial play and a new key player.

For that reason, newspaper staff writers frequently cover hometown teams quite differently. Premium is placed on unique and colorful angles for leads and insightful—at times, critical—analysis of teams, players and coaches, all written in much greater detail that sometimes runs into three or four *columns*, not three or four grafs.

Reaching for the Unusual

Guaranteed lots of newshole and expected to find unusual writing angles, newspaper reporters frequently slip into dramatic, almost impressionistic realms when covering the hometown team.

Sometimes, it seems the outcome—the score—is of secondary importance. Note this story in *The Atlanta Journal-Constitution*:

HOUSTON—John Rocker looked at catcher Eddie Perez with fear in his eyes. Houston's Ken Caminiti had just hit a pitch to deep center field in the bottom of the ninth inning with a runner on second and the Braves clinging to a 7-5 lead.

Rocker didn't realize Andruw Jones was camped under the ball a few yards shy of the warning track. He didn't realize the Braves were about to wrap up their eighth consecutive trip to the National League Championship Series.

"I grabbed my hat, like 'Gah ball, please come down,'" Rocker said. "I didn't get a chance to celebrate. I was still gasping for air when Andruw caught the ball."

Jones' catch provided the final out of another nerve-racking victory against the Astros, who battled valiantly again Saturday but lost the best-of-five series three games to one.

The Braves will open the NLCS on Tuesday night at Turner Field against the New York Mets, who also wrapped up a 3-1 first-round victory Saturday by beating Arizona 4-3 in 10 innings.

You'll note that the writer holds the outcome to the fourth graf, obviously assuming all reader-fans in Atlanta saw the game on television or at least heard of the outcome well before the story hit the *Journal-Constitution*'s sports front (under the banner, "Rocker Closes the Deal," and the sub-head, "Braves Dispose of Astros, Get Mets in NLCS").

The writer's assumption—probably justified—enables her to capture *The Moment* in the lead, reaching for the drama of that key play.

And because she reports for a morning paper, the writer has the luxury of waiting for post-game interviews, then plugging a colorful quote into the third graf.

AP writers, racing against newspaper deadlines across the nation, in all time zones, sometimes don't have such luxuries. Their stories are written immediately following the final out and filed via laptops long before the stadium empties of fans.

Now, before we proceed, look again at the previous lead graf. Note anything questionable? How about this: Can a reporter, particularly one sitting up in the press box, see *fear* in the eyes of a pitcher, way down there on the mound?

That is, reaching for the unusual or stretching for dramatic color can take you into journalistically dangerous territory. If you *can* see what's in their eyes, can you be certain it's fear? Maybe it's "stunned disbelief," "eager anticipation," "amazement" or another of the clichés found in so many similar stories and in so many sports pages.

Also note how the writer moves quickly, in the fourth and fifth grafs, to position the game within the wider context of the Braves' drive toward the NLCS. That structure is chosen because the story serves as a section-front *wrap-up* or quick summary. For game detail, fans are directed to four inside pages where other writers offer sidebars, analysis, color and columns of stats.

The wrap-up nature of the story becomes clear when the writer, after presenting context in the fourth and fifth grafs, makes a transition not into hard news but, rather, "softer" color angles. The following are the sixth through eleventh grafs:

> When the game ended, the Braves didn't hug, jump around or make a human pile when they gathered on the mound. They just let out a collective breath and did their usual high-fives down a line.
>
> "Relief," echoed Perez, Rocker, manager Bobby Cox and any other teammate who was asked to express his post-game sentiment.
>
> "I don't think I've ever been this tired after a four-game series," Chipper Jones said.
>
> The Braves lost Game 1, but came back to win Game 2 on Kevin Millwood's one-hitter, Game 3 with the help of a 10-inning escape from a bases-loaded, nobody-out jam, and then Game 4 with four outs from Rocker to kill a serious last-gasp effort from the Astros.
>
> For this, they get the Mets, who come back to Turner Field for an NLCS many anticipated.
>
> "I think people knew we were a force [before this series]," Chipper Jones said. "I don't know if people have really taken us seriously as far as being a contender."

Now the writer concludes with a quick look from the losing Astros' viewpoint and one (just one) hard-news graf on play highlights:

> There's a fine line between winning championships and heading home. Just ask the Astros, who just lost their third consecutive Division Series in the most excruciating of ways.
>
> After losing Friday night's 12-inning heart-breaker and trailing 7-0 against John Smoltz on Saturday, the Astros should have been finished. But they had something left for the final game in the Astrodome.
>
> Caminiti's three-run homer, his third of the series, cut the Braves' lead to 7-4 in the eighth inning. Another RBI hit by Tim Bogar, and the Braves were begging Rocker for more heroics.
>
> Carroll Rogers
> *The Atlanta Journal-Constitution* [10]

A couple things to remember for the day when *you* join colleagues in similar team coverage of a single event:

- Obtain from your editors precise delineation of your writing assignment. If your editors aren't precise—and, often they cannot be—sort out with your writing colleagues who will write what. Front-page wrap-ups aren't written like detailed play-by-play stories destined for inside pages, or vice versa. Avoid overlap.

- If you draw the *color assignment* look for the featurish angles—indeed, look deeply into their eyes. But be careful how you describe what you see.

Sometimes, of course, overlap is inevitable, as it is for two *Boston Globe* writers, one writing the straight hard-news lead and the other a sidebar column, on the same game. First, the game lead:

> SEATTLE—The philosophy remains unchanged, from Denton T. "Cy" Young, the first to win 20 games for the Olde Towne Team 98 years ago, to the skinny Dominican who yesterday became the Red Sox' newest 20-game winner. This is what stoppers do.
>
> "It's really important for me to set the tone, to bring the team back to life," Martinez said after he struck out 15, held Seattle to two hits in eight innings, and combined with Rod Beck to shut out the Mariners, 4-0, to become Boston's first 20-game winner since Clemens went 21-6 in 1990.
>
> Gordon Edes
> *The Boston Globe*[11]

Now, 20-game winners don't come along every day, so Edes' colleague at the *Boston Globe*, columnist Dan Shaughnessy, justifiably takes the same angle in his column (played side-by-side with Edes' piece).

> SEATTLE—It's a pretty impressive group, this private club that includes Cy Young, Babe Ruth, Smoky Joe Wood, Lefty Grove, Jim Lonborg, Luis Tiant, Dennis Eckersley and Roger Clemens.
>
> All of the above had at least one 20-win season for the Boston Red Sox, and yesterday at dangerous Safeco Field, Pedro Martinez earned lodge membership with eight innings of two-hit, 15-strikeout pitching in a 4-0 victory over the Mariners.
>
> Martinez becomes the first 20-game winner in the majors this season and Boston's first since Clemens turned the trick way back in 1990. ...
>
> Dan Shaughnessy
> *The Boston Globe*[12]

Inside, on a full page devoted exclusively to the game, *Globe* editors give readers hundreds more words from both Shaughnessy and Edes, plus a lengthy sidebar in which Edes disgorges from his notebook a huge number of tidbits—chatty, informal writing that gives fans much to discuss over a beer or coffee. Also on the page: a game photo, box scores and columns of batting and pitching stats.

Double-Play: Spot News Plus Analysis

When they "single-staff" a game—assign just one writer—editors expect spot news *and* analytical angles to be woven into a game lead.

Here's Henry Schulman going both ways for the *San Francisco Chronicle*:

> D-Backs 12
> Giants 3
>
> PHOENIX—There is never a good time to go into an offensive funk. Nor is there a good time for Barry Bonds to be sitting on the bench injured. That both events have converged bodes ill for the Giants, who left Bank One Ballpark yesterday on the short end of a 12-3 thrashing.
>
> Bonds missed the game with inflammation in his left elbow, which affects his ability to hit certain pitches. He was examined by Phoenix-area orthopedist Dr. Rob Meislin yesterday and will undergo an MRI in the Bay Area today. His status for tonight's home game against the Florida Marlins is questionable.

Note, above, the writer's quick turn, in the second graf, to Bonds' injury and, in a superbly placed *look-ahead angle*, how the writer analyzes the seriousness of the injury for the team's fortunes.

To the almost total exclusion of game details, the look-ahead and analytical drift of the writing continues:

> Needless to say, for the Giants, a lot will be riding on that test. Bonds is having a terrific start, batting .366 with four homers and 12 RBIs in 12 games. He owned the team RBI lead until Rich Aurilia reached 14 yesterday with his three-run homer off Armando Reynoso, the only Giants runs.
>
> If Bonds has to go on the disabled list for the first time as a Giant, he would join starting pitcher Mark Gardner, who was placed there Saturday with inflammation in his pitching shoulder.
>
> In the wake of their rubber-game defeat to the improved Diamondbacks yesterday, the Giants pondered the possibility that Bonds will be missing, or at least physically limited, in the days ahead.
>
> Henry Schulman
> *San Francisco Chronicle*[13]

Lesson: Sometimes, the news peg you select for your lead graf—a key play, star's performance or, as above, an injury—is so overwhelmingly important that it must dominate your entire story.

Knowing when that all-important development has arrived requires reporting judgment. Knowing how much detail to include requires writing judgment.

Developing that judgment, both as a reporter and a writer, takes intimate understanding of the game, keen appreciation of reader-fans' wants and needs and experience. Until you develop experience, read great writers for how they handle such dilemmas. You might even listen to editors. Some know what they're doing.

Among experienced journalists, striking unanimity frequently emerges on what the news is when a big story breaks in baseball. Note the following:

> In an improbable setting, David Cone performed an improbable feat Sunday.
>
> He pitched the Yankees' second perfect game in little more than a year, playing in front of Don Larsen, who pitched a perfect World Series game for the Yankees in 1956.
>
> Larsen was at Yankee Stadium to help celebrate Yogi Berra Day, and after Larsen threw the ceremonial first pitch to Berra, Cone took command of the mound and retired all 27 Montreal batters he faced as the Yankees beat the Expos, 6-0.
>
> Murray Chass
> *The New York Times*[14]

> David Cone tossed a perfect game on a perfect day at Yankee Stadium yesterday.
>
> The rapier-sharp Cone mowed down 27 straight Montreal Expos to win, 6-0—joining the exclusive club that includes Yankees Don Larsen and David Wells—on a day the Bombers honored Yogi Berra.
>
> Virginia Breen, Bill Egbert and Dave Goldiner
> *New York Daily News*[15]

> On a day Don Larsen was celebrated at Yankee Stadium, David Cone pitched a perfect game of his own.
>
> Cone dazzled the Montreal Expos with a wide assortment of pitches Sunday, throwing the 14th perfect game in modern baseball. The Yanks won 6-0.
>
> On the very same field where Larsen pitched a perfect game against Brooklyn in Game 6 of the 1956 World Series, Cone struck out 10 to do the same. Cone, who got his first shutout in exactly four years, didn't go to a three-ball count all day.
>
> The Associated Press[16]

Lesson: When you are on a story and big news breaks (and that *will* happen to you in a sportswriting career), don't try to be fancy and don't reach to the heavens for writing help. Just *focus intently on the news* and write it simply and clearly.

But where, precisely, *is* the news?

How the Pros Spot News

Top baseball writers generally seek the news in any game by looking first at four obvious categories: batting, pitching, baserunning and fielding.

Let's look at how *The Atlanta Journal-Constitution* does that. Here's the scenario:

It's mid-August, and the Atlanta Braves (75-49) can aspire reasonably to making the playoffs and, perhaps, the World Series. Fan interest is high, and the *Journal-Constitution* gives major coverage to each game.

The San Diego Padres are in Atlanta for three games. Atlanta takes the first, 4-3; coverage dominates Page One of the sports section, then jumps inside with sidebars, features and stats.

One sidebar—"Game Report"—examines the game with reporting that focuses on those top new categories: batting, pitching, baserunning and fielding. However, the writing by Thomas Stinson, opens with a fifth concept, a general "scene-setter" graf:

> **ABOUT LAST NIGHT**: Atlanta opened a six-game homestand on an adrenalin rush, Ozzie Guillen bringing home Andruw Jones with a shallow grounder in the infield grass as the Braves won in the 11th, their second straight extra-inning win. Jones had opened the inning with a double, took third on an outfield error and scored to complete the comeback. The Braves bullpen pitched three more innings of scoreless relief.

With that overview established, writer Stinson moves to batting. Note carefully what he prioritizes as *news*:

> **AT THE PLATE**: With the bases loaded in the eighth and the Braves down 3-2, Brian Jordan, who had gone 0-for-3 and stranded a pair of runners, fell behind 1-2 to Dan Miceli before sending a routine double-play grounder to shortstop Chris Gomez. But second baseman Damian Jackson's throw to first was wide and though first baseman Wally Joyner appeared to hold the base, umpire Bill Hohn called Jordan safe, allowing the tying run to score. Bret Boone's first-inning double was his eighth in 11 games.

Now to the news in pitching:

> **ON THE MOUND**: When Trevor Hoffman inherited a bases-loaded situation from Miceli with no outs in the ninth, he struck out Randall Simon looking. He then got ahead of Gerald Williams 0-2 before Williams' grounder to short forced Andruw Jones at the plate. Hoffman then got Bret Boone to foul out to third baseman Phil Nevin to end the inning. Glavine started the third by walking pitcher Matt Clement to open the inning and walking Reggie Sanders with two out. Glavine then got ahead of Nevin 0-2 before he laced a 2-2 fastball into the left field seats.

And the single most important development in baserunning:

> **ON THE BASES:** Boone misread a Chipper Jones line drive to center in the first inning and took off for third base. The ball was caught by Eric Owens, who turned it into an 8-4 double play.

Finally:

> **IN THE FIELD:** Nevin allowed a Boone grounder to bounce off his glove into shallow left field in the eighth, scoring pinch-runner Walt Weiss. With men on first and third and one out in the fifth, Eddie Perez sent an apparent double-play grounder toward third. Nevin's throw to second retired Jose Hernandez but umpire Hohn ruled Perez safe on Jackson's throw, allowing Andruw Jones to score. Replays showed Perez arrived after the ball.
>
> Thomas Stinson
The Atlanta Journal-Constitution [17]

Still, Stinson is not finished. He turns now to even more detail, in a sidebar slugged, "How They Scored." It's several hundred words, starting with the Padres' half of the third inning:

> **PADRES THIRD:** Clement walked. Owens grounded out, third baseman C. Jones to first baseman Klesko, Clement to second. Gwynn grounded out, shortstop Hernandez to first baseman Klesko, Clement to third. Sanders walked. Nevin homered to left on a 2-2 count, Clement scored, Sanders scored. Gonzalez grounded out, shortstop Hernandez to first baseman Klesko. Padres 3, Braves 0. [18]

Stinson also does a box score, then a look-ahead to the third game in the Braves-Padres series (reporting where, when, probable starting pitchers and so forth).

In a feature titled, "Braves Notebook," Stinson wraps up a full column of those tidbits so beloved by baseball fans ("Sporting a new goatee and strumming Rudy Seanez's guitar, catcher Javy Lopez made his first visit to the clubhouse Friday, walking with just a slight limp 3½ weeks after knee surgery.")

Clearly, if you want a career in big-league journalism reporting baseball you must have an eye for the larger picture—the context of a season, a team's overall status and *still* be able to catch the nitty-gritty (and *all* of it).

How can any reporter do that? *By methodically* recording and analyzing each play as the game unfolds.

Scoring the Game

Your writing on a baseball game must flow from firm understanding of each play and its meaning, if any, for the outcome.

Play-by-play action in football and basketball generally is recorded by reporters in their own personalized shorthand. In baseball, reporters—and many fans—use a standardized *scorecard* to record details that, to the practiced eye, present a clear picture of the contest.

Scorecards and, particularly, the notations reporters scribble on them, don't lend themselves to photo-reproduction in this book. But let's look at the types of information Carroll Rogers of *The Atlanta Journal-Constitution* kept on her scorecard as she covered the first game of the 1999 World Series between the Atlanta Braves and New York Yankees.[19]

Rogers' notes illustrate the types of information you should examine during a game for top-priority news angles you'll need to write your story.

Atop the scorecard, Rogers notes, "49°, 8:11 (p.m., when the game starts), wind chill 34°"—important because, of course, weather conditions frequently are crucial to the outcome of games. Also noted: "Attendance 51,342."

Baseball has its own notation system. For example, each position carries a number: the pitcher is No. 1; catcher, 2; first baseman, 3; second baseman, 4: third baseman, 5; shortstop, 6; leftfielder, 7; centerfielder, 8; rightfielder, 9.

The top half of Rogers' scorecard is devoted to the Yankees. Batters are listed in the order in which they go to the plate—the "batting order." For this game, Chuck Knoblauch, Yankee second baseman, leads his team's batting order.

In vertical columns on the scorecard, Rogers lists this information for Knoblauch (and, of course, all other Yankees batters who follow him):

—Errors (none)

—Uniform number (11)

—Position (4, which, again, means second baseman)

—Batting performance inning by inning. For example, in the column for the third inning, Roger notes, "F8." That means Knoblauch "flied out"—hit a fly ball to centerfield, which is position No. 8. The ball was caught for the out. Other examples of this notation system: "L3" means a line drive was hit to the first baseman, who caught it for the out; "F7" followed by a circled 2 means the batter flied out to leftfield, for the second out of the inning.

—AB (at bats—the number of times Knoblauch batted, which was four in this game)

—BB (bases on balls; none)

—R (runs scored; one)

—H (hits; none)
—RBI (runs batted in; none)
—Extra Base H (hits; none)
—Other (stolen bases and so forth; none)

For all Yankee batters, Rogers totals 30 at bats, 6 bases on balls, 4 runs, 6 hits, 4 runs batted in, no extra-base hits and 2 stolen bases—information that quickly gives Rogers her writing angle on Yankee batting.

Now, the scorecard lists Yankee *pitchers*. The starting pitcher is Orlando Hernandez. He's pulled from the game after pitching seven innings, and three teammates follow him to the mound before the game ends.

For each pitcher, a completed score card presents this information:

—W/L (pitcher's season won-lost record)
—IP (innings pitched)
—H (hits given up)
—AB (total of batters faced, *minus* the number walked, hit with a pitched ball and so forth)
—BF (total batters faced)
—R (runs given up)
—ER (earned runs—those scored against the pitcher through hitting and not defensive error)
—HR (home runs hit off the pitcher)
—S (stolen bases)
—SF (sacrifice flies)
—BB (bases on balls given up by pitcher)
—I (intentional walks given by pitcher)
—HB (hit batters—batters struck by pitched balls)
—SO (strikeouts)
—WP (wild pitches)
—BK (balks)

In just that manner, Rogers methodically notes play-by-play action through-out the World Series (which the Yankees sweep, 4-0) so at the end of each game she rapidly can write fact-filled stories containing *essential statistical substance*.

Regardless of any keyboard magic you can unleash, with colorful descriptive or analytical insights, your baseball writing must communicate the stats—and lots of them.

Other Stats Your Readers Need

In addition to stats you plug into your game stories, you must prepare *linescores*. Here's one from *USA Today* on a New York Mets and Baltimore Orioles game:[20]

New York..................200 033 000 - 8
Baltimore..................100 000 410 - 6

As you can see at a glance, the linescore shows *scoring by inning* and that New York won, 8-6.

Box scores are individual batting performance and other details. To illustrate, here is the first line for New York batters:

Batting	ab	r	h	bi	bb	so	lo	avg.
NEW YORK								
Henderson lf	4	3	3	1	1	0	1	.319

Information presented above, from left: Henderson, a leftfielder, has 4 at bats, 3 runs, 3 homeruns, and bats in one run. He walks one base on balls, has no strikeouts ("SO") and is left on base once. His *season* batting average is .319.

This information is followed by three grafs in "agate" (small type) that details action in *batting, baserunning* and *fielding*.

Next, the box score presents information on pitching. The first line for New York:

Pitching	ip	h	r	er	bb	so	bf	era
NEW YORK								
Yoshii W, 7-7	6 1/3	8	4	4	2	2	27	5.06

From left, the box score information above: New York pitcher Yoshii, whose season record is 7 wins and 7 losses, pitches 6 1/3 innings against Baltimore. He gives up 8 hits, 4 runs. The "4 ER" means the four runs are "earned" by batters with hits, not scored through defensive errors by Yoshii's teammates. Yoshii gives up 2 bases on balls and strikes out 2 batters among the 27 he faces. "ERA" means earned run average—that is, so far this season, batters have earned 5.06 runs on average from Yoshii per game.

This section of the *USA Today* box score is followed by more "agate" that details, among other things, how many pitches each pitcher throws and how many are strikes. Also noted: pitchers face five-mile-an-hour winds blowing "left to right."

A true fan will "re-play" a game by reading information in linescores and box scores. And, if that fan spots a crucial play or key development you have not mentioned in your game story, your writing will be judged incomplete.

Be aware, also, that fans are cross-checking as you write about overall team performances or league play during a season. Fans do this by consulting stats published periodically in all major sports sections.

USA Today, for example, devotes entire pages to team and league stats. Under the headline, "American League Team-by-Team Statistics," *USA Today* provides this:[21]

— The "AL Beat," an analysis by Mel Antonen on strengths and weaknesses of AL teams, trades being discussed and so forth.
— For *each* batter on *all* American League teams, *17* categories of stats—batting averages, games played, at bats, strike outs and so forth.
— For *each* pitcher on *all* teams, *16* categories of stats—won-loss records, earned run averages, innings pitched, hits given up and so forth.
— Attendance records for all teams, at home games and away games.
— Each team's won-lost record against every other team in the league.
— A *batting* comparison that presents *19* categories of information for each team, including how many bases a team has stolen, how many times its players have been caught stealing and so forth.
— A *pitching* comparison that presents *16* categories of information.
— An "AL Team Victory Breakdown" that illustrates, among other things, whether wins and losses were on the road or at home, at night or in day games, on grass or artificial turf.

Here, young writer, is the lesson: To write successfully about baseball for people who love it, you must love the game yourself. You must write in an incredibly detailed and nuanced style that combines overarching understanding with grasp of the nitty-gritty. Players who can bat lefthanded *and* righthanded are "switch hitters." Successful baseball writers are "switch hitters," too.

Summary

— Reporting successfully about baseball is a year-round effort that requires a conversational style of writing for reader-fans about news items large and small.
— Baseball writing often is more even in tone than writing about other sports because the baseball season is long and the games played many.
— Major newspapers, such as *USA Today*, report baseball 12 months a year, even with football and basketball seasons under way.
— With spring training, newspapers broaden their coverage to include stories that wouldn't meet standard definitions of news in other journalistic categories.
— When the season starts, writers are challenged to cover scores of games, yet maintain—day after day—writing with vigor and freshness.

—AP writers cover every game, every day, and learn to prioritize news carefully, placing truly important developments high in their stories so editors can cut them from the bottom up, to get maximum numbers of stories in limited newshole.

—Many spot-news stories written by AP focus on communicating who won, the score and who was a key player—and don't attempt to be featurish or particularly colorful.

—Writing directly, in minimalist language, can cause a terrible sameness to settle over stories. So, many newspaper writers try for unique and colorful angles.

—Newspaper writers, unlike AP writers, usually are guaranteed lots of newshole for covering hometown teams and are freer to slip into dramatic, almost impressionistic writing realms.

—Featurish writing presents dangers—such as "reading" what's in somebody's mind or describing what the reporter "sees" in their eyes.

—Writers who "single-staff" a game—that is, cover it alone—often are required to report spot news *and* write insightful analysis requiring expert knowledge of the game.

—Successful baseball writers look for news first in four areas—batting, pitching, baserunning and fielding.

—Using a standard scorecard to record play-by-play action enables you to identify key factors you must return to at game's end when writing your lead story.

—Expert reader-fans seek understanding of a game by studying linescores and box scores, so your writing must reflect all key factors recorded in such stats or your writing will be judged incomplete.

Exercises

1. Read *USA Today*'s sports section (or another your instructor designates) for five consecutive days. In 350 to 400 words, comment on a) the newspaper's spot-news, straightforward baseball coverage, b) its analytical/interpretive writing and c) (if in season) its statistical presentation. Is the newspaper's emphasis on colorful, insightful analysis or hard-news, factual reporting? Or, do you see another pattern of coverage?

2. Read three consecutive days of AP game-story writing in a newspaper your instructor designates (or, if it's off-season, in a designated archival source). In about 350 words, comment on reporting techniques and writing styles you see represented therein. What do the AP's writers seem to take as their reporting/writing mission? What are the strengths and weaknesses of their styles? Importantly, what would *you* do differently?

3. Analyze baseball game coverage in the national edition of *The New York Times* for a period designated by your instructor. In 300 words, describe how the reporting and writing differ (if they do) from the AP stories you studied in

Exercise 2. In terms of what you perceive the *Times'* journalistic mission to be, do you think its writers succeed? Identify strengths and weaknesses of the *Times'* writing.

4. Your instructor will provide you with the linescore, box score and other "agate" published by a newspaper on a baseball game. By analyzing the stats reported therein you should be able to "see" the game. Using only these stats, write a game story of about 300 words.

5. Report and write about a baseball game your instructor will designate. Use a standard scorecard to record play-by-play action. Write a game story of about 400 words. Include interviews with winners, losers and coaches.

Recommended Reading

For further reading of straightforward spot-news baseball writing in minimalist language, see Associated Press game coverage in any newspaper sports section. Much AP writing is a model of how to do it quickly, completely, accurately—and game after game.

You'll be the gainer also if you study writing by staffers of major newspapers—among them, the *New York Times, Boston Globe, Washington Post, Chicago Tribune, Atlanta Journal-Constitution, Dallas Morning News* and *Los Angeles Times*.

Among magazines, note *Sports Illustrated, Baseball Weekly* and *Sporting News*. For help on stats, see the baseball section in *The Associated Press Stylebook*.

And, of course, for listings of *thousands* of books on baseball, go to *www.amazon.com*.

Notes

1. "In Focus: Baseball's Winter Meetings," *USA Today*, Dec. 10, 1999, p. C-3.
2. March 14, 1999, p. D-12.
3. "Phillies Notes," March 12, 1999, p. D-7.
4. "Yankee Ends Real Corker of a Mystery," April 11, 1999, p. A-1.
5. "Mets Rally to Beat Phillies," May 16, 1999, p. E-4.
6. "National League," May 16, 1999, p. E-4.
7. Ibid.
8. Ibid.
9. Ibid.
10. "Rocker Closes the Deal," Oct. 10, 1999, p. E-1.
11. "For Martinex, It's 20 Won," Sept. 5, 1999, p. C-1.
12. "He Decks Seattle, Joins Elite Boston Club," Sept. 5, 1999, p. C-1.
13. "D-Backs Club Slumping Giants," April 19, 1999, p. E-1.
14. Dispatch for morning papers, July 19, 1999.
15. "Cone Is Perfect!" July 19, 1999, p. 2 of a special wrap-around.

16. Dispatch for morning papers, July 19, 1999.

17. "Game Report," Aug. 21, 1999, p. C-5.

18. Ibid.

19. My thanks to Carroll Rogers and her *Journal-Constitution* sportswriter colleague Marc Schlabach for their assistance in providing this scorecard. In the spirit of journalistic openness, Schlabach is a former student of mine.

20. This material is drawn from "Major League Baseball," *USA Today*, July 20, 1999, p. C-4.

21. Drawn from *USA Today*, July 20, 1999, p. C-6.

9

Covering Basketball

BASKETBALL, DICTIONARIES say, is "a game played . . . on a rectangular court having a raised basket at each end, points being scored by tossing a large, round ball through the opponent's basket."

True, of course. But, oh, how limited! So, I must add:

- Basketball is an incredibly complicated game requiring of consistent winners a unique physical agility and stamina plus mental discipline and team-oriented "game smarts."
- Throughout the United States (and in much of the world), the game is an obsession for millions, many of whom play it or watch it being played virtually anywhere, from blacktop playgrounds to driveways, where garages are backboards, to huge arenas, where the backdrop is a huge sports business (and lots of money).
- At every level—prep, college and pro—newspapers devote enormous newshole and staff resources to informing readers about which teams toss that "large, round ball" through baskets with the most success.

In all of that, of course, is huge career potential for the aspiring sportswriter, and we turn in Chapter Nine to some hints on how you can develop the reporter's eye and writer's touch needed in covering basketball.

We'll start where it all starts for virtually every big-time basketball writer—covering a high school game.

On the Prep Beat: A Case Study

For Jon Gallo of *The Washington Post*, covering prep basketball is his most difficult sports assignment.

"It's a hundred times easier to cover a college game," he says, because at that level [and in the pros], sports information officials provide what a writer needs—background on teams, players and games played, season statistics on every aspect of the game *and*, importantly, interviews with players and coaches.

"On the prep beat," Gallo says, "you get no backup on statistics, no guaranteed interview time with anyone and, most of the time, not even a table to put your laptop computer on. You sit with everyone else, keep your own stats, then rush around, trying to find a telephone line so you can file your story back to the office."[1]

And you do this a lot.

During basketball season, Gallo is one of 6 full-time and 15 part-time *Post* reporters assigned to prep games played by teams in 27 boys' leagues and 16 independent boys' schools plus 25 girls' leagues and 11 independents. Gallo covers three or four games weekly at District of Columbia and suburban schools and also reports swimming and gymnastics.

Let's follow Gallo through a Beltway game between Montrose Christian and Riverdale Baptist.

Getting Ready

Before the game, Gallo "sets up" his reporter's notebook with key data. ("You really have to get in good with coaches, or you won't get this stuff.") His first page has the following penciled notations, which he will use immediately when he starts writing at game's end *and which he then will store in his desk for future references*:

> Rockville, 7:30
> > No. 5 Montrose Christian (8-2, 1-0 Belt)
> > Mustangs
> > Bob Monroe 3
> > Drew Hall 10
> > Levi Watkins 21
> > Marvin Lewis 24 [Georgia Tech]
> > Mohamed Diakite 44 [St. John's]
> > Josh Hutchinson 43
> > (and so forth)

Translation:

The game starts with tip-off at 7:30 p.m., in Rockville, Md., home court of Montrose Christian Academy. Montrose is ranked No. 5 in suburban boys' basketball, with 8 wins and 2 losses overall, and one win and no losses in the Beltway League. The team's nickname is "Mustangs."

Players are listed with jersey numbers and, in brackets, the names of colleges if they have agreed in writing (with signed "letters of intent") to attend.

On the second page of his reporter's notebook, Gallo notes:

> No. 10 Riverdale Baptist (19-3, 1-0 Beltway)
> Coach Walter Webb
> Crusaders
> Won 6 straight
>
> Patrick Atanagana 00
> Greg Harrison 4
> Wayne Gibson 22
> Kevin Bell 24 [American]
> Emmanuel Witherspoon 50
> (and so forth)

Translation:

Riverdale is ranked No. 10 in boys' basketball, with 19 wins and 3 losses overall, and one win and no losses in the Beltway League.

For Riverdale, Gallo lists the coach's name (Gallo is "in good" with coach Webb), the team's nickname ("Crusaders") and a salient fact—the team is on a roll, having won six straight games.

Whatever note-taking system you develop, *make certain it's legible and understandable*. It's frustrating to flip back through your notes under deadline pressure at game's end (or months later, when writing an end-of-season wrap-up) and find you can't read what you jotted down in the heat of play!

Gallo's system for keeping game stats is designed to highlight key plays, turnovers and other pivotal moments. Let's look.

After the Tip-Off

Each page of Gallo's notebook is divided into two halves, with a rule down the middle. His game stats on the Montrose-Riverdale game look like this:

	M	R	
Riverdale wins tip			
R4 for 3 LW	0	3	7:07
M10 layup	2	3	6:01
R24 for 3 RW	2	6	5:48
M over/back			5:43
R24 J (15)	2	8	5:29
M3 for 3 RW	5	8	5:22
R00 2 FT 0-0	5	10	5:08
PF 50 M off.			4:40
PF 50 M			4:30
R3 put-back	5	12	4:17
PF21 M 23R 0-0	5	12	4:09
R22 for 3 TK	5	15	4:00
(and so forth)			

Translation:

Riverdale's center bats the tip-off to a teammate, and they're off and running.

With 7:07 minutes remaining in the eight-minute quarter, Riverdale's No. 4 (Greg Harrison) scores with a shot from the left wing of the court (that's from the far left, as you face the backboard, outside the center lane). Gallo enters three points on the Riverdale side of his notebook.

At 6:01, Montrose's No. 10 drives in for a layup, and scores two points for his team.

Riverdale's No. 24 hits for three points from the right wing, and the score is Riverdale 6, Montrose 2, with 5:48 remaining.

Montrose commits an "over and back," which means the team moves the ball across mid-court, into Riverdale's half of the court, but then moves it *back* into Montrose territory. Montrose has to turn over the ball to Riverdale.

At 5:29, Riverdale's No. 24 scores on a jump shot taken 15 feet from the basket, and the score is 8-2.

Montrose's No. 3 hits for three points from the right wing, taking the score to 8-5, and, after being fouled, Riverdale's No. 00 (Patrick Atanagana, you'll recall from Gallo's pre-game jottings) gets two free throws. He makes both, taking the score to 10-5.

Under Gallo's system, two free throws are noted as "0-0." The zeros are *blacked in* if the free throws are made; the zeros are *left empty* if the free throws are missed.

At 4:40 and 4:30, Montrose's No. 50 is charged with two personal fouls—one while playing offense ("off.") and one on defense.

At 4:17 left in the quarter, something all coaches want to see their players do: Riverdale's No. 3 gets a "put-back"—a rebound and score.

Next pivotal play: Montrose's No. 21 commits a personal foul, and Riverdale's No. 23 gets two free throws—and misses both. Score stays at 12-5.

With 4:00 remaining, Riverdale's Wayne Gibson, No. 22, scores three points with a shot from the "tip of the key"—just outside the semi-circle at the outer end of the free-throw lane.

Until the final buzzer, Gallo continues his careful notations, thinking simultaneously of possible writing angles for his story.

Picking Your Story Angle

With his notes and ongoing analysis as the game is developing, Gallo is identifying crucial factors he'll highlight in his writing.

First, Gallo says, he examines *turning points* in the game and, importantly, the plays—the how and why—that led up to them.

Second, Gallo turns to the *biggest single play* and, he says, "what that means beyond the game, beyond the score." (As we'll discuss later, the biggest single play in the Montrose-Riverdale game means an upset.)

Third, Gallo notes *star-player performances*. You'll recall his pregame notations included references to stars who have signed with colleges. Their performance is watched particularly closely.

Fourth, Gallo watches for "runs"—those sometimes startling moments in a basketball game when a team does everything right and quickly scores on successive plays to run up its total points. Such runs can set the tempo for a game, even throw the entire momentum one way or another.

Fifth, Gallo studies coaching strategies and game plans. "Some teams play 'half-court' strategies, meaning they walk the ball up the court, slowly dribbling the ball around, then move in with strict ball control to score. It's sometimes slow and dull, but beautiful to watch when it works right. Other teams may play the 'fast-break,' often called, 'run-and-gun,' and that means running up and down like crazy, shooting a lot and trying to put a lot of points on the board very quickly to build momentum."

Sixth, at game's end, Gallo quickly notes fan reaction or player and coach quotes that shed light on the outcome.

Let's look at the story Gallo wrote on Riverdale vs. Montrose.

Riverdale Baptist Upends Montrose Christian

Under that three-column headline on Page 7 of its sports section, *The Washington Post* reports to its many reader-fans news of the upset in Beltway League boys basketball.

Gallo's lead focuses on one key play:

As he stood at the free throw line in front of a near-capacity crowd at Montrose Christian Academy, senior guard Wes Key did not need to think about what would transpire in the next 10 seconds.

In his second graf, Gallo goes to a quote from the star of the evening:

"While everyone in the building was wondering what was going to happen next, I knew what was going to happen—I was going to make it and the game would be over," said Key, whose two free throws helped No. 10 Riverdale Baptist secure a 71-68 victory over No. 5 Montrose Christian in a Beltway League contest last night in Rockville.
"I knew this game was over."

Gallo turns in his next graf to fan reaction. "It was unusual," he said later, "to see visiting fans storm the home team's court."

Key's sixth and final free throw of the evening swished the net—just as the previous five did—and moments later, he found himself at the free throw line again, mobbed by teammates and fans who came from the Upper Marlboro area and stormed the court in revelry following Riverdale's seventh straight victory.

Now, the reporter's patient cultivation of coach Walter Webb as a news source pays off in a post-game interview:

"To come in here to their house and beat Montrose is one of the most emotional victories I ever had as a player or a coach," said Riverdale coach Walter Webb, who could not stop the tears of joy running down his face. "We believed we had a chance to come in here and win. We weren't intimidated."

At this point, Gallo's laborious notetaking provides essential statistical substance for a two-graf examination of key moments in the game:

Trailing 49-38 with 2 minutes 17 seconds remaining in the third quarter, Montrose Christian (8-3, 1-1) closed the period on an 8-0 run capped by guard Marvin Lewis' three-pointer at the buzzer. Lewis and Drew Hall led Montrose with 21 points apiece.
Montrose tied the game at 57 on two free throws by Ali Berdiel with 5:56 remaining and took the lead on a short jump shot by Mohamed Diakite. But Riverdale (20-3, 2-0) maintained its composure. Guard Greg Harrison (12 points) made back-to-back three-pointers to regain the lead for Riverdale, 63-59, with 3:34 remaining.

Gallo's story concludes with a "kicker"—a quote that ends the story on a strong note. (Don't let your stories simply trail off to a fuzzy, meaningless end.)

"That's when I knew this game was over," said senior guard Kevin Bell, who scored a game-high 22 points. "From that point on, I knew there was no way we were not going to win this game."

Jon Gallo
The Washington Post[2]

"I wrote more," Gallo said in a later interview. "But they (desk editors) chopped it down."

Again: In real-world sportswriting you *will* be edited down—unless you learn to write tightly, without excess wordage or redundancies, *and to write only to the news merits of your story*. Don't overwrite, attempting to carry the length of your story beyond its news merits. At first sight of such excesses, editors will move in on your copy—and chop it.

Even though Gallo's story is edited down, additional—and crucial—details on the game are included in a box score. This is how it looks in *The Washington Post*:

> **No. 10 RIVERDALE BAPTIST 71,**
> **No. 5 MONTROSE CHRISTIAN 68**
> R (20-3, 3-0)—Atanagana 5, Harrison 12, Gibson 14, Bell 20, Whitherspoon 5, Key 13. **Totals 21 19-30 71.**
> M (8-3)—Monroe 6, Hall 21, Watkins 6, Lewis 21, Diakite 6, Berdiel 5, Smallwood 3. **Totals 24 12-19 68.**
> **Halftime:** Riverdale Baptist 40-31.
> **Three-point goals:** R 10 (Harrison 4, Gibson 3, Bell 2, Key); M 8 (Hall 3, Lewis 3, Smallwood, Monroe).[3]

Note the box score focuses on scoring by individual players, particularly those who score three-point goals. Focus your writing on those statistics too.

Incidentally, some basketball writers keep "shot charts." These visually illustrate from which places on the floor shots are taken and made or missed. Gallo pays no attention to shot charts.

"I don't see what they add to my understanding," he said. "There is no chronological representation of when those shots were made or how they influenced momentum or the outcome of the game."

On the College Level: Write Short or Long?

Three realities must drive your writing about college basketball:

No. 1: A great many teams, in both men's and women's competition, play a great many games during what inevitably becomes a jam-packed season. Only in baseball is there similar day-to-day, game-story pressure.

No. 2: However, newspapers (or any other medium) have only finite newshole for basketball because they are inundated with news from more than the hard court; other sports, particularly football and baseball's spring opener, overlap.

No. 3: You therefore must develop keen news instincts that pinpoint your reporting on truly pivotal developments in a game. Then focus your writing to pack the most crucial factors into early grafs of what might end up as an edited—almost truncated—story.

You'll find no better masters of the detailed yet snappy basketball story than AP reporters, who write for newspapers near and far, for editors who may want to go short on a particular game or go long.

How AP Goes Both Short and Long

California is a major basketball state, and *San Francisco Chronicle* editors must give their reader-fans coverage of important games, both at home and nationwide. Most coverage of distant games comes from AP.

With plenty of action on home courts, *Chronicle* editors have newshole for only short stories on even major games elsewhere. But AP writers can pack amazing amounts of information in those short versions—and still write in an open, engaging style.

Note this four-graf version published by the *Chronicle* (emphasis added on key points):

> *Kevin Freeman and Jake Voskuhl each had 16 points* as *No. 6 Connecticut* beat Fordham 94-75 yesterday for the Huskies' *seventh straight victory.*
>
> Connecticut (7-1) *shot 57 percent* from the field (36-for-62), including 6-for-8 by Freeman and 5-for-6 by Voskuhl, *while holding Fordham to 37 percent* (26-for-70).
>
> *Fordham (4-4) played without second leading scorer and rebounder Bevon Robin. He was suspended for the game by coach Bob Hill for violating team rules. Jason Harris led the Rams with 15 points.*
>
> "It happened last night, almost today," Hill said without giving details of the *apparent curfew violation.* "The most disappointing thing about this game was that we didn't have everybody. We put this together by the seat of our pants."
>
> The Associated Press [4]

Obviously, that AP version leaves true basketball fans thirsting for more details. But in the West, editors have newshole only to give reader-fans just a sip. A long drink—running, perhaps, into hundreds of words—would be published by papers in the East, where Connecticut is a hugely important team.

Here's the point: Just as AP's writers face enormous competition for *Chronicle* newshole, so will you, writing for your hometown newspaper, face competition—and drastic editing—if you write long, without discipline and without focus.

However, there is major danger in writing this type of tightly disciplined spot-news lead. You can concentrate so intently on packing in important statistical information that you end up with a dry, numbers-laden accountant's report.

However, note again, in the previous example, how AP's (anonymous) writer gets the stats in, all right, *but* does so in open, readable fashion *and* let's you know why Fordham's star, Bevon Robin, was absent. *And, the writer does it in just 118 words!*

Below, an AP story on women's basketball "goes long" because the writer (also anonymous) is guaranteed larger newshole in papers across the nation— *guaranteed* because a) women's basketball is major news, after decades of struggling for recognition, and b) the nation's No. 1 team is on a 30-game winning streak.

Note the story (fronted in *The New York Times'* sports section) opens with a look-ahead angle that, as *The Washington Post's* Jon Gallo says, goes beyond the game and beyond the score.

> NORMAL, ILL.—Purdue once again showed its mettle when things got tense, and now the Boilermakers are taking their No. 1 ranking and 30-game winning streak to the Final Four.
> Seniors Ukari Figgs and Stephanie White-McCarty, Purdue's leaders all season, led a strong finish that sent the Boilermakers to a 75-62 victory over Rutgers in the Midwest Regional final tonight.

Now, quickly, one more graf on the game, then a graf on Purdue's well-known coach.

> Urged on by several thousand of their fans in the crowd of 8,844, the Boilermakers (32-1) did not panic after falling behind by 10 points in the first half, scored the first 7 points of the second half to get back in the game and then relied on their two seniors down the stretch.
> The victory gives Carolyn Peck at least one more game as the coach at Purdue. She is leaving to become coach and general manager of the new Orlando franchise in the Women's National Basketball Association.

Then, back to the look-ahead angle, the meaning beyond the game and beyond the score:

> Purdue, which made its only other trip to the National Collegiate Athletic Association's Final Four in 1994, will play the West Regional champion—either Louisiana Tech or UCLA—in the national semifinals in San Jose, Calif., on Friday.

Note how smoothly AP's writer weaves salient factors into the story: Purdue takes No. 1 ranking to Final Four (first graf), Purdue shows mettle under tension (first), two seniors lead strong finish (second), Boilermakers don't panic despite being behind (third), victory gives Peck another game as coach (fourth) and Purdue's likely Final Four opponents (fifth).

This story could be chopped at this point. But because the game is so significant, AP's writer—and the *Times*, which published the story—let it run long, with seven grafs of play-by-play. AP's writer obviously reported the game using a note-taking system similar to that of *The Washington Post*'s Gallo. (Emphasis added to illustrate how a superb writer can weave in crucial material.)

> Rutgers (29-6), *which has never been to the Final Four*, held Purdue *in check for much of the second half* behind Shawnetta Stewart, *who led all scorers with 24 points*. But the Scarlet Knights *could not hold on* after leading by 4 with less than six and a half minutes left.
>
> *White-McCarty, named the outstanding player* in the regional, *scored nine* of her 22 points in the final 4:12, *while Figgs had 13 of her 18* in the final 6:33. *Camille Cooper, Purdue's main inside threat, kept the Boilermakers in it early with a career-high 20 points* on 8-of-9 shooting.
>
> Rutgers was leading 53-49 when *Figgs and White-McCarty took over.*
>
> *First Figgs hit a 3-pointer* and sank three free throws to put Purdue ahead 55-53 with 4:59 left, its first lead since midway through the first half.
>
> Then *it was White-McCarty's turn.* She scored seven straight Purdue points as the lead grew to 66-55, including *a three-point play with a basket that probably had no business going in.*
>
> White-McCarty stumbled as she was fouled by Tammy Sutton-Brown while driving to the basket, threw the ball up underhanded and it dropped through the hoop. *She then sank the free throw, completing a play that seemed to insure that Purdue would win.*
>
> *Purdue finished 30 of 46 at the free-throw line.* Rutgers was 7 for 15.
>
> The Associated Press[5]

How to Use Other News Pegs

Like *The Washington Post*'s Gallo, the *Chicago Tribune*'s Alan Sutton knows a *turning point* in a game when he sees one. He also knows how to write engagingly about it:

> NORMAL, ILL.—The turning point in Marshall's 52-44 victory in the Class AA girls basketball quarterfinals Friday may have come with 51.7 seconds left in the first quarter.
>
> That's when Waubonsie Valley's Stacey Byrd hit a three-pointer from, oh, about as far away as Aurora to give the underdog and second-ranked Warriors a 17-6 lead.

"She was toasting us in the first half," Marshall coach Dorothy Gaters said of the 5-foot-8-inch senior.

From that point on, it was No. 1 Marshall's defense and sophomore Cappie Pondexter who turned up the heat. Pondexter's 25 points powered the six-time state champions into Saturday's 11:15 a.m. semifinal in Redbird Arena against Glenbard West.

Allan Sutton
Chicago Tribune[6]

Incidentally, if you don't know Illinois' geography, you may have missed the wry second-graf reference above to Aurora, which is *miles* from Normal. Mark of a real pro: writing jewels hidden nicely in all the verbiage, just waiting to be discovered by delighted readers!

The Boston Globe's Joe Burris pulled me in with this one (I'm a sucker for a *question lead*):

DENVER—Got answers?

Ninth-seeded New Mexico could have used a few yesterday in its NCAA Tournament West Regional second-round game against top-seeded Connecticut. Over the first 7:12, its players seemed dazed and confused, puzzled as to why they fell behind, 17-0, against an up-tempo team playing in a halfcourt set.

Most everyone figured if the Lobos slowed down the high-octane Huskies, they would have a chance at an upset. Instead, UConn's pressure defense and exceptional outside shooting gave New Mexico problems it never solved.

That left UConn a clear path to its fourth Sweet 16 appearance since 1994. The Huskies led by as many as 18 points in the first half and cruised to a relatively easy 78-56 victory.

Joe Burris
The Boston Globe[7]

Question leads are effective because they force your readers to switch from passive information-absorption to active involvement in answering a question. But write question leads carefully. Note above, for example, how the *Globe*'s Burris quickly details precisely what puzzled New Mexico and why the team needed help in coming up with answers. You can't simply drop a question in your lead, then walk away from it—or the answer.

Steve Kirk of Knight Ridder Newspapers catches basketball fans with imaginative use of the *you lead*.

CLEMSON, S.C.—You are Clemson, and your emotions are at war.

You just watched your four seniors taken out of the game, one-by-one, to loud ovations during a nearly perfect, 92-64, Senior Day mauling of Georgia Tech.

You witnessed a team having so much fun inside Littlejohn Coliseum on Sunday afternoon that center Tom Wideman tried his first 3-point shot in his 123rd college game and walk-on guard J.D. Powell made his first in his fifth game.

So, do you bask in the glory of a student section gone mad, storming onto the court to celebrate a glorious regular-season ending for four senior starters? Do you revel in late optimism over the final three home games, during which the Tigers beat Tech, Virginia and Florida State by a combined 84 points?

After two more grafs in this vein, writer Kirk casts the "you" question several ways:

If, you're (Clemson coach Larry) Shyatt, you pause to resist tears in the press conference and tell the room how proud you are of a team that might have finished tied for seventh in the nine-team ACC but didn't quit despite a 1-7 start in the conference.

If you're (Clemson center) Wideman, you utter the first semblance of acceptance that the Tigers might indeed be headed to their first NIT since 1995.

Steve Kirk
Knight Ridder Newspapers[8]

Below, Earl Gustkey of the *Los Angeles Times* focuses on a *star performer*. Lesson: In a lead pegged to a star performer you must flesh out details to support the lead's peg (emphasis added):

The UCLA women's basketball team, still without senior point guard Erica Gomez because of shoulder surgery, *got an All-American second-half performance by forward Maylana Martin* Saturday in a 86-67 victory over Pepperdine at Malibu.

Martin, working inside, scored 21 points on eight-of-16 shooting as she benefited from a season-best three-point shooting (eight of 17) by her teammates that softened up Pepperdine's zone defense.

UCLA (4-2) started fast, but the Waves' collapsing zone made it an even game for the last five minutes of the first half.

"In the first half, they sagged on me and blocked me out, too," Martin said.

But when Kaz [Nicole Kaczmarski] and Michelle [Greco] starting hitting those three, it opened things up inside for me."

Kaczmarski, the highly touted freshman recruit from New York, made four of nine three-point shots, and Greco made four of five.

Earl Gustkey
Los Angeles Times[9]

We write *news* for *news*papers, but a bit of history works occasionally, as in this *contrast lead* (emphasis added):

> ST. PETERSBURG, FLA.—*In 1990*, Duke gave the University of Connecticut the greatest basketball heartache in its history when it beat the Huskies at the buzzer for a spot in the Final Four. *Monday night*, in a game that will go down as one of the NCAA Tournament's greatest upsets, UConn returned the favor in stunning fashion, beating the seemingly unbeatable Blue Devils 77-74 to win the NCAA championship.

Important: If you dip into history for a lead, *move very quickly back to the news* as does the writer in his second and subsequent grafs:

> UConn (34-3) snapped Duke's 32-game winning streak with a determined performance for the ages.
>
> Duke, which was going for its third national title of this decade, had its chances in the closing seconds. Down 75-74, the Blue Devils got the ball back after a miss by Khalid El-Amin with 20 seconds left. That's when Duke coach Mike Krzyzewski picked senior Trajan Langdon to go one-on-one with Augusta's Ricky Moore. Langdon forced a shot and was called for traveling with 5.4 seconds left.
>
> El-Amin then made two three throws with 5.2 seconds remaining. Langdon tried to get off a final 3-point shot but ended the game sprawled on the floor as time ran out.
>
> Tony Barnhart
> *The Atlanta Journal-Constitution* [10]

Incidentally, note above that Barnhart, a *real* pro, referred in his lead to "*one of the ... greatest upsets,*" and avoided the mistake of amateurs, which is to write about "*the greatest upset ever*" or "a moment in sports that will be remembered *forever*" or, indeed, to write with confidence about the *fastest, largest, highest, greatest. ...*

Believe it: Coming soon, in a game tomorrow, next week or next season, is somebody who is faster or larger, who can jump higher and will be remembered—for a day or two, at least—as the greatest!

And Watch for College Features

Covering just basketball game stories alone is a huge task for any newspaper. (Remember: Gallo and his *Washington Post* colleagues cover *52 prep leagues* and *27 independent* prep schools, along with college and pro sports!)

So, during basketball season, many newspapers publish fewer features than during football season, when far fewer games must be covered and more time is available to find off-beat features.

But when you see a *newsfeature*—an offbeat but topical story close to the news—*grab it!*

Kevin Tatum of *The Philadelphia Inquirer* saw a newsfeature that beautifully captures the emotion of college basketball. Emotion erupts in pro ball, too, of course, but on the college and prep levels, emotion often is a game-turning factor and, thus, a dimension you must consider in your writing. Here's Tatum's introduction:

> PRINCETON—Whenever Spencer Gloger catches the ball on the wing, the Princeton faithful at Jadwin Gym leap to their feet in unison and make the "whoosh" sound.
>
> Rarely does the spindly 6-foot-6 freshman guard from Santa Margarita, Calif., disappoint. With the game on the line against Texas Christian on Thursday, Gloger nailed two straight three-pointers from the corner to give the Tigers a 63-57 lead.
>
> And when the Horned Frogs forced overtime, Gloger made the key plays down the stretch to secure the 77-72 triumph. He handled the ball effectively against the press, grabbed key rebounds, and, with 19.5 seconds left, calmly sank a pair of free throws to give Princeton the victory.
>
> Gloger, who finished with a team high of 18 points after compiling 20 the game before, is just beginning his career at Princeton, which is 5-4. But already he is being talked about as if he could be the second coming of Bill Bradley.
>
> Kevin Tatum
> *The Philadelphia Inquirer*[11]

Although the writing above reads like a *game lead* (and was published in December, in basketball season), it in fact is the intro to a lengthy feature on Princeton's Gloger, headlined, "Star in Stripes." (Princeton's Tigers wear stripes—get it?)

With this story, the *Inquirer*'s Tatum faced fierce competition for space in his paper's sports pages. But he got prominent display on sports' Page One, and his story was "jumped" inside, where it ran for nearly two full columns. His Page One competition: Philadelphia Eagles football, then in full swing; a huge story on off-season baseball trades (the *beautiful* lead of which, by Jayson Stark, was, "It wasn't a trade. It was more like a four-franchise pileup."); and the abrupt resignation of the Phoenix Suns' coach.

So, how does writer Tatum elbow his nongame, nonspot *newsfeature* onto Page One, against that *spot-news* competition? *He writes his way on that page!* Look again at the four grafs reprinted above. Tatum catches emotion, action and, importantly, narrows his story to something all basketball fans can "see" as they read—a single dramatic performance by a young star.

Hooking readers with his action lead, Tatum broadens his story to how this "blue-chip player" was recruited against bigger basketball powers and why experts think he's destined for greatness. The *news* angle: Reader, dear reader, watch this young fellow the rest of the season, the rest of his career; he'll be a great one.

Tom Friend of *The New York Times* puts a wonderfully deft touch on a news-feature when he discovers that after a long, dry period, basketball is improving at the University of California-Berkeley:

> BERKELEY, CALIF.—The graduate students here are on strike, the under-graduates dodge the picket line and a male student walks unclothed to class every day—though, on cold days, he throws on a knapsack. Berkeley has always been the 1960s in microcosm, and now that even includes the basketball team.
>
> Tom Friend
> *The New York Times* [12]

Hard Hitting on the Pro Level

Reflect on the tone of writing we've seen so far in this chapter. It generally accents the positive—applauds, really—in reporting how boys and girls race up and down prep courts in the wholesome game of basketball, and, at the college level, how young men and women give their all to achieve wonderful things for the old alma mater.

Now, note the tone of this *pro-level* lead by Tim Kawakami of *The Los Angeles Times* (emphasis added):

> Wow, are the Lakers going to be hurt in the strength-of-schedule rankings after this one or what?
>
> The Lakers did not have to exert their will against the Clippers on Tuesday night as much as simply show up and watch the *Clippers spontaneously combust.*
>
> There weren't statistics to review after the Lakers' 95-68 victory before 18,719 at Staples Center, *it was more like rubble.*
>
> *Where you thought a team stood, there were only fragments.*
>
> *Where there might have been a semblance of pride there was a swift surrender.*
>
> The Lakers had little to do with it, other than grabbing all the rebounds, driving down the uncrowded lanes and accepting the Clipper *clanks* with open arms and open shots.
>
> "I don't know if we were star-struck or what," said Clipper swingman Tyrone Nesby. "Nobody came to play. I hope everybody's as embarrassed as I am."
>
> The centerpiece of *this grandiose, gruesome tragic-comedy* was the second quarter, when the Clippers made only one of their 18 shots and scored a total of three points (only one short of the NBA record low).

Adding in their final scoreless 3:50 of the first quarter, the Clippers came up with 15:50 of *the silliest, most unbelievable basketball an NBA team can produce.*

> Tim Kawakami
> *The Los Angeles Times* [13]

Tough stuff, huh? Try this one:

Just when it appeared the Bulls were ready to make that quantum leap from horrible to mediocre, they stubbed their toe against one of the league's worst road teams Friday night at the United Center.

The Atlanta Hawks, off to their worst start since the 1976-77 season, prevailed 89-83.

> Fred Mitchell
> *Chicago Tribune* [14]

Yes, sports fans, we're now in the big leagues, where sportswriters feel no obligation to avoid the humiliation of children on the hard court and no compulsion to buy into the old alma-mater romanticism of the collegiate circuit. That sense of obligation and that compulsion *do* soften the critical tone of much writing at the prep and college levels (although *coaches* get gloves-off coverage).

However, here in the big leagues, in the NBA, basketball is a hard-eyed game played for big money by tough public-figure, multimillion-dollar athletes. And, that's the way many sportswriters cover it.

Here's Skip Bayless of the *Chicago Tribune* on the Washington Wizards: "In Washington, fewer and fewer fans are off to see the Wizards, who are viewed as aging and boring and disgustingly overpaid." [15]

Alluding to their multimillion-dollar team payroll, Steve Brandon of the *Portland Sunday Oregonian* writes that the Trail Blazers, in losing to the Phoenix Suns, "more closely resembled a bounced check than a $73.9 million juggernaut." [16]

Obviously aghast at their lousy play, Jeffrey Denberg of *The Atlanta Journal-Constitution* refers to the "bottom-feeding Chicago Bulls." [17]

To Curtis Bunn, the Vancouver Grizzlies "have been ghastly this season" and Selena Roberts of *The New York Times*, normally the home of journalistic discourse that's terribly civilized, sees the New York Knicks as "an elite franchise sliding toward mediocrity and on the fringe of disarray." [18]

Even AP writers, who normally seek authoritative sources and full attribution for anything even slightly subjective or opinionated, get into the hard-knocks spirit in covering professional basketball. The Knicks in one account are "lethargic" and, in another, Toronto is "abysmal." [19]

So, writers at the pro level take a tough, sometimes almost adversarial approach to a game that, at prep and college levels, is covered much more gently.

What else distinguishes pro coverage? *Enormously detailed stories and stats.*

For that Blazers-Suns game cited earlier (Steve Brandon had the Blazers resembling a "bounced check," you'll recall), the *Sunday Oregonian* ran two side-by-side stories across the top of Page One of the sports section, then jumped both inside, where they ran on for hundreds of words.[20] Also inside:

- A "Notebook" sidebar focusing on, "Clifford Robinson had 23 points and six assists in the Phoenix Suns' 110-102 win Friday night over the Trail Blazers."
- Quarter-by-quarter summary of key plays, points scored and rebounds.
- "At-a-glance" examination of three factors: "Why The Blazers Lost," "Top Performers" and "Injury Report."
- A boxed schedule charting every game the Blazers have played and are yet to play—complete with times and which games will be televised.

As in covering prep or college basketball, writers at the pro level must include key stats—individual scoring, personal fouls, turnovers and so forth—in their stories. *But,* in the big leagues, writers can wing it, confident that much of the nitty-gritty demanded by fans is in the box scores, which at the pro level normally present much more information than is found in box scores at the prep and college level.

This is how the *Sunday Oregonian*'s box score looks:

PHOENIX 110

Player	M	FG	3Pt	FT	Reb O-T	A	P	S	T	Blk	Pts
Gugliotta	39	6-13	0-1	5-8	3-14	2	2	0	1	0	17
Robinson	45	9-17	4-6	1-1	0-2	6	1	2	2	1	23
Miller	30	6-9	0-0	0-0	1-6	2	4	0	1	3	12
(etc.)											

PORTLAND 102

Player	M	FG	3Pt	FT	Reb O-T	A	P	S	T	Blk	Pts
Pippen	40	7-12	2-5	3-5	2-10	6	4	1	3	0	19
Wallace	40	8-14	0-1	0-0	2-6	2	0	1	3	1	16
Sabonis	20	2-7	0-0	0-0	2-7	1	1	0	1	2	4
(etc.)											

Translation (for the first player in the Phoenix box):

Gugliotta played 39 minutes, scored 6 field goals out of 13 shots taken; missed the one three-point shot he took, and made 5 out of 8 free-throw attempts.

Gugliotta grabbed 14 rebounds, 3 on offense. He had 2 assists, 2 personal fouls. He had no "steals" and one turnover. He blocked no shots taken by opponents and scored 17 points himself.

But there's even more in the *Sunday Oregonian*'s box score: team scoring by quarters and detailed information such as percentages of field goal attempts that scored, how many rebounds each team grabbed, what technical fouls were committed, turnovers—the detail runs on and on.

Why so much detail?

For one thing, reader-fans demand it so they can virtually replay games in their heads. For another, sports editors serve fans who play "fantasy" basketball—internet games in which fans "coach" teams they put together through "drafts" and "trades." It's a huge hobby among fans of basketball (and other sports), and newspaper stats are read eagerly by fantasy "coaches" plotting their strategies!

Summary

—Covering basketball, which has millions of fans nationwide, is a major reporting assignment at many U.S. newspapers.

—Particularly when reporting at the prep level, you must develop your own individual shorthand techniques for keeping stats during a game.

—First, "set up" your reporter's notebook to include background on teams, players and coaches you'll need quickly when writing under deadline pressure.

—Second, ensure your "short-hand" records key plays, turnovers and other pivotal moments in a game.

—When picking a story angle, seek your lead among turning points, key plays, star-player performances, high-scoring "runs" and coaching strategies.

—Shot charts are kept by some reporters to graphically illustrate points on the floor from which shots are taken (and made or lost), but not all reporters agree such charts are meaningful.

—At the college level, your writing must be driven by three realities: the large number of games played, the limited newshole newspapers can accord basketball and, thus, the need for you to develop keen news instincts on what is important. Then write as tightly as possible.

—Watch Associated Press writers for hints on how to pack amazing amounts of information into stories that can be edited to four or five grafs and still be readable.

—There's major danger, however, in tightly disciplined, spot-news stories packed with information. Unless crafted carefully they read like dry, numbers-laden accountant's reports.

—Highly-talented writers peg basketball leads to turning points, or use question leads, "you" leads or other imaginative angles to make their stories open and engaging.

—College-level basketball is rich with features, so even though you're hard pressed to cover spot news, watch for feature angles.

—Reporting on pro basketball often takes a stronger, even adversarial tone, compared to prep and college coverage, which often avoids humiliating children who play the prep game or buys into the "old alma-mater" romanticism of the collegiate circuit.

Exercises

1. Your assignment is to develop your own shorthand for keeping stats during a basketball game. Use Jon Gallo's method from Chapter Nine as a guide and "set up" a reporter's notebook as if you were covering your college team at play. Note the types of information—nicknames for both teams, coaches' names and so forth—that you would record for later reference when writing your story. Then, jot down the shorthand symbols and techniques you would use *during* a game to record field goals, free throws, rebounds, personal fouls and all other key stats and turning points necessary for a game story. Your instructor will judge how complete, logical and understandable your system is.

2. Examine basketball stories in a newspaper designated by your instructor (or in examples your instructor will provide) and, in about 350 words, discuss the story angles selected by writers. Did they focus on turning points or big plays or star-player performances? Were they successful from the reader's viewpoint?

3. Study four AP stories that are "run short"—in four or five grafs—in a

newspaper designated by your instructor (or in examples provided by your instructor). In about 300 words, analyze the success of the writers in including operative information and, yet, maintaining readability. Did the writers highlight truly important facts? And, are the stories open, engaging and readable?

4. Cover a basketball game designated by your instructor. Keep detailed play-by-play notes, using the shorthand described in this chapter. In the appropriate wordage, translate their meaning and present both your notes and the translation to your instructor, who will judge the professionalism of your reporting techniques.

5. Cover a game designated by your instructor and write a lead story, scoring summaries and a box score. Explain in a cover note why you selected your lead's angle. Do the facts of the game, as revealed in the box score, support your choice of a lead angle? For example, if you peg your lead to a star-player performance, does the box score show the performance indeed was that newsworthy?

Recommended Reading

Strong basketball coverage runs regularly in the *Los Angeles Times, Chicago Tribune, Boston Globe* and the national edition of the *New York Times* (good on newsfeatures and player/coach profiles). You could spend time profitably studying college and pro coverage in those papers, along with many other metropolitan newspapers throughout the country.

For quick access to coverage in scores of papers, go to www.executivelibary.com/#News.

Virtually all aspects of basketball are covered in the more than 3,100 books on the game listed by amazon.com alone. If you're a beginner in covering the game, there are basic explanatory books for you. If your understanding of the game is sophisticated, there are books on highly technical subjects.

Notes

1. My thanks to Jon Gallo, who contributed to this chapter in a series of interviews in January 2000. In the spirit of journalistic disclosure, Gallo is a former student of mine.
2. "Riverdale Baptist Upends Montrose Christian," Jan. 11, 2000, p. D-7.
3. "Boys Basketball Box Scores," Jan. 11, 2000, p. D-6.
4. Dispatch for morning papers, Dec. 13, 1999, p. C-12.
5. Dispatch for morning papers, March 23, 1999, published in the *Times* as "No. 1 Purdue Reaches Final four by Pulling Rank on Rutgers," *The New York Times* that day, p. C-25.
6. "Commandos Still Toast of Tourney," March 7, 1999, Section 3, p. 1.

7. "UConn's on a Mission," March 14, 1999, p. D-1.

8. Dispatch for morning papers, March 1, 1999.

9. "Martin Leads UCLA Past Pepperdine," Dec. 12, 1999, p. D-11.

10. "UConn Believe It, Huskies," March 30, 1999, p. E-1.

11. "Star in Stripes," Dec. 14, 1999, p. C-1.

12. "Even Without the Smile, Kidd's Game Has Become Pure Magic," Dec. 13, 1992, p. S-3.

13. "It's a Low-Out for Clippers," Dec. 15, 1999, p. D-1.

14. "Bulls Fumble a Chance," Jan. 16, 2000, Section 3, p. 1.

15. "In the Wake of the News," Jan. 16, 2000, Section 3, p. 1.

16. "Phoenix, Kidd Outplay Blazers," Dec. 19, 1999, p. F-1.

17. "Hawks See Bulls Game As Must-Win," Jan. 25, 2000, p. F-5.

18. Bunn's quote is in, "Abdur-Rahim Frustrated," April 3, 1999, p. C-4, and Roberts' in, "Knicks Grab a Ledge; Now They Will Test Their Nails," March 29, 1999, p. 37.

19. Dispatches for morning papers of Dec. 19, 1999, and Jan. 12, 2000, respectively.

20. This *Sunday Oregonian* material is drawn from Blazers coverage on pages 1 and 9, Dec. 19, 1999.

PART FIVE

Covering the Others

Where, outside football, basketball and baseball, can you find a satisfying and meaningful career in sportswriting?

Virtually anywhere.

Throughout the nation, there is exploding interest—and participation—in a widening range of sports: soccer and hockey, of course, and tennis and golf, but also lacrosse, gymnastics, running, jogging, walking . . . and how about bass fishing or deer hunting? Or rock climbing and surfing?

In covering such sports, even those that attract relatively few fans, you cannot relax your reporting vigilance or your efforts to write clearly and, above all, accurately and with authority.

No matter how narrowly focused—how *esoteric*—a sport may be, newspaper editors will require you to meet the news needs of discerning readers who know the sport intimately.

Magazine editors meet reader demands for expert reporting with specialty publications that focus narrowly, but in depth, on a sport. Note *Climbing* or *Wind Surfing*, for example, or *Snowboarding* and *Transworld Surf*.

So, if you have interest and expertise in a specialty sport, there are many good possibilities you can find a newspaper or magazine that needs you.

We turn now to some of these possibilities (no book can cover them *all*) in Part Five's single chapter, The Wider World of Sports.

Sports we'll discuss in detail—hockey, soccer, tennis, golf—are so popular that in some sections of the country they are major sports, right along with baseball, basketball and football. However, and unfortunately, the space limitations of book publishing prevent focus on many other sports.

Nevertheless, our discussion of reporting and writing techniques will illustrate the opportunities and challenges available for you in that much wider world of sports outside football, baseball and basketball.

10

The Wider World of Sports

This is why editors define "sports" as much more than what happens on the gridiron, baseball diamond or hard court:

- More fans (78,972) jammed into Giants Stadium in New York City for the opener of the 1999 Women's World Soccer Cup than ever showed up for any Giants or Jets football game. More than *90,000* packed the Rose Bowl in Pasadena, Calif., to watch U.S. women battle China's team and win the championship.[1]
- Even in the sunny South, ice hockey is the favorite sport of millions, and the game's all-time high scorer, Wayne Gretzky, is regarded by many as one of the greatest athletes of our time, if not *the* greatest.
- Americans spend far more on fishing and hunting than to attend *all* professional sports events ($40.9 billion annually vs. $5.9 billion a year, according to a U.S. government study in the past decade).[2]

Obviously, you are not exiled to a quiet backwater of the sports department if assigned to cover sports other than the Big Three.

Hockey

As in any organized sport, it's teamwork that creates success in ice hockey. But, it's dazzling play by individual players that frequently captures the attention of fans—and writers.

At the prep level, here's Jon Gallo of *The Washington Post* focusing on an offensive play by one young star, Brian Adams, in a game between Landon School of Bethesda, Md., and the Churchill High School Bulldogs of Rockville:

> Adams went out and personally picked apart the Bulldogs' defense, scoring two goals and assisting on four—including three by freshman Peter Lamade—to lead the Bethesda private school to a 7-1 victory.
>
> Jon Gallo
> *The Washington Post*[3]

At the college level, Bob Monahan of *The Boston Globe* sees a *defensive* play as pivotal in a game:

> DURHAM, N.H.—Merrimack College staged a major upset here last night when it battled the University of New Hampshire to a 2-2 tie before a capacity house in Hockey East action. It was Merrimack's fourth straight overtime game, a school record.
>
> Warriors' goalie Tom Welby of West Roxbury was fantastic while making 31 saves, three in the final 30 seconds of overtime.
>
> Bob Monahan
> *The Boston Globe*[4]

At the pro level, you'll see two now-familiar writing approaches:

- AP writers, covering *every* game, *every day*, write directly and tautly, often at the expense of color and descriptives, to ensure their stories communicate the essentials even if newspaper editors chop them to a graf or two.
- Newspaper writers, guaranteed sufficient newshole by their own editors, stretch for unique and colorful angles and *frequently write in conversational style that communicates analysis and interpretation.*

First, here is how the AP covers hockey:

> Goalie Bill Ranford won his first start for Detroit and the Red Wings extended their winning streak to five games with a 5-3 win over the visiting Chicago Blackhawks Friday night.
>
> Ranford, starting for the first time since Detroit obtained him in a trade with Tampa Bay, made 27 saves for his first win since Jan. 21.
>
> Wendel Clark, Vyacheslav Kozlov, Larry Murphy, Martin Lapointe and Brendan Shanahan scored for Detroit. Sergei Fedorov, Igor Larionov and Steve Yzerman each had two assists.
>
> Eric Daze, Jean-Pierre Dumont and Reid Simpson scored for the Blackhawks.
>
> The first-place Red Wings moved nine points ahead of idle St. Louis in the Central Division race. Detroit has seven games left and the Blues eight.
>
> The Associated Press[5]

Red Wings 2, Kings 1

Todd Gill, coming back from a broken forearm, scored in his first game in two months to help host Detroit win its fourth straight.

Sergei Fedorov also scored for the first-place Red Wings, who move nine points ahead of St. Louis in the Central race.

The Associated Press[6]

Now, *The Los Angeles Times'* Elliott Teaford, blessed with huge newshole, *talks with readers*:

> PITTSBURGH—The Mighty Ducks were equal parts lucky and good Saturday against the mighty lifeless Pittsburgh Penguins.
>
> No question, the Ducks were due for a game like their 7-1 rout of the Penguins before a sellout crowd of 17,124 at Mellon Arena. They played a strong skating game and capitalized on shoddy Pittsburgh goaltending that resulted in some rather fortunate goals.
>
> But the Ducks created their luck by playing with a passion that has often been absent during a month-long slump that dropped them to 10th place in the Western Conference.

Here, a quick graf of context:

> All things considered, the Ducks' first victory at Pittsburgh in their seven-season history was the perfect way to start a four-game East Coast trip.

Now, quotes that explain the why and how:

> The Ducks left nothing to chance against the struggling Penguins, who are 2-7-1 in their last 10 games. The Ducks clicked twice on their power play, silenced the Penguins on theirs and muzzled league-leading scorer Jaromir Jagr.
>
> "We all knew we blew one the other night against New York," captain Paul Kariya said, referring to the Ducks' 4-2 loss Wednesday against the lowly Islanders.
>
> Instead of moping about Wednesday's loss, the Ducks took the ice Saturday with a mission.
>
> "We all know our predicament," Coach Craig Hartsburg said. "We've got to be ready to play every night."
>
> Sounds simple enough, but the Ducks have been guilty this season of starting games with their hearts and minds seemingly elsewhere. That was not the case Saturday night, however.

Note we're hundreds of words into the *Times* story, and so far it focuses principally on analysis and context. Only now does the writer turn to play-by-play action, which continues for hundreds more of words:

A Duck victory was never in doubt after Teemu Selanne split two Penguins at the blue line, raced ahead on a breakaway and scored 3:19 into the game.

Jean-Sebastien Aubin, Pittsburgh's rookie goaltender, deflected Selanne's shot with his glove, but the puck tricked into the net.

It wouldn't be the last time the Ducks would score on a shot Aubin mishandled. Aubin flubbed two other goals ...

Antti Aalto's power-play goal, on a quick turn-and-shoot from the left faceoff circle, gave the Ducks a 2-0 lead at 12:12. Martin Straka countered for Pittsburgh at 13:23.

But the first of Kariya's two goals put the Ducks in command again 40 seconds later. Kariya also scored on a wicked third-period backhander for his team-leading 28th goal.

Elliott Teaford
The Los Angeles Times[7]

Neither writing style—AP's taut and direct or the *Times'* expansive and analytical—delivers all the information hockey fans need. So *summaries* are published for every game. Here's the AP's on a National Hockey League game between Los Angeles and Detroit:

National Hockey League

Los Angeles	0	0	1 - 1
Detroit	1	1	0 - 2

Game Summary:
First Period: 1, Detroit, Fedorov 23 (Murphy, Holmstrom), 15:47.
Second Period: 2, Detroit, Gill 4, 11:57.
Third Period: 3, Los Angeles, Robitaille 34 (Stumpel, Norstrom), 15:58.
Shots on Goal: Los Angeles 15-6-7: 28. Detroit 12-16-9: 37.
Power Plays: Los Angeles 0 of 2; Detroit 0 of 4.
Goalies: Los Angeles, Fiset 14-18-1 (37 shots-35 saves). Detroit, Osgood 32-23-4 (28-27).
Attendance: 19,983.

This is how you translate the summary:

—In the *first period*, the first score was by Detroit's Fedorov, who now has 23 goals for the season. In this score, Fedorov was assisted by teammates Murphy and Holmstrom, who brought the puck down the ice and passed to him so he could shoot it into the net. He scored with 15:47 minutes elapsed in the period.

—*Shots on goal* means Los Angeles players shot the puck 15 times in the first period, 6 in the second and 7 in the third.

—In *power plays*, a team has the advantage because all its players are on the ice while the opposing team is disadvantaged with one or more players in the penalty box, out of action. Los Angeles had two such opportunities but didn't score on either.

—The summary's reference to *goalies* shows that goalie Fiset of Los Angeles now has a season record of 14 wins, 18 losses and 1 tie. In this game, Detroit players shot at his goal 37 times; he "saved" 35—but two got past him, and Detroit won.

Reflect on this hockey writing at prep, college and pro levels as you develop *your* writing style. Lessons:

- As in all team sports, *highlight star performance*, defensive and offensive.
- *Characterize individual play and the game outcome.* Recall the *Globe's* Monahan characterized his game as a "major upset" and goalie Tom Welby's play as "fantastic."
- *Ensure your early grafs communicate the essentials.* In the AP's Detroit-Chicago game story, star performance, score and winning streak all were in the first graf.[8] And, look again at *The Los Angeles Times'* Ducks-Penguins story. Despite the writer's more leisurely, conversational style, he also weaves the essentials into early grafs.
- *Include analysis and interpretation.* Recall *The Washington Post's* Gallo pointed out a star player "personally picked apart" the opposing team's defense. *The Los Angeles Times'* Teaford, an experienced hockey writer, virtually devoted his first four grafs to his own personal observations.

Incidentally, you'll note no reference above to hockey's violence—rough but legitimate body checking but, as well, all-too-frequent fistfights and brawls. Violence is a given in hockey, and it rarely figures in lead writing unless pivotal in a game's outcome.

Violence and the penalties it draws usually are left to summaries. The following is the form, drawn from an AP summary on a Dallas-Tampa game.

Penalty: Hogue, Dal (roughing), 15:22 [9]

Translation:

With 15:22 minutes elapsed in the period, Dallas' Hogue was penalized for roughing an opponent. Other penalties are levied for such things as fighting (a major penalty) and cross-checking (minor). Offenders must sit in the penalty box for 2, 4, 5 or 10 minutes, depending on the seriousness of their offense.

Golf

In covering golf, understand that you're writing about a sport that's an *obsession* for millions.

In fact, the London-based *Economist* magazine signals that golf is more than an obsession; it's a *disease* or *religion*:

> ST. ANDREWS, SCOTLAND—For those afflicted with the disease of golf, St. Andrews is a place of pilgrimage. Golfers regard the place with the sort of reverence Catholics reserve for Lourdes. About 300,000 of the faithful trek from all across the world to the little Scottish town every year, some to play on the venerable turf of the Old Course, many more just to gawp or to hope that, inspired by seeing where the game was born, their handicap will be magically reduced.
>
> *The Economist*[10]

Now, you really need not look for medical or theological angles in writing golf. But leading golf writers *do* look for certain themes.

- Player vs. player, particularly dominance of a star over all other players or an unexpected victory by a challenger.
- Player vs. the rigors of a course or hole, usually represented by reporting whether a player is over or under par but sometimes by reporting how a player fights sand traps, trees and other obstacles fiendishly designed into a course to frustrate players.
- Players vs. weather and course conditions. Rain, wind and whether fairways are lush and greens are "fast" all influence play, and for readers sophisticated in the game, you'll need to provide expert commentary on those factors.

In the following, an AP writer captures a player vs. player battle in the Ladies Professional Golf Association *and*, by comparing strokes to par, the drama of player vs. course:

> NASHVILLE, TENN.—Michelle McGann shot a seven-under-par 65 to take a one-shot lead over Annika Sorenstam after the second round of the $750,000 Sara Lee Classic.
>
> In a tournament in which breaking records has become almost routine at the 6,242-yard Hermitage Golf Course, McGann's two-day score of 16-under-par was the lowest 36-hole total in LPGA history. Judy Dickinson's previous record of minus-15 at the S&H Golf Classic had stood since 1985.
>
> The Associated Press[11]

Covering the Professional Golfers' Association, Harry Blauvelt of *USA Today* finds his angle not in the tournament leader but, rather, in the drama of a man who is of small stature among professional athletes but who plays very big golf:

> Diminutive Jeff Sluman, the PGA Tour's little big man, was standing tall after the opening round of the Colonial Tournament in Fort Worth.
>
> Small wonder. The 5-7, 140-pound Sluman has all the shots.
>
> He fired a 3-under-par 67 Thursday to trail leader Steve Flesch by one stroke. Sluman is tied with Vijay Singh in second.
>
> "I love the par-70s for my type of game," Sluman said.

Writer Blauvelt continues his focus on Sluman—and moves to his battle with another opponent, weather:

> The field had to contend with difficult, windy conditions.
>
> "If you caught the wrong gust," said Sluman, 41, "you weren't going to be rewarded, not even with a good shot."
>
> He was especially pleased with the way he played the back nine, with three birdies and a bogey for a 2-under 33.
>
> "I thought I did everything pretty good today," he said. "It's very difficult in the wind to put up a good score."

Now, another reason to focus the story on Sluman: He's a big money winner in a sport whose professionals are measured in large part by dollar signs.

> Unless Sluman quits the tour this weekend, he's a cinch to enjoy his best year.
>
> He earned $1,148,375 (last year), good enough to rank 21st, even though he ranked 138th in driving distance at 266.5.
>
> This week, he's ninth at $1,019,945.

> Harry Blauvelt
> *USA Today*[12]

Incidentally, note above that *USA Today*'s writer quotes the golfer extensively on questions reader-fans would ask.

Again: When good quotes surface, plug them into your story and get out of the way. Let newsmakers talk directly to your readers.

A course's physical layout is critically important to reader-fans because golfers *play against terrain* as in no other sport. Your writing must catch the drama in that.

True golfing mystique shrouds the course design and its challenges at Augusta National in Georgia, where the Masters tournament is held annually. Each year, *The Atlanta Journal-Constitution* devotes pages to describing the course. As an example of the *technical nuances your writing must capture*, here is the newspaper's description in 1999 of Augusta National's 18th hole, a par-4, 405-yard challenge nicknamed "Holly":

Holly

'98 avg. 4.139 (11th)

— Description: A narrow chute through which to drive. A gentle fade on this tough, uphill hole is the ticket, with enough distance to leave a short enough iron for the approach. Sandy Lyle's 7-iron from the left fairway bunker, to 10 feet for what evolved as a winning birdie in 1988, was a famous moment here.

— Changes: 1958—Mounding built left of green. 1967—Double bunker constructed on left in fairway landing area.

— Comment: "I generally play for position with a 3-wood, playing to the right of the bunker and just short of it, leaving myself a 5- or 6-iron to the green. It's really important to get the ball on the right level; if you do, you'll always have a birdie put."

Jack Nicklaus[13]

For every hole, the *Journal-Constitution* presents a description, each with an artist's drawing of the hole and approach and, as above, a comment by a famous golfer.

Note the *history* of this par-4 hole is described, including the fact that golfers in the 1998 Masters averaged 4.139 strokes to get into the cup, making Holly the 11th most difficult hole that year. And, the description includes changes made—and when—in the hole's green and bunkers.

The beautiful "kicker" is the description of the approach to the hole—the challenge—and Jack Nicklaus' strategy for beating it.

The *Chicago Tribune* provides technical—and detailed—coverage of the 81st PGA Championship at Medinah Country Club outside Chicago, including "Hardest Hole of the Day," the "Easiest" and "Shot of the Day."

Again as an example of technical strengths you must weave into your writing, here is one *Tribune* report:

Hardest Hole of the Day

No. 9

Par 4

439 yards

Eagles: 1

Birdies: 11

Pars: 87

Bogeys: 52

Double bogeys or worse: 2

Avg: 4.287

Stuart Appleby made this hole look easy by holing a shot from the rough for an eagle. Otherwise, the players had trouble getting through the dogleg in four. This hole is one of the tougher driving holes on the course.

Chicago Tribune[14]

For major tournaments, newspapers carry extensive stats, the most significant of which you must weave into your writing.

For example, on the PGA Championship, the *Chicago Tribune* lists leaders in driving distance, driving accuracy, greens reached in regulation strokes, putting averages and birdie leaders. Each golfer's strokes on each hole are compared to par.

For most tournaments, however, newspapers limit stats to listing leaders. Here's how AP does that for the BellSouth Classic:

> Duluth, Ga.
> Par-72 (36-36), 7,259-yd. T.P.C. Sugarloaf course
> First-round scores
> Duffy Waldorf............31-32—63   -9
> Grant Waite...............32-32—64   -8
> David Duval...............35-31—66   -6
> (and so forth)

Translation:
The leader, Duffy Waldorf, shot 31 on the first nine holes, 32 on the second nine for a day's total 63, which was 9 strokes under par.[15]

Soccer

Soccer at the professional level in the United States struggles for fan support.

Soccer at the college level is one of those "nonrevenue-producing" sports subsidized mostly by football.

Soccer at many metropolitan newspapers is a story consigned to pages inside—frequently deep inside.

And, soccer is an extremely important sport for a beginning sportswriter to master.

A contradiction? No. Here's why:

At the community level, in those small towns where most sportswriting careers begin, soccer is exploding in popularity in kiddie, high school and recreational leagues. Hundreds of thousands of youngsters are out there, kicking the ball around in a sport favored by parents for its relative lack of physical contact and violence.

And at college and national levels, pulling along a new generation of reader-fans, are teams that are improving rapidly in a game that is the world's leading spectator sport—except in the United States.

The momentum in the United States is being built particularly by women. The U.S. women's team won the World Cup Championship in 1999 and established nationwide recognition for some of its players, such as Mia Hamm, Julie Foudy, Briana Curry and Brandi Chastain. Such was their success that the Women's United Soccer Association, the only professional, full-time women's soccer league in the world, was launched.

Nevertheless, American interest in soccer doesn't approach the near frenzy of fans in Europe or Latin America (or the Ivory Coast, where the military leader charged the national team "behaved unworthily" in losing the African Nations

Cup; he put the players in military detention for two days and threatened to draft them into the army if they had another bad game).[16]

Zak Ivkovic, soccer writer for *Newsday*, charges not enough U.S. journalists understand the game:

> Major League Soccer commissioner Doug Logan was absolutely right to blast the media for its indifference in covering D.C. United's 2-0 win over Brazil's famed Vasco da Gama in the Interamerican Cup title game. It just goes to show how uneducated most media people are about the significance of such a win for a 3-year-old professional league in this country.
>
> "We managed to achieve a success in splendid secrecy in this country," Logan said days after the victory. "Sports editors should hold their heads in shame."
>
> Zak Ivkovic
> *Newsday*[17]

Some major papers, however, *do* have knowledgeable soccer writers, and give them newshole to report the game. Among them are the *New York Times*, *Washington Post*, *Boston Globe*, *Chicago Tribune*, *USA Today* and *Charlotte Observer*.

But with soccer not yet a leader on the U.S. scene, many reporters frequently write generally descriptive stories designed to introduce the game and its nuances to the American heart and mind.

Here's George Vecsey of *The New York Times* describing the U.S. women's team, victors in the 1999 World Cup:

> America's newest sensations are going back on the road, not as the national team, but as instant celebrities. They are going out to strut their stuff the way Babe Ruth and Lou Gehrig used to barnstorm back in the 20s, to make a few extra dollars and take their game to the hinterlands.
>
> "They are a cult," mused Keith Cooper, the director of communications for the world soccer body known as FIFA. "But most cults take longer to develop than this one."
>
> The women came from way off the pop-culture map. A month ago, when I tried to tell colleagues and friends about these American women, I would be aware of them casting discreet glances at their watches and shuffling their feet.
>
> Now the American women are hot.
>
> George Vecsey
> *The New York Times*[18]

Covering the men's teams, Steven Goff of *The Washington Post* reports Major League Soccer (MLS) officials in 1999 are hopeful attendance, around 14,000 per game, may increase:

However, caution remains the theme.

"Every year is crucial until we establish ourselves in the hearts and minds of the paying public and in the culture of the United States," New England Revolution General Manager Brian O'Donovan said. "That's a very difficult thing to do. We've got to realize we're still struggling for our survival. We've got to continue to work very, very hard. If we lose sight of that, we're done for, we're finished."

MLS has lost about $20 million a year since its launch, but key investors have guaranteed financial support for the next five seasons. In that time, league officials agree, the crucial numbers need to rise, starting with attendance for the New York/New Jersey, Kansas City, Dallas, Miami and Tampa Bay franchises.

Steven Goff
The Washington Post[19]

Peter Brewington of *USA Today* does a major takeout on U.S. star Mia Hamm to inform readers that, well, she *is* a star and *is* an American, facts obviously unknown to many readers:

Mia Hamm claims not to remember her first international goal. For the record: It came July 25, 1990, against Norway. She was 18.

Hamm, now 27, won't forget her next goal.

If she scores Saturday against Brazil at the Citrus Bowl in Orlando, she will reach 108 goals. She will break the world mark of 107 she shares with retired Italian star Elisabetta Vignotto. The men's record, held by Brazilian legend Pele, is 77, although scoring is more difficult.

Peter Brewington
USA Today[20]

So, the first lesson in covering soccer is *set the scene, explain the game and build interest*. You cannot assume a generally high level of understanding among readers only recently introduced to soccer (a disadvantage not encountered by European writers covering England vs. Scotland in 1999, the *127th annual game* in their rivalry).

In game coverage, writing styles vary from the AP's hard-news, straight-in approach to featurish intros. Examples of the AP's soccer writing:

FORT LAUDERDALE, FLA.—Roy Lassiter's goal in the sixth round of a shoot-out gave D.C. United a 1-0 victory over the Miami Fusion yesterday, completing their sweep of a first-round Eastern Conference playoff series.

United secured the victory when goalkeeper Tom Presthus stopped Miami's Tyron Marshall on his shoot-out attempt.

Now, a brief single graf of context:

D.C. advanced to the Eastern finals, where it will meet the Columbus Crew, who beat Tampa Bay in the opening round.

And back to game action:

Marco Etcheverry and Diego Sonora also scored shoot-out goals for United. The Fusion's shoot-out scorers were Jim Rooney and Saul Martinez.

Despite both teams being down to 10 players—each saw a starter ejected late in the first half—there were few scoring chances in the second half. D.C.'s Carey Talley launched a shot from 25 yards out that was stopped by Miami goalie Jeff Cassar. The Fusion's best scoring opportunity in regulation came when Eric Wynalda had a clear path to the D.C. goal area after receiving a pass from Nelson Vargas in the 82nd minute. Presthus kicked away Wynalda's point-blank shot.

The Associated Press [21]

Note above that AP's writer focuses on the game-winning penalty kick, a "shoot-out," and in the second graf, a key play by a goalkeeper.

Next, an AP writer reports more expansively on *key plays*:

COLUMBUS, OHIO—Stern John scored two goals in a seven-minute span Sunday and the Columbus Crew beat the Tampa Bay Mutiny, 2-0, in the first game of the best-of-three Major League Soccer Eastern Conference semifinals.

John's first goal came in the 77th minute on an assist from Brian West, who had kicked it toward Brian McBride. The ball landed at McBride's feet, but he never touched it as John scored from 12 yards, beating Mutiny goalkeeper Scott Garlick on the left side.

John, whose 18 goals in the regular season tied him for the league lead, used the bottom of his foot to redirect a free kick by Robert Warzycha past Garlick in the 84th minute. ...

Tampa Bay had an edge of 17-13 in total shots—11-5 in the second half—but Columbus had a 5-2 lead in shots on goal. The Mutiny was called for 22 fouls, compared with eight for the Crew.

The Associated Press [22]

As in covering other sports, newspaper correspondents writing soccer try to go beyond the AP's bare-bone style and to combine featurish intros with analytical angles and the news—who won.

Steven Goff of *The Washington Post* does all that *and* weaves in context and the outcome of another important game:

LAS VEGAS—There were several reasons for D.C. United's 3-1 semifinal loss to Necaxa of Mexico late Friday night in the CONCACAF Champions Cup, but none was as glaring as goalkeeper Tom Presthus's misadventure.

"It obviously wasn't the best game I've played and it was an awful time for it to happen," Presthus said this morning. "I could have done better—much better."

Presthus' mistakes resulted in Necaxa's first and third goals and left United in Sunday's third-place match against the Chicago Fire at Sam Boyd Stadium. Later Sunday Necaxa plays Alajuela of Costa Rica—which beat Chicago in a penalty kick tiebreaker Friday—for the North American title and a berth in the inaugural world cup championships early next year in Brazil.

United Coach Thomas Rongen said he would start several reserves against the Fire, but hadn't made any final decisions. Leading scorer Roy Lassiter, who injured his calf in the first half Friday, will not play and probably will miss United's Major League Soccer game against Tampa Bay Wednesday at RFK Stadium.

Now, back to goalkeeper Presthus (and note the writer's obvious understanding of soccer):

> As for Presthus ...
> With United leading 1-0 on Carey Talley's volley in the 26th minute, Presthus made his first critical error late in the first half. A corner kick that had been flicked along the end line caught Presthus by surprise and bounced off his hands, allowing Sergio Almaguer to easily nod the ball past him.
> Early in the second half, Presthus had little chance of stopping Agustin Delgado's hard shot that gave Necaxa a 2-1 lead, but 11 minutes later he misjudged a corner kick and let the ball soar past him for Edgar Oliva to head into an open net.
>
> Steven Goff
> *The Washington Post*[23]

USA Today's Peter Brewington displays an equally strong grasp of the game in reporting how Yuri Lavrinenko and Aleksey Korol led Indiana to a 1-0 win over Santa Clara and a second consecutive NCAA Men's College Cup title:

> Lavrinenko carried the ball almost 50 yards, dished it to Korol, who deftly touched it twice and fed it back to his countryman for a sharp finish.
> "We know each other so well we rarely have miscommunication," said Lavrinenko, the Cup's outstanding offensive player.
> Korol said: "They covered me, and I dropped it back to Yuri. His move was the key to the goal."...
> In the 30th minute, (Indiana) defender John Swann was standing at the goal all alone when he cleared a ball over the goal with his head.
> In the 77th minute, forward Shawn Percell had a clear shot from 10 yards, but Hoosier's goalkeeper T.J. Hannig forced him to misfire to the right.
>
> Peter Brewington
> *USA Today*[24]

As in all sportswriting, know your game! But in soccer, write for a wider audience that might *not* know it. Note how John Powers of the *Boston Globe* produces soccer copy even non-fans can understand:

> U.S 5
> Ireland 0
>
> FOXBOROUGH—It was a class reunion that turned into a tutorial.
>
> The U.S. women's soccer team hadn't been together on a soccer field since the players were love-bombing Brandi Chastain on the floor of the Rose Bowl. But they got back into celebratory mode quickly yesterday afternoon, taking overmatched Ireland to school, 5-0, before 30,564 at Foxboro Stadium.
>
> Tiffeny Milbrett scored two goals, and Julie Floudy, Kristine Lilly and Joy Fawcett each added one as the Americans breezed past their green-clad visitors, who got an unaccustomed taste of life at soccer's upper level.
>
> It was the first time the Americans had played together since they defeated China on penalty kicks in the Women's World Cup final eight weeks ago, and their mood was decidedly more relaxed. "It'll be fun," Milbrett said. "No restraints. The reins are off of us."
>
> The Irish, who hadn't even qualified to try to qualify for the Cup, were happy just to be invited into the same playpen with the world champions. "Lambs to the slaughter," coach Mick Cooke joked.
>
> John Powers
The Boston Globe[25]

Soccer stats are simple, compared to, say, baseball's. Here are the *Globe*'s on U.S. vs. Ireland:

Soccer: United States 5, Ireland 0, Foxboro Stadium

Ireland	0	0 - 0
United States	2	3 - 5

Game Summary:
Tiffeny Milbrett (Cindy Parlow) 25th minute; Julie Foudy (Milbrett) 38th; Milbrett (Sara Whalen) 59th; Joy Fawcett (Brandi Chastain) 72nd; Kristine Lilly (unassisted) 75th.
Saves: 1, Emma Byrne 5; U.S., Saskia Webber, Sonya Maher 0.
Shots: 13; U.S. 26.
Corner Kicks: 10; US 17.
Referee: Nancy Lay (US).
Attendance: 30,564.

Translation is simple, too. In scoring, Tiffeny Milbrett scored first, with an assist from Cindy Parlow, with 25 minutes elapsed in the match. Ireland's goal-keeper, Emma Byrne, had five saves (but, obviously, missed five U.S. shots, which scored). Incidentally, note the attendance—30,564, a respectable crowd in most leagues, for most sports.

For MLS games, *USA Today* presents more detail:

Soccer: Colorado 1, Chicago 0

Colorado Rapids	1	0	1
Chicago Fire	0	0	0

Game Summary:
Col–DiGiamarino (Harris, Paule) 12.
Col—Shots on Goals: 6 (Bravo 2); Fouls: 11 (Limpar 3); Offside: 4; Corner Kicks: 3; Saves: Hahnemann 9; Possession Pct.: 44%
Chi—Shots on Goals: 9 (Wolff 3); Fouls: 17 (Nowak 7); Offside: 0; Corner Kicks: 14; Saves: Thornton 5; Possession Pct.: 56%.
Attendance: 25,201.

Translation:

In scoring, Colorado's DiGiamarino, with an assist from Harris and Paule, scored his 12th goal of the season. Note also fouls, corner kicks and possession—all factors you must weave into your writing. And, again, note the attendance—25,201, drawn by Chicago Fire, defending MLS champions at the time.

In league standings, the following is what fans want to know.

Major League Soccer Standings

Eastern	W	L	SW	Pts	GF	GA
Columbus	6	2	2	14	9	7
D.C.	5	3	2	11	18	15
NY-NJ	4	4	2	8	8	9

Translation:

Columbus has 6 wins, 2 losses. Two wins were "SW"—shoot-out wins—won on a penalty kick. In soccer, a win earns three points in the standings. A shootout win, however, earns one point. Columbus has 14 points under such scoring. It has nine "goals for"; seven have been scored against the team.

Tennis

For writers, the dynamics of covering tennis closely resemble those of reporting golf.

Both sports revolve principally around the individual rather than team performance. Both are wildly popular participatory sports played by millions. Both create star personalities at the pro level through intense press coverage. Both are driven at the pro level by big money—*huge* money.

But, despite the money and hype, readers are attracted by the impressive athleticism and grace displayed often in both games.

Tall order, young writer, but you must capture all that in reporting tennis—and simultaneously keep your perspective. It's a *business*, as well as a game.

The AP demonstrates such a balanced, discerning view:

> Boosters of women's professional tennis could deny that the future of their sport depends on the glamour of the game's biggest stars. These are the best female athletes in the world, they could argue, and then they can go on to cite their grace, their power and their speed.
>
> Who wouldn't want to watch, especially with several intriguing rivalries budding and the caliber of play rising?
>
> So, OK, Ann Kournikova stirred interest with her looks. And, OK, Venus and Serena Williams were seen styling in *Vogue* and popping off like Charles Barkley to the media. But, ah, the game, that was the thing.
>
> Until, that was, last year. Right there on the cover of *GQ*, wearing a flashy white dress, was the world's No. 1 player and the sweetheart of the women's game, Martina Hingis, smiling under the headline: "The Champ Is a Vamp."
>
> Apparently, the girl was loving it. And so, too, perhaps, were those involved in the business side of women's tennis, the companies and promoters who hope to use the appeal of Hingis, Kournikova, the Williams sisters and other stars to create a powerful marketing machine for the millennium.
>
> "In this day and age, sports has to be viewed as entertainment," said Joe Favorito, the vice president of the Women's Tennis Association. "These are women who look pretty good and who are products of their generation."
>
> The Associated Press [26]

In writing big-time tennis, you must satisfy reader interest in players as star personalities and, especially, the intensity of man-against-man and woman-against-woman competition. AP captures that in a *feature story*:

> NEW YORK—A few years after cynics claimed tennis was dying, record crowds are expected at the (1999) U.S. Open amid the blossoming of new players and the renewed rivalry between Pete Sampras and Andre Agassi.
>
> The U.S. Open starting Monday closes out a sizzling summer that began with Agassi and Steffi Graf triumphing on the French clay, moved on to

wins by Sampras and Lindsay Davenport on Wimbledon's grass and winds up on the hardcourts of the National Tennis Center.

The game is full of talented and personable young players: Alexandra Stevenson and Jelena Dokic, the latest in a long parade of talented teens making their mark; Marat Safin and Dominik Hrbaty, breaking through on the men's side.

Patrick Rafter, tennis' GQ cover boy, comes into the Open as the two-time defending champion and is giving the men's game the feeling of the late '70s and early '80s, when three great players—Connors, Borg and McEnroe—vied for big titles.

Everything is looking up for the sport these days, from soaring TV ratings to climbing sales of tennis balls and rackets as more kids and weekend hackers take to the courts. The rise of Venus and Serena Williams to prominence had as much to do with that as anything else.

Steve Wilstein
The Associated Press [27]

Even in *spot-news coverage* of match competition, the AP's tennis writers display featurish styles sometimes absent from, say, their hockey writing, which can get almost mechanical in packing everything—the entire Five Ws and How—into the first graf. Note this featurish tennis intro:

NEW YORK—Neither seven double-faults by Venus Williams nor a whipping wind that sent shots flying as wildly as Wiffle balls in Martina Hingis' match could keep them from their inevitable rematch at the U.S. Open.

Two years after Hingis thrashed the inexperienced Williams in the final of her Open debut, the two will meet again in Arthur Ashe Stadium, this time in the semifinals.

"Last time, I honestly did not know what I was doing," Williams said of her 6-0, 6-4 loss to Hingis for the 1997 title. "I'm a different player now."

"The key for me is definitely to abandon all unforced errors. In order not to play her and myself, I have to stop making errors."

Note how AP's writer draws a word picture of double-faults and "whipping wind" to pull readers in, but quickly turns, still in the first graf, to a *look-ahead angle*—the woman vs. woman competition ahead in the "inevitable rematch."

Also note we're four grafs into the story and we *still* don't know the outcome of the match at hand. Here's how the writer gets back to that:

From 0-2 Tuesday, the top-ranked Hingis won 12 straight games amid stiff gusts to stroll into the semis with a 6-2, 6-0 victory over Anke Huber.

The wind died down a bit after a brief shower in the evening, and the No. 3 Williams unleashed an all-court attack that enabled her to overcome serving woes in a 6-4, 6-3 win against No. 12 Barbara Schett.

Williams dominated at the net and the baseline in the slugfest against the hard-hitting Schett, punctuating the first set with an overhead that caromed into the stands on set point. She broke Schett's service three times in the second set, the last time closing out the match with a backhand return that Schett couldn't touch. ...

Hingis couldn't quite get a bead on the balls Huber was sending her way during the first couple of games, and she couldn't tame the shots she was sending back.

Hingis' befuddlement didn't last long, though, as she demonstrated her talent for adjusting to difficult conditions and outthink opponents.

Players have complained about the wind in the stadium since it opened two years ago. But the remnants of tropical storm Dennis have buffeted the court for several days, making this year's conditions the worst so far.

The Associated Press [28]

So newsworthy are some of tennis' stars (not to say, *flamboyant personalities*), that their mere presence can dominate spot-news coverage of a match:

HARARE, ZIMBABWE—The crowd rocked to the rhythm of tribal dancers.

Spectators did the wave.

The din was so loud the umpire could barely be heard.

And John McEnroe wanted nothing more than to pick up a racket.

But McEnroe, making his debut as Davis Cup captain could only stalk the sideline Friday as the United States split its opening singles matches with Zimbabwe.

"I wasn't able to get up and play," McEnroe said.

Andre Agassi, helped by some questionable line calls, won the opener by overpowering Wayne Black, 7-5, 6-3, 7-5.

Then Black's brother, Byron Black, defeated Chris Woodruff 7-6 (7-2), 6-3, 6-2 to even the best-of-5, first-round series.

Andrew Selsky
The Associated Press [29]

Note in the two previous examples these three points:

- It's the drama of one-on-one competition that drives vigorous tennis writing.
- Your writing must catch the *atmosphere* of tennis—the crowd, the noise, the "Wiffle balls."
- As in golf, playing conditions and weather are crucial (recall AP's "whipping wind" and player complaints).

And, don't forget the money. The AP focuses on that in one competition:

This time both Williams sisters did their part setting up a family showdown in the most lucrative tournament in the world.

Serena Williams, the U.S. Open champion, beat Lindsay Davenport 6-3, 6-4 after older sister Venus defeated top-ranked Martina Hingis 6-2, 6-7 (6-

8), 9-7 in yesterday's semifinals of the $6.7 million Grand Slam Cup in Munich, Germany. ...

Tomorrow's final will add $1.3 million to the family budget, with $800,000 going to the winner.

It will also give Serena, at 18 one year younger than Venus, the chance to gain her first victory in the historic sister-sister series. She also collects a $100,000 bonus for her U.S. Open title, win or lose.

"Not bad," Serena said of the money the sisters will earn. "I'm going to hate to see my tax return."

The Associated Press [30]

Some newspaper writers stretch for original intros:

MELBOURNE, AUSTRALIA—He is an unrelenting pit bull. If he is across the net from you in a tennis match, he is unflinching, unbending, unstoppable. He is Andre Agassi men's single champion of the Australian Open.

He won that title, yet another in his current march through men's tennis, by beating defending champion Yevgeny Kafelnikov of Russia on the fast center court at Rod Laver Arena today, 3-6, 6-3, 6-2, 6-4.

Bill Dwyre
The Los Angeles Times [31]

NEW YORK—It was a New York kind of day at Arthur Ashe Stadium. Too much traffic (blimps, jets and skywriters clogged the blue skies above the court), wall-to-wall people (20,000-plus fans including Jimmy Carter and Donald Trump) and the usual loudmouths ("C'mon, Andre, send dis clown back to St. Petersburg!").

Appropriately, in their U.S. Open semifinals yesterday, Americans Andre Agassi and Todd Martin couldn't have been ruder to a couple of out-of-towners.

Agassi, the doe-eyed, pigeon-toed No. 2 seed from Las Vegas, advanced to his third straight Grand Slam final, thrashing third-seeded Russian Yevgeny Kafelnikov, 1-6, 6-3, 6-3, 6-3.

Earlier, No. 7 seed Todd Martin, graying, often injured and without a major on his lengthy resume, destroyed unseeded Frenchman Cedric Pioline, 6-4, 6-1, 6-2.

Frank Fitzpatrick
The Philadelphia Inquirer [32]

And some newspaper writers stretch (I think) too far (emphasis added):

WIMBLEDON, ENGLAND—Boris Becker, *the war horse who put himself out to pasture* two years ago but decided to *tackle* Wimbledon one last time, today *pawed and pounded* his way out of a two-sets-to-none deficit against Scotland's Miles Maclagan and into the second round.

On Court Two, this facility's renowned and reviled Graveyard Court, Becker recovered his poise, erased three match points, and secured his 69th victory at Wimbledon. Becker's 31st ace clinched the 5-7, 6-7 (7-9), 6-4, 7-5, 6-2 comeback.

> Robin Finn
> *The New York Times*[33]

What do *you* think? Did Finn stretch too far?

Newspapers generally don't report stats for tennis, but on important matches, *The Atlanta Journal-Constitution* breaks out numbers that reveal to reader-fans *how* a match was won. The following illustrates key factors *you must weave into your writing:*

How Agassi Won

	Agassi	Martin
1st serve percentage	64	60
Aces	7	23
Double faults	4	8
% 1st serve points won	75	71
% 2nd serve points won	66	59
Winners	39	74
Unforced errors	23	60
Break points	5-10	0-8
Net points	16-19	62-97

Translation:

—Andre Agassi got the ball into play (without hitting it into the net or out of bounds) with his first serve 64 percent of the time.

—On seven of his first serves, Agassi placed the ball where his opponent could not hit it (an "ace").

—Four times, Agassi failed on both his first and second serves to get the ball properly into play. (He hit it out of bounds or into the net twice in a row.)

—Agassi won the point on his first serve 75 percent of the time, 66 percent on his second serve. (Both are high rates of success.)

—On 39 occasions, after the serve, Agassi put the ball into his opponent's half of the court and won the point because the ball was unreturnable.

—Unforced errors are those made by a player who should—but doesn't—return a ball. Agassi committed 23 such errors.

—On 10 occasions, when his opponent was serving, Agassi could have won the game by scoring the next point. He did so five times.

—Net points are scored when a player moves forward to the net to return the ball, rather than playing it from deeper in the court, near the "base line." Agassi moved to the net 19 times and scored 16 times. (Note his opponent,

Todd Martin, played a different strategy—moving to the net 97 times and scoring on 62 occasions.)[34]

Covering Outdoor Sports

The numbers are stunning, according to John Morton, a leading newspaper analyst:[35]

- 40 million people 16 or older were spending on average more than $1,000 annually in the past decade on fishing and hunting (or $40.9 billion total).
- *Bird watching* attracted 65 million adults who were spending about $5.2 billion on seed, feeders, books and binoculars; other forms of wildlife watching generated $12.9 billion in retail spending.
- 73.5 million Americans 6 or older fished in 1993, 25.4 million fired a gun, 20 million hunted.

Against those numbers, American were spending only a relatively paltry $5.9 billion annually to attend professional sports events.

Yet, many newspaper sports editors cover outdoor news only sporadically and, when they do, often tuck it deep in back-of-section pages. Nevertheless, if you are passionate about hunting, fishing, backpacking, skiing or any of those other sports that draw millions of people to field, stream and mountainside, be encouraged! Major newspapers *do* provide jobs covering outdoor sports, although they are relatively few in comparison to jobs covering major sports.

Many magazines focus exclusively on outdoor sports. *Outdoor Life*, for example, has covered hunting, fishing and other outdoor sports since 1898. *Climbing, Snowboarding* and other "niche" magazines focus even more narrowly on a single outdoor sport.

I turn now to writing columns and opinion pieces. (And, I do so with apologies to you who want to cover lacrosse, field hockey, arena football, gymnastics ... the list is long and, indeed, inviting. But "newshole" is limited for books, as for newspapers and magazines!)

Summary

—Meaningful careers await sportswriters in covering soccer, hockey, golf, tennis and other participatory sports exploding in popularity across the nation.

—In covering sports that are narrowly focused or, even, esoteric, you must use expert reporting and writing techniques to meet the news needs of discerning readers who know the sports intimately.

—In ice hockey, covering every game, every day, Associated Press writers frequently write directly and tautly to ensure their stories communicate essentials even if edited down to a couple paragraphs.

—Newspaper writers, guaranteed sufficient newshole by their own editors, often stretch for unique angles and write longer stories in conversational style.

—Much outstanding hockey writing highlights star performance, characterizes individual play and includes analysis and interpretation.

—In covering golf, understand you cover a sport that's an obsession for millions who watch it or play it.

—Good golf writing reports player vs. player action, player vs. rigors of a course or hole and player vs. weather and course conditions.

—Weave into your golf writing the leaders in driving distance, driving accuracy, greens reached in regulation strokes, putting averages and birdie leaders.

—Soccer draws fewer fans than "big-money" sports in America but beginner writers must learn to cover the game because of its exploding popularity among young people.

—Many soccer writers write generally descriptive stories designed to introduce the game and its nuances to Americans because soccer is not yet a leader on the U.S. scene.

—In tennis, the dynamics of coverage resemble those of golf because both sports revolve principally around individual play and both are wildly popular participatory sports surrounded in huge hype and money.

—Nevertheless, tennis and golf attract many readers because of the impressive athleticism and grace displayed often in both games, all of which your writing must capture.

—Your tennis writing should reflect the drama of one-on-one competition, plus the atmosphere of the match (crowd and noise) and playing conditions and weather.

—Although Americans spend billions of dollars on outdoor sports, editors give relatively little attention to fishing, backpacking, hunting or other "field" sports; nevertheless, newspapers and, particularly, magazines do offer job opportunities in outdoor reporting.

Exercises

1. Your instructor will provide summaries for a National Hockey League game. Analyze the stats, then, in about 250 words, discuss highlights you would feature in a spot-news story about the game. Pay particular attention to defensive and offensive factors and, as discussed in Chapter Ten, individual play, shots on goal, power plays and goalie performance.

2. Interview a well-known golfer or the golf coach at your university or a "pro" at a local golf club. The purpose is for you to gain understanding of the player vs. course element of golf, as discussed in this chapter. For a newspaper audience, write about 300 words on the interviewee's explanation of such

things as driving distance, driving accuracy and putting skills needed to "beat" a local course. As guidelines, use *The Atlanta Journal-Constitution* and *Chicago Tribune* examples in this chapter.

3. Interview a college soccer player or coach on the physical demands of the game, the athleticism required to play it and how all that contrasts with the demands of team sports more familiar to Americans, such as basketball and football. Write this in about 350 words. The purpose is to familiarize yourself with soccer and learn how to "translate" nuances of the game for readers.

4. Interview a tennis player or coach on the training and lifestyle required for success in hotly competitive tennis. Structure your story to reveal to readers the self-discipline and hard work needed to win on the court. Write this in wordage required to get a complete picture before your readers.

5. Depending on the season, cover a hockey, tennis, golf or soccer contest. Using reporting and writing hints from Chapter 10, write *two* intros of about five grafs each—one in direct, taut AP style and another in the expansive, descriptive and analytical style of newspaper writers whose work we saw in this chapter.

Recommended Reading

Sports cited in this chapter are covered extremely well by the *New York Times, Atlanta Journal-Constitution, Philadelphia Inquirer, Boston Globe, Chicago Tribune, Los Angeles Times, Charlotte Observer, Dallas Morning News.*

Sports Illustrated is strong in all sports. Magazines too numerous to cite individually cover hockey, soccer, tennis and golf in depth. *Sporting News* and *ESPN Magazine* present excellent overviews.

Beginner sportswriters will find a treasure of helpful books on *www.amazon.com* (1,579 were listed at last report on hockey alone, 2,991 on golf, 1,618 on soccer and 1,376 on tennis!) But the following might be especially helpful:

On hockey, see Dan Diamond (editor), James Duplacey (editor) and Igor Kuperman, *Total Hockey: The Official Encyclopedia of the National Hockey League* (1998) and, if you're new to the game, John Davidson and John Steinbreder, *Hockey for Dummies* (IDG Books Worldwide, 1997.)

To see how tennis *should* be played, note Tina Hoskins, *1001 Incredible Tennis Games, Drills & Tips* (Hoskins Publishing, 1997.)

Soccer is explained in Dan Herbst and Bobby Howe (editor), *Soccer: How to Play The Game: The Official Playing and Coaching Manual of The United States Soccer Federation* (Universe Publishing, 1999.)

For golf, if you are a beginner in covering it, see Gary McCord, John Huggan and Alice Cooper, *Golf for Dummies*, 2nd ed. (IDG Books Worldwide, 1999.)

Notes

1. Jere Longman, "Crowd, On and Off Field, Forced Scurry to Scramble," *The New York Times*, June 21, 1999, p. D-4.

2. John Morton, "Charge the Error to Sports Editors," *American Journalism Review*, July-August 1995, p. 52.

3. "Adam's Six Points, Lamade's Hat Trick Give Landon a Boost," Jan. 29, 2000, p. D-8.

4. "Warriors Play UNH to a Tie," Feb. 5, 2000, p. G-7.

5. Dispatch for morning papers, April 3, 1999.

6. Dispatch for morning papers, April 1, 1999.

7. "Ducks Look Like a New Team," Jan. 30, 2000, p. D-8.

8. Drawn from AP dispatch for morning papers, April 1, 1999.

9. Drawn from AP dispatch for morning papers, April 1, 1999.

10. "A Surfeit of Golf," July 17, 1999, p. 53.

11. Dispatch for morning papers, May 6, 1999.

12. "Sluman Still Going Strong," May 21, 1999, p. C-8.

13. "Masters '99," April 4, 1999, p. E-8.

14. "Leader Board," Aug. 13, 1999, Section 4, p. 7.

15. From AP dispatch for morning papers, April 2, 1999.

16. "Ivory Coast's Chief Gets Tough After Early Loss," *Chicago Tribune*, Feb. 2, 2000, Section 3, p. 2.

17. "Ignorant Media Draws Red Card," Dec. 20, 1998, p. C-11.

18. "Sports of the Times," July 12, 1999, p. D-1.

19. "MLS Set for 'Year of No Excuses,'" March 19, 1999 p. D-10.

20. "Hamm on Verge of Scoring Record," May 21, 1999, p. C-10.

21. Dispatch for morning papers, Oct. 25, 1999.

22. Dispatch for morning papers, Oct. 18, 1999, p. C-15.

23. "Presthus Ponders Mistakes," Oct. 3, 1999, p. D-8.

24. "Ukrainian Connection Stays Tight at Indiana," Dec. 31, 1999, p. C-17.

25. "Lesson Plan: Five Easy Pieces," Sept. 5, 1999, p. C-4.

26. Dispatch for morning papers, March 28, 1999.

27. Dispatch for morning papers, Aug. 29, 1999.

28. Dispatch for morning papers, Sept. 8, 1999.

29. Dispatch for Sunday papers, Feb. 6, 2000.

30. Dispatch for morning papers, Oct. 2, 1999.

31. "Agassi Gets His Year Off to a Grand Start," Jan. 30, 2000, p. D-1.

32. "Agassi, Martin Blow Through Semis, Set Up All-American Final," Sept. 2, 1999, p. D-4.

33. "Becker Stretching Out His Final Wimbledon," June 23, 1999, p. D-5.

34. From "Open: Agassi Stronger at the End," *The Atlanta Journal-Constitution*, Sept., 13, 1999, p. D-3.

35. John Morton, "Charge the Error to Sports Editors," op. cit.

PART SIX

Columns:
The Winner's Circle
in Sportswriting

Nothing in sports reporting gives you the journalistic *elbowroom* that comes from writing a column.

Nothing matches a column for opening the world of sports to *your* personal definition of what news is and *your* analysis of what it means.

And, if your analysis is sound and your writing strong, there's nothing like a column for gathering thousands of devoted readers who will flip pages eagerly every day, looking for you.

Small wonder, then, that for many sportswriters a column is a career destination, a coveted goal, the *winner's circle* hoped for after years in basic reporting and writing on the daily news beat.

No wonder, either, that sports editors have their pick of the *very best* writers as columnists.

You, of course, can aspire to be among those very best, if you first master the reporting and writing fundamentals we've discussed in this book.

There are more column-writing jobs available in sports than in any other sector of journalism. Major newspapers have many sports columnists. Even small papers have several because editors know columns are great reader attractions.

Make no mistake, however, if you hope to write a column, you are aspiring to join really great writers in the winner's circle.

Pulitzer prizes for commentary have gone to four sports columnists (Jim Murray of *The Los Angeles Times* and Red Smith, Dave Anderson and Arthur Daley of *The New York Times*).

And among sportswriters today, some columnists are legends— Mike Lupica, Tom Boswell, Tony Kornheiser, Furman Bisher, Bob Ryan, Murray Chass, George Vecsey and Frederick C. Klein, among them.

As you'll see in pages ahead, two characteristics specially mark these great columnists: truly insightful understanding of the sports they cover and mastery of the written language that at times carries a sheer beauty matching any prose anywhere, in or out of journalism.

We'll examine column writing in two parts.

In Chapter Eleven, Writing Game Columns, we'll look at columnists who tie their writing to spot-news developments, combining old-fashioned reporting with informed opinion on a single game or other current sports event.

In Chapter Twelve, In This Corner . . . , we'll look at fixture columns—those scheduled generally for the same days and "anchored" in the same spot in a newspaper. Though often found in the same corner of a page, these columns free writers to roam the world of sports and follow their writer's muse wherever it leads, sometimes into the news and sometimes out of it, and down memory lane.

11

Writing Game Columns

ALTHOUGH MUCH spot-news writing in sports is (and should be) analytical, it's in column writing that you can examine and interpret—with special microscopic intensity—a key development in a game, a personality or dramatic moment.

And, it's in a column that you can get truly creative as a writer without the restraints that do (and should) tie spot-news *reporting* to journalism's tradition of striving for objectivity.

In column writing, you can say it your way, in your words.

Thus, columnist Ian O'Connor of the *New York Daily News* watches the New York Giants whip the Dallas Cowboys 20-7, and, while others write spot-news stories on the game, O'Connor uses his column to focus intently on a personality:

> IRVING—Occasionally, the coach moved down the sideline with purpose, whispering into his headset, acting like he was about to split the atom. Mostly, Barry Switzer stood there with hands in pockets, doing his best to look dumb. He ran a morally bankrupt program in college, and was proud to do the same in the pros. Yesterday, the Giants granted him a perfectly appropriate farewell. They used second-team players to close down his third-rate act.

After that stunningly direct opener, O'Connor weaves in detail that will make his column *a stand-alone narrative*. Remember: Even though others write spot-news stories, *your column must enable readers to under-*

stand the news event, as well as your commentary on it. O'Connor accomplishes that although he focuses on a *personality*:

> The Cowboys quit in their final game, the signs as clear as Switzer's fate. Troy Aikman did everything but walk off the field, a trick he had already performed in practice. Michael Irvin was seen crying near the bench, even before he refused to break up Jason Sehorn's interception. Erik Williams spent the afternoon delivering illegal jabs to Michael Strahan's helmet, looking more for a brawl than a measure of consolation.
>
> There were silly penalties—three on the first possession alone—and unforced fumbles, helping the Giants rest their playoff-bound starters, helping the Cowboys honor their retirement-bound coach.
>
> "I'm personally responsible," Switzer said after watching the Giants complete a 20-7 victory, a clean sweep of the NFC East and a 10-5-1 season. "There will be lots of changes made in lots of areas."

Now, with context established (with the 20-7 score and Giant's 10-5-1 season), O'Connor refocuses his microscope on Switzer (and note the beautiful writing touch in the last graf):

> One change, in one area, is of paramount concern. For the first time, Switzer said he didn't know if he wanted to return as coach and acknowledged having talks with Jerry Jones about the possibility of remaining in a diminished role. Jones would claim he had no recollection of these discussions.
>
> It's all moot now. A worn coach goes home, a fresh team goes forward. The Giants eased their way into the playoffs, taking a 20-0 halftime lead and then deploying Dave Brown and a procession of reserves for the game's balance. *Across the field, Dallas was left a physical, ethical and emotional wreck. The Titanic made less noise as it headed for bottom.*
>
> Ian O'Connor
> *New York Daily News*[1]

In the following, a columnist recounts a *moment* when it became clear to him the Baltimore Colts should start a young Tim Couch, not the veteran Ty Detmer, at quarterback:

> After Sunday, the answer is easy.
> I knew it when I saw the young man taking one hit after another. Yet

Couch continually popped right up and beat his linemen back to the huddle as if nothing worse happened to him than he dropped a penny on the sidewalk.

I knew it when I saw the red welt near his right eye, the scratches on his cheek, the sweat pouring down on his forehead—and this was during his postgame news conference. Yet, he vowed to keep running the ball if that's what it takes to get a first down.

I knew it when Baltimore coach Brian Billick said: "Couch is a good athlete who can stretch a defense because he's good on his feet and handles himself well."

Terry Pluto
Akron Beacon-Journal[2]

Key plays—quarterback sacks and pass defense—are examined by columnist Tom Powers of the *St. Paul Pioneer-Press*:

MINNEAPOLIS—The Vikings got bullied on their own playground.

Singularly unimpressed by Minnesota's reputation as a squad for the ages, the Oakland Raiders beat up the home team.

"It was like a heavyweight fight," running back Tyrone Wheatley said. "We knocked them out."

I'll say. They tossed Vikings blockers aside as if they were rag dolls, sacking Randall Cunningham six times and deflecting a handful of passes.

Tom Powers
St. Paul Pioneer-Press[3]

There are brief examples of columnists using keen powers of observation to focus on personalities, plays or moments, then writing with vigor and imagination.

Let's look at some things to keep in mind as you venture into such column writing.

Cover the Five Ws and How

Your mission as a columnist is not to write a game story with a spot-news lead, but 1) your column must contain enough basic reporting so it stands alone, yet 2) not duplicate the game lead that a colleague might write.

For example, the *Dallas Morning News* assigns Chip Brown to report NCAA Tournament play in Boston, and he produces this *spot-news* account:

BOSTON—Purdue, loser of five of its last six games and seven of its last 11, was supposed to be the fragmented team that didn't deserve a berth in the NCAA Tournament.

But it was Big 12 regular-season champion Texas that played like a jittery team with no confidence Friday night.

The Longhorns failed to take advantage of a huge size advantage and made countless mistakes, particularly down the stretch, in a 58-54 loss to the Boilermakers in the first round of the East Region.

> Chip Brown
> *The Dallas Morning News*[4]

Displayed next to that game lead is this column:

BOSTON—Even during their shoot-around less than half an hour before tipoff, when there was nothing between them but air and space, balls crashed off the rim. Some careened to the left. Others ricocheted to the right.

And the only person in the Fleet Center gym Friday evening with a helmet on was that blockhead Purdue mascot, Boilermaker Special. Under a gold construction helmet, he wielded a sledgehammer with less possibility of hurting someone than the masons masquerading as Texas Longhorns basketball players.

In the end, however, everyone but the Longhorns escaped without injury. The Longhorns didn't do damage to anyone but themselves.

The Gang That Couldn't Shoot Straight from Austin only shot themselves in their collective foot in losing a very winnable game, 58-54.

They pulled up and shot airballs. Pulled up and hit the side of the backboard.

> Kevin B. Blackistone
> *The Dallas Morning News*[5]

Note that Blackistone opens with free-ranging imagery and hard-hitting commentary, not who won, who lost. *But* he also neatly weaves in the who, what, where, when, why and how.

Whatever angle your commentary takes, *get the basic ingredients of the news story—the facts—into your column.*

Provide Added Value

Clever writing will attract readers to your column and even hold them—for a while.

But to pull them all the way through your column and, importantly, keep them coming back to you day after day, you must give them *substantive added value*—new facts, new understanding—as a reward for reading you.

Next, for example, is a columnist who combines clever writing with substantive added value. At issue is Ken Griffey Jr., and his jump from the Seattle Mariners baseball team to the Cincinnati Reds, in a complicated maneuver involving free agentry, league regulations, salary caps. ...

First, there's the come-on with clever writing:

> These are now the two single most important numbers in all of sports: 10 and 5.
>
> Ten years in the major leagues, five years with the same team.
>
> Carrying around 10 and 5 is better than being armed with a .38 or a .45. Plus, you don't have to wait for a license and you don't need to get fingerprinted.
>
> Ken Griffey Jr. pointed 10 and 5 at his employer and cocked the hammer. The Seattle Mariners had no more choice than passengers on a hijacked airliner.
>
> So in the most lopsided transaction since the island of Manhattan was purchased for $24 worth of beads, Junior jilted Seattle and forced the Mariners to hand him over to the Cincinnati Reds.

That's Bill Lyon of the *Philadelphia Inquirer*, and he's got me hooked (you, too?), particularly because I don't understand how Griffey, under a Mariners' contract, could pull off the switch. And *that* is what Lyon proceeds to explain and *that* is the added value in his column:

> Having coldly stripped the Mariners of all bargaining leverage, having purposefully driven down his market value and scared away all suitors, Junior watched without apparent regret as, in return for the best player in baseball they received ... well, not even the Reds' best player.
>
> What, exactly, did Junior fetch? Youth, the Mariners said, hopefully, trying to muster the faintest sort of positive spin. Specifically, four youths. They may or may not ever be heard from again.
>
> It was more an extortion than it was a transaction, and if ever a deal screamed that it is not in the best interests of baseball, this one does.
>
> And that's the magic phrase, isn't it? *In the best interests of baseball.* Isn't that the catchall, the rationalization that the commissioner and the Lords of Baseball always use either as a bugle charge to battle or a shield to hide behind?

Now, Lyon swings into a *call for action*—a characteristic of strong column writing because it not only outlines a problem but also points toward a solution:

> So, where are they now, with their trumpets and their outrage?
>
> Who in charge is going to stand up and call a hijacking a hijacking, and then void it?
>
> The rules against tampering were violated. The new commissioner has

only recently been granted authority and power beyond even that of the Boss of Bosses. When does he bring down the hammer?

There was a time, and not so long ago, when the owners had all the power and the players were, essentially, chattel. That wasn't fair and it wasn't right. Now the world has turned upside down, the inmates hold the keys, 10 and 5 is more convincing than anything made by Colt or Smith & Wesson, but that isn't any more fair or right, either.

Bill Lyon
The Philadelphia Inquirer[6]

Well, on goes Lyon, explaining in colorful detail how Griffey did a number on the Mariners. His column is *good reading*, and it's packed with *added value reporting*.

Another example: Suddenly, the complicated point system used in auto racing to determine the NASCAR Winston Cup championship goes awry. Ed Hinton of *Sports Illustrated*, in his column, "Inside Motor Sports," establishes the change in the first graf:

> NASCAR's Winston Cup championship, which only two weeks ago looked as if it had been locked up by Dale Jarrett, has turned into a crap-shoot with 10 races left in the season. Jarrett hemorrhaged more of his points lead on Sunday by finishing 16th in the Southern 500 at storied Darlington Raceway.

But, *why* did Jarrett do so poorly at Darlington? In superb added value reporting, the *SI* columnist explains:

> Jarrett was doomed in Darlington when a flat tire caused his Taurus to spin out during last Friday's first-round qualifying, which meant he would start 36th in the 43-car field.
>
> "The qualifying effort just killed us. We didn't realize how much of a disadvantage that would be," Jarrett said after the race.

Ed Hinton
Sports Illustrated[7]

Added value writing frequently flows from watching a sports event and thinking in broadly analytical terms far beyond the outcome—the score.

Note this day-after reflection on what *really* happened in a football game:

> TAMPA, FLA.—For much of July and August, Giants fans heard Coach Jim Fassel talk about the new-fangled, high powered, wide-open offense he was ready to unleash in his third year on the job. This Giants offense would be versatile, volatile and unpredictable.
>
> During the preseason, the Giants offered tantalizing morsels of wide-open things to come, and fans, hungry for a change, bit. It turns out that

the newfangled Giants offense everyone has been talking about is its defense.

On a day when the Giants' offense and Tampa Bay's offense fought a duel of ineptitude, the Giants' defense made it clear that until further notice the team's foundation is what it has always been: defense. The new offense mustered four first downs and 107 yards; the defense accounted for 14 points and set up a field goal in the Giants' 17-13 victory over the Buccaneers.

> William C. Rhoden
> *The New York Times*[8]

Note the authoritative tone of a day-after analysis by a writer who has covered pro football for *40 years*:

> CLEVELAND—Small Ball might get you respect, but not a victory.
>
> The expansion Browns played the kind of game they needed to beat the New England Patriots yesterday, but couldn't finish the job.
>
> Drew Bledsoe and Terry Glenn were just too much for them.
>
> When you are a second-division team in the NFL, the best way to try to pull an upset is to play Small Ball. The idea is to avoid giving up the big play on defense and keep the clock moving while on offense.
>
> The Browns were doing well on the defensive part of the plan until Glenn blew the game open with a 54-yard touchdown reception at the start of the fourth quarter.

> Will McDonough
> *The Boston Globe*[9]

In a more philosophical approach to added value reporting, Jon Saraceno of *USA Today* spends time with heavyweight boxer Mike Tyson (walking with him in a graveyard!), trying to unlock the puzzle of his personality and moods. And, columnist Saraceno lets us *see*:

> At 33, he remains the wild, wondrous man-child, full of insight and insecurity, an impulsive, moody fatalist tortured by his past and present. He's introspective; his philosophical ruminations would surprise you. Flecks of gray peek around his temple. His millions have evaporated; the scar tissue won't. He looks more like an aged fighter trying to scale Mount Comeback. He's often surrounded by people but always looks alone to me.

> Jon Saraceno
> *USA Today*[10]

When readers leave your column with such images in their minds and when readers exclaim, "I didn't know *that!*"—then, you've added value to your writing.

Stay Close to the News

Truly big news stories create waves of reader interest, and you dramatically increase your chances of being read if your column is timely and on the tip of a news wave. An example:

For weeks, sports pages carry precedes on the approaching Kentucky Derby. It's the biggest horse race each year. Fan interest is intense.

And *there*, smack in the middle of that fan interest, and positioning his column on the tip of the news wave, is Furman Bisher of *The Atlanta Journal-Constitution*. The race will be run on Saturday; *the day before*, on Friday, Bisher looks ahead:

> LOUISVILLE, KY.—Take my word for it, this is a cockeyed Kentucky Derby coming up, and let me give you a quick clue: A horse named Answer Lively was two-year-old champion last year, and he sewed it up by winning the Breeders Cup Juvenile here on the Churchill Downs track. The track handicapper had Answer Lively opening at 50-1 for the Derby.
>
> Furman Bisher
> *The Atlanta Journal-Constitution* [11]

Incidentally, note that Bisher quotes the *track handicapper* on odds for that long shot. Setting odds yourself—or predicting the outcome of *any* sports event—is dangerous business.

Looking *backward* a day, Steve Campbell of the *Albany (N.Y.) Times Union* examines, in his Saturday column, a Friday night game—and *looks ahead* (emphasis added):

> NEW YORK—The score was tied in the fourth quarter, and the ball was in the hands of Tim Hardaway. He was so open on the right wing, behind the 3-point arc, he had almost no choice but to shoot the ball.
>
> The way things have been going, the New York Knicks had the Miami Heat right where they wanted it.
>
> Swish.
>
> The Heat was in the lead. The Heat would stay in the lead from there, building on it until it had an 87-72 victory Friday night at Madison Square Garden. The best-of-five Eastern Conference series is tied at two games apiece, *but the advantage definitely has shifted in the Heat's favor.*
>
> *For one thing*, Game 5 will be in Miami. *For another*, the Heat finally detected indications that Hardaway is alive, if not necessarily well. While 14-points on 5-of-14 shooting isn't going to conjure comparisons to Michael Jordan, it almost qualifies as a resurrection in Hardaway's case.
>
> Steve Campbell
> *Albany (N.Y.) Times Union* [12]

Note that columnist Campbell interprets the situation ("advantage definitely has shifted in the Heat's favor") *and* gives readers his evidence for that interpretation ("For one thing" and "For another").

Make it a rule: Call the shots as you see them, analyze and interpret in your own personal way, *but* always show your readers the logic of your thinking. You'll strengthen enormously your credibility—your *authority*—if you base your opinions on sound reporting and careful examination of facts, then present your interpretation in considered (but nonetheless vigorous and colorful) writing, *and let readers see the process.*

Demonstrating the strength of game columns that are *timely,* columnist C.W. Nevius of the *San Francisco Chronicle* jumps right into a breaking spot-news story:

> Backup quarterback Jeff Garcia was everything the 49ers wanted yesterday—calm, quick and error-free. But do they want to see him again in six days in St. Louis?
>
> There's this week's storyline, and you might as well get used to it. Starting quarterback Steve Young, who sat out yesterday's game after sustaining a concussion last Monday night, says he will visit his neurosurgeon, Dr. Gary Steinberg, today or tomorrow and will make a decision about next Sunday as quickly as possible. And for those of you assuming that you couldn't drag Young out of the game with a team of wild offensive linemen, don't be so sure.

Now, columnist Nevius *chats* with readers, much as fans chat with each other, about what's ahead:

> This is not the same guy who ran full-tilt back on the field after suffering three concussions in an 11-month period beginning two years ago. Does he take concussions with more gravity now?
>
> "Much more seriously now," Young said after the win over the Titans. ...
>
> It is going to make for an interesting little choice for what can literally be called the 49ers' "brain trust," this week. In the past, it wouldn't be much of a decision. The Rams were terrible, and four games into the season the 49ers would have already had a nice cushion in the NFC West.
>
> But now, against all odds, the Rams are hot, the 49ers need the win and you have to wonder if you want to risk Young on the plastic grass in St. Louis.
>
> C.W. Nevius
> *San Francisco Chronicle* [13]

There is much room in newspapers for reflective, featurish columns with no timely news pegs, and we'll discuss them in the next chapter. But with game columns, stay close to the news.

Take Readers With You

You've probably tumbled to it by now, but a great joy in journalism is that we writers get to go places that most people can't—and we are envied for it.

So, you'll do your readers a favor if you take them on your jaunts onto the field and into the locker room, where only we insiders go. Let them see what only we insiders and the athletes themselves see; let your readers hear, smell and touch.

For example, the Boston Red Sox travel to Oakland to play a hot series with the Athletics, and *Boston Globe* newswriters cover the *spot-news* action. Not columnist Dan Shaughnessy. He takes his readers behind the scenes:

> OAKLAND, CALIF.—The 1999 Oakland A's appear to be direct descendants of the old Oakland Raiders of Ken Stabler, John Matuszak and Ted Hendricks.
>
> Before last night's game against the Red Sox, the first of a crucial two-game set, the A's locker room was a study in chaos. Nirvana blared from a clubhouse stereo, volume set on 11. Guys with mustaches and tattoos dressed in front of their lockers, or slouched on sofas eating burgers and fries from McDonald's. Young players wore their caps backward, and autographed photos of pro wrestlers dotted the walls. This must be what it looks and sounds like when the Hell's Angels pull into a truck stop.
>
> Dan Shaughnessy
> *The Boston Globe*[14]

Can't you *see* it? Can't you *hear* it?

Note how effective a column can be when it lets the reader "see":

> Peter O'Malley looked out the window of his ninth-floor downtown office Wednesday toward a grassy patch of Chavez Ravine.
>
> A splendid view. A sickening view.
>
> "I was about to say it's clear out, but maybe it's a little bit murky," he said, laughing.
>
> The real story of why Los Angeles lost its third professional football team in five years Wednesday is not found in Houston, which threw us through the ropes, or Atlanta, where owners kicked us in the ribs.

But, what does the *view* have to do with it? The columnist, Bill Plaschke of *The Los Angeles Times*, explains:

> The real story is found in that view.
>
> Where our new stadium should have been sitting. Where our new team should be playing.
>
> Chavez Ravine, next to Dodger Stadium, is where football would have returned to Los Angeles long before Houston even lost its *first* team, but for a shortsighted mayor and the mild-mannered leader who would not fight him.

"Today, we would be about to be playing football in Los Angeles in a new, extraordinary, finest-ever football stadium," O'Malley said. "It's sad."

A beloved site. A trustworthy owner. Public funds only for access roads. At the very least, sad.

Still, isn't there a *factual story* to be told, despite all this emotional imagery? Yes, and columnist Plaschke tells it:

The real story of why Los Angeles lost a bid for an expansion team is the old story of how, no matter how many thousands of citizens pledge allegiance to sports, they are never a match for the personal agendas of those few who control politics.

Bill Plaschke
Los Angeles Times [15]

That is, take your readers along, all right, but *show them something meaningful when you get to the destination.*

Also, don't think the "come-along-with-me" column need be limited to a trip, physically, into a locker room or executive suite high above Los Angeles. Your column can be built around a trip behind the scenes of a news story or one that, for example, extends into the heart and soul of a baseball team. Thomas Boswell, widely recognized as one of the finest baseball commentators, shows how to do that:

The most valuable player of the 1999 World Series may have been Mariano Rivera but the most valuable person was Yankees Manager Joe Torre.

Without Rivera, as well as Derek Jeter and Bernie Williams, there would be no Yankees dynasty. They're the indispensable players. But Torre is the irreplaceable person. He's the heart of the Yankees—the franchise that, for generations, was supposed to function quite well without that particular organ. The manager with the kindest ferocious face in sports makes these Yanks everybody's team, not just New York's.

As the Yankees burst from their dugout to celebrate their World Series triumph on Wednesday night, tears streamed down Torre's face. He's so happy to be alive these days—he claims to feel everything so much more intensely since his return from prostate cancer treatment this spring—that emotions just pour out of him.

Thomas Boswell
Washington Post [16]

Write for Intimacy With Readers

You've seen it in spot-news stories: A source "told a reporter" or "told the Daily Bugle," as if a reporter is a nonhuman instrument and a newspaper a machine that listens.

There's a tradition in American newswriting of avoiding the personal pronoun "I," and that creates a distant, even cold tone some reporters adopt in mistaken belief that dehumanizing their writing somehow shows dispassionate objectivity.

When you turn to a column, there's no need to write in impersonal, dull and leaden language. Indeed, you should strive for a warm, highly personal style that *reaches out to each reader individually*, as you would reach out with conversational informality in a chat with a friend.

There is no better vehicle for communicating individually with readers than a column written in a "we-and-us" tone. Note this example (emphasis added):

> If recent history has taught *us* anything, it is to not get too excited about what happens once one of *our* local pro football teams falls out of the play-off race, mathematically or logically.
>
> A year ago, for instance, *we* had the Giants finishing up an 8-8 season to a warm round of applause, with five victories in their last six games. They ruined Denver's bid for an undefeated regular season. They slaughtered Kansas City. They anointed Ken Graham, career backup, as the man to lead them, while they waited till next year.
>
> Next year came. The Giants right away went into punt formation.
>
> This is something Bill Parcells has often warned against—the notion that the conclusion of one season has much to do with the next. Next year will bring the inevitable changes in personnel, for all. It will bring a fresh batch of injuries, the possibility that this season's leaks will be plugged only to have others suddenly spring up. It will bring, week after pressurized week, a game that must be won, as opposed to the spoiler's brand of victory the Jets and their young quarterback, Ray Lucas, have earned in six of the last eight weeks.
>
> Harvey Araton
> *The New York Times* [17]

Believe it: New York fans talk about "our" Giants and what "we" can accomplish in the new season. The *Times'* Araton gets on that wavelength with his we-us-our tone, which runs throughout his column.

Another *Times* columnist, George Vecsey, gets *very* personal in commenting on settlement, the day before, of a dispute between NBA players and owners:

> Having seen coal miners crawl back into the 36-inch seam at the end of a strike, convinced they had been done dirty by the coal operators, I have the tiniest bit of trouble seeing the basketball players as an oppressed class.
>
> Having seen schoolteachers trudge back into the classroom at the end of a strike, fearful they had been hammered by the school board, I have the slightest difficulty brooding about our tall friends.
>
> On the other hand, I don't think the National Basketball Association players want our condescension or our sympathy at the end of the lockout dispute. I can hardly wait until tomorrow when they flaunt their fur cloaks

and their gold accessories at us, because then I will know things are back to normal.

The players deserve what they make, as talented performers. They also have mouths to feed, just like coal miners and school teachers, even though it may not look that way to the public.

It is not clear to me that the players got whacked that badly in the settlement, which was ratified by the league's board of governors yesterday. And as the son of two union pioneers, far be it from me to tell the players they should have stood up to the big bullies from ownership, and stayed out all year.

George Vecsey
The New York Times[18]

Aside from the perpendicular pronoun "I" that strides through the column above, note these characteristics:

- This column *hits hard*, implicitly stating it is "we"—the fans—who have been disadvantaged in all this.
- The column is *balanced*, criticizing players and owners alike.
- There is *no hero worship* here; instead, the subject is a bunch of arrogant rich guys who play for big money paid by other rich guys, who are "bullies" to boot.
- There is *true, deep emotion* in this column, clearly born of bitter life experience, and Vecsey draws fully from what obviously were angry childhood moments—watching a disappointed coal-miner father, perhaps, and an underpaid schoolteacher mother labor under a brutish school board.
- There is *fundamental honesty* in Vecsey's approach, a tone of "let me tell you where I'm coming from" as he reveals up front that he is dipping into his personal past to put the NBA dispute into perspective for his readers.

Honest. If nothing else, columnist Vecsey is honest—even when stumped. Note below his charming admission in another column that, Well, Dear Reader, I frankly don't know. ...

After staring at my screen saver for the past hour, I still cannot come up with an argument why the Knicks absolutely cannot beat the San Antonio Spurs in the finals.

I want to clear my throat authoritatively and pretend I'm a hoop maven and declare that the Knicks cannot possibly match the Twin Towers.

But all I know is what I have seen for the last month: Sprewell and Houston bonding on the court, Camby coming on in the stretch as Lemon Drop Kid did in the Belmont.

By the way, this is hardly a triumphal bleat from some giddy Knicks fan. I have no emotional attachment to them or their organization, plus they are bad for my health—late hours, indoor games, stale air at their dismal practice gym.

But they made the Garden rock last Friday, and I am not so sure they cannot do it again when they come home next Monday.

This team is a work in progress. The sum is greater than the parts. This is not a normal season. An eighth-seeded team is in the finals. Ignore their chaos at your own peril.

George Vecsey
The New York Times[19]

That's how to achieve intimacy with readers: Let them know your daddy was a coal miner; write authoritatively when you can but cheerfully acknowledge your inadequacy when you can't.

However, I think Vecsey makes one mistake: He writes in sports "shorthand," understood easily only by confirmed sports fans. And, this denies entry into his column by readers who don't follow *two* sports closely. You must know basketball to catch his reference to the "Twin Towers" and the last-name-only mentions of Sprewell, Houston and Camby. And, if you're not a horse-racing fan would you *really* know Lemon Drop Kid came on in the stretch at Belmont?

Now, here's a lead that many students of literature will understand:

CLEVELAND—Terry Glenn proved Thomas Wolfe was wrong. You can go home again. Or at least within 142 miles of home.

The Columbus, Ohio, native and one-time Cleveland Browns fan made his hometown proud and his boyhood team miserable yesterday by not only beating them with a Patriots-record 13 receptions and a backbreaking touchdown, but by embarrassing them as well when he gained more yards on his own in the first 45:09 (214) than the Browns did (190).

Ron Borges
The Boston Globe[20]

But do you think *all* reader-fans will know the saying, "You can't go home again," came from Thomas Wolfe, a novelist who died in 1938?

That is, get intimate with readers, yes. Chat with readers as with a circle of friends, yes. But don't close the conversational circle against less-well-informed outsiders.

Write to Balance the News

Our *news* reporting covers stories as they break. But sometimes they break in patterns that distort public perceptions. You can write columns to balance spot-news stories and how the public perceives them.

For example, NFL players are involved in violent off-field incidents. Every week or so, it seems, a player punches up a girlfriend or breaks up a bar. Then, police say two players are involved in killings.

By sheer weight of coverage—justifiable and necessary coverage, of course—
our *news pages* make it very easy for readers to perceive all NFL players as hoods.

Quickly, while this public image is fresh, Kevin Blackistone of the *Dallas Morning News* writes a column to put the news in perspective:

> Ray Lewis and Rae Carruth are professional football players.
> Ray Lewis and Rae Carruth are murder suspects.
> Therefore, all professional football players can be suspected of being murderers.
>
> Nothing could be further from the truth, no matter its apparently logical deduction. But in the wake of last week's news concerning Lewis, the All-Pro Baltimore linebacker who was jailed without bail on charges of killing two men in Atlanta, there are people who will syllogize and reach that very conclusion.
>
> There were others who work in the media last week talking and writing about "athletes" when discussing the problems of Lewis and Carruth, as opposed to discussing Lewis and Carruth as mere individuals.
>
> But as Rosalyn Dunlap, a former All-America sprinter who now studies such problems, is quoted in an upcoming edition of the journal *Issues of Society*:
>
> "Perpetrators are not limited to any category or occupation. The difference is that athletes who rape or batter will end up on TV or in the newspapers."
>
> Kevin Blackistone
> *The Dallas Morning News*[21]

You'll note, incidentally, that Blackistone doesn't hesitate to blame "others who work in the media" for what he considers erroneous public perceptions. The honesty in that statement won't escape Blackistone's readers.

Honest—and balanced—discussion of hockey violence leads Bill Reynolds of *The Providence Journal* to throw the net of blame more widely—to cover not only the media, but also fans and the larger society. Reynolds writes his column immediately after an NHL player is struck from behind with a stick and knocked unconscious (His attacker is suspended for the season.):

> The surprising thing is not that Marty McSorley took a stick to Donald Brashear's head; it's that it doesn't happen more often.
>
> For don't we have a double standard when it comes to violence in sports, whether it's boxing, hockey fights or a good hit in football? Aren't we always tiptoeing along some fault line, both glorifying violence and then supposedly being shocked by it? Isn't the lure of violence—and the promise of it—one of the reasons both NASCAR and professional wrestling are so popular?
>
> Just asking.
>
> But if violence runs through both sports and the culture like some rampant virus, the NHL has nurtured an environment for it: players fighting

without a whole lot of repercussions; too many guys whose sole job is to be enforcers; an entire hockey culture that worships the big hit. Is there any wonder someone snaps once in a while?

Bill Reynolds
The Providence Journal[22]

Keep in mind: A column is not a license to stab and wound indiscriminately or write unfairly and without balance. Rather, a column is a *solemn responsibility* because it gives you added strengths—the *firepower*—of analysis, interpretation and opinion. You're still a *journalist* when you move into column writing, and still obliged to strive for accuracy, fairness and balance.

Write to Have—and Give—Fun

Yes, sports is serious—and big—business. Yes, games are life-or-death for millions of fans.

But, hey! Can't we have a little fun around here?

Yes—and by *having* fun, we can *give* fun to our readers.

David Steele of the *San Francisco Chronicle* sure had fun commenting that prospects for the NBA's Golden State Warriors improved with a trade the day before:

They have youth. They have a plan. And they have hope, real hope. Now, when someone asks you, "What the hell are the Warriors doing?" you no longer have to shrug, roll your eyes and stutter incoherently.

David Steele
San Francisco Chronicle[23]

Imagine the chuckles Furman Bisher drew in a column the day after Bobby Cremins resigned as Georgia Tech's basketball coach:

When he came, Georgia Tech basketball was in the dumpster. What he inherited was like the tatters of an army fleeing in retreat. It was good for laughs, but poor comedy. Playing North Carolina at Chapel Hill, one of his big men got the second-half tipoff and was so surprised that he broke into the clear and scored a basket at the Tar Heels' end of the court.

Furman Bisher
The Atlanta Journal-Constitution[24]

The *Journal-Constitution*'s Steve Hummer draws belly-laughs in a column on a forthcoming fight in London between Mike Tyson and a fighter he describes as a "well-used" pug (who I will call "Fred Smith," to protect the victim):

> It has been reported that the (Fred Smith) camp has been paid the equivalent of $30,000 for the right to place advertising on the soles of its man's boxing boots. Of course, the only way the sponsor—reportedly a London tabloid—gets fair value is if (Smith) spends a good deal of time off his feet. The standing eight-count is a hindrance to commerce.
>
> Steve Hummer
> *The Atlanta Journal-Constitution*[25]

Dave Hyde of the *Sun-Sentinel* in south Florida, where, the chamber of commerce brags, the sun always shines, ventures north to Atlanta for the Super Bowl and finds, of all things, an ice storm shut down the city and ... well, this is how Hyde describes it in a dispatch to folks back home:

> As I look out my hotel window, it's hard to tell whether that's freezing rain falling to the ground or Chamber of Commerce members jumping to it.
> I mean, Hot-lanta?
> Ha-ha-lanta?
> This isn't just a Super Bowl that furthers Atlanta's hopes for the Winter Olympics. It's one where teams will ride to the game on a Zamboni. It's a game where (last one, OK?) the Weather Channel has the most relevant broadcast rights.
>
> Dave Hyde
> (South Florida) *Sun-Sentinel*[26]

And (last one, OK?), a renown writer watches his beloved Philadelphia Eagles really boot a game:

> PHILADELPHIA—We're accustomed to train wrecks in this city. We're used to the bizarre and the incalculably stupid and the unforgivingly hideous.
> But Sunday the beloved Iggles, who long ago mastered the art of the ignominious pratfall, outdid even themselves.
> It wasn't so much that they lost again. It was that the Birds did something that caused people to stop and think and then say: "You know, I don't believe I've ever seen that before."
>
> Bill Lyon
> *The Philadelphia Inquirer*[27]

The Game-Column Checklist

Now, before we move, in Chapter Twelve, to a different form of column writing, run down a final checklist for the spot-news game column:

✓ You need strong reporting skills to strengthen your writing with *added value* facts and insights. Your writing, clever though it may be, won't attract readers unless your column contains substantive information.

✓ You must know your game, your sport and your beat. Columns exude authority only if their authors are serious students of sports, as well as whizzes at the keyboard.

✓ You must cultivate authoritative sources whose background information, news tips and analytical interpretations will give your column added credibility and newsy freshness. Simply sitting in a corner and pondering the world of sports—writing "thumb suckers"—won't do. Like good newswriting, good column writing is mostly strong reporting, except that good columns have a top dressing of informed opinion and clever writing spin.

✓ Stay close to the news; comment today on last night's game; write tomorrow about the forthcoming weekend contest. There's room in opinion writing for timelessly moving your muse far afield—but not in game columns.

✓ Recognize the power of a column and the impact you can have—for good or bad. Take to column writing the same search for accuracy and sense of fairness and balance that should drive your basic newswriting.

✓ Have fun; give fun. A quip here, a hilarious graf there, a funny column—all can pull readers to your byline and give us at least momentary relief from the doom and gloom that sometimes dominate the news.

Summary

—Nothing in sports reporting gives you the journalistic *elbow room*—the freedom—of writing a column of your analysis of the news.

—But your column on a game or spot-news event should be well reported so it is a stand-alone narrative readers will understand.

—Game columns can focus on personalities, key plays or dramatic moments that sometimes are not emphasized enough in spot-news reporting.

—Your mission is not to write a game story, but to weave the Five Ws and How into your column.

—Clever writing alone won't attract readers, so offer added value reporting—new facts, new understanding—as a reward for reading you.

—Your column will be strengthened if you include a call for action—not only an outline of a problem but possible solution, too.

—Truly big news stories create waves of reader interest, and you dramatically increase your chances of being read if you position your column on the crest of that reader interest; stay close to the news.

—Your credibility—your authority—is enhanced if you base your opinions on sound reporting and careful examination of the facts, and let readers see the logic of your thinking.

—Game columns are particularly effective if timely, in a news sense, and written in a conversational, chatty tone.

—Readers love to see what's behind the scenes, on the field and in the locker

room, so you do them a great favor if you take them there in your writing.
—Write for intimacy with readers by using the perpendicular pronoun "I" and creating a "we" and "us" tone they can identify with in your column.
—Don't write in sports "shorthand" that excludes from your column any prospective reader who isn't an expert in your sport; translate terms and interpret meaning.
—Certain news coverage, such as repeated stories on crimes by athletes, can create an imbalanced perception in the public mind; a column can show the other side of such stories and present a balanced view.
—Although sports is serious business, you can have a little fun—and give some to readers—by writing humorously.

Exercises

1. Examine today's "Sports of the Times" column in the national edition of *The New York Times* (or another column your instructor designates) and discuss, in about 250 words, the apparent intent of the writer. Is this a game column that focuses on a key play in a sports event, a dramatic moment or a personality? Is the column a stand-alone narrative from which you can understand the Five Ws and How of the event being discussed?

2. Study your choice of a column from a nearby metropolitan newspaper (or a column designated by your instructor) and discuss, in about 300 words, two dimensions of the writing: 1) opinion and analysis, and 2) added value reporting. Does the writer present new facts and insights that reward readers, or is the column built solely on the writer's opinions and interpretations?

3. Cover a local sports event approved by your instructor and write, in the length required, an added-value column. Be certain to give your readers facts and insights beyond what would be presented in a straight-news account of the event. Look for key plays, moments or personalities that might be pegs for your insights.

4. Write a sports column that includes a *call for action*. This could be a column, for example, calling for a new coach of a college team, or perhaps proposing more funding of intramural sports on your campus. Do a responsible reporting job, consult authoritative sources and let your writing show readers how you reached your conclusions. Write this in the appropriate length, but use no more than 450 words.

5. Write a column that takes your readers with you behind the scenes of sports on your campus. That could be a visit to a locker room, a training session, an interview with a coach or a visit to any place or person not normally accessible to reader-fans but open to "insiders," such as sportswriters. Do this column in the wordage required.

Recommended Reading

The columnists cited in this chapter are available for your daily reading on their newspapers' individual Web sites. Reading them—and others—daily undoubtedly is the best "recommended reading" you can find.

The longer writing structures used in columns are addressed in Conrad C. Fink and Donald E. Fink, *Introduction of Magazine Writing* (New York: Macmillan Publishing Company, 1994), and Conrad C. Fink, *Writing Opinion for Impact* (Ames: Iowa State University Press, 1999).

Notes

1. "Switzer a Goner, But Boys Quit First," Dec. 22, 1997, p. 56.
2. "What They're Saying, *Atlanta Journal-Constitution*, Sept. 27, 1999, p. G-3.
3. "What They're Saying," *Atlanta Journal-Constitution*, Sept. 20, 1999, p. D-3.
4. "Texas Eyes Aren't Smiling," March 13, 1999, p. B-1.
5. "It Looked Winnable, But UT Had No Shot," March 13, 1999, p. B-1.
6. "Griffey Did a Job on Seattle," Feb. 12, p. E-1.
7. "Inside Motor Sports," Sept. 13, 1999, p. 104.
8. "Sports of the Times," Sept. 13, 1999, p. D-7.
9. "One Small Problem: Offense is Lacking," Oct. 4, 1999, p. D-7.
10. "Keeping Score," Oct. 22, 1999, p. C-3.
11. "Derby Seers Face Enigma," April 30, 1999, p. D-1.
12. "New York Starting to Sweat," May 15, 1999, p. C-1.
13. "Give Garcia the Ball Again Next Week," Oct. 4, 1999, p. C-1.
14. "These A's Were Born to Be Wild," Sept. 8, 1999, p. E-1.
15. "DefLAted," Oct. 7, 1999, p. D-1.
16. "All Together Now, Yankees," Oct. 29, 1999, p. D-1.
17. "Sports of the Times," Dec. 29, 1999, p. D-1.
18. "Sports of the Times," Jan. 8, 1999, p. C-19.
19. "Sports of the Times," June 15, 1999, p. D-1.
20. "Home Where the Heart Is for Glenn," Oct. 4, 1999, p. D-1.
21. "The Buzz," *Columbus (Ga.) Ledger-Enquirer*, Feb. 7, 2000, p. B-2.
22. "The Buzz," *Columbus (Ga.) Ledger-Enquirer*, Feb. 28, 2000, p. B-2.
23. "Finally, There Is Reason for Hope," Feb. 17, 2000, p. E-1.
24. "Cremins' Departure Graceful," Feb. 19, 2000, p. H-2.
25. "Budge's Death Deserves More Than Passing Shot," Jan. 29, 2000, p. D-3.
26. "The Buzz," *Columbus (Ga.) Ledger-Enquirer*, Jan. 31, 2000, p. B-2.
27. "What They're Saying," *Atlanta Journal-Constitution*, Sept. 20, 1999, p. D-3.

12

In This Corner ...

YOU'VE NOW learned to report sports news and to write columns explaining a game or illuminating other spot-news events.

Is that it? Are we finished?

Not yet. We must discuss columnists who roam free of any timely spot-news "peg," who range far beyond a single game or event and who critique, not merely report or explain—columnists who criticize and, yes, *crusade*.

Columnists given such freedom by major newspapers have enormous journalistic muscle, so normally only the most seasoned, skilled and responsible writers reach this coveted second-level column assignment.

And those who do get the assignment frequently become the sports section's principal attraction for large numbers of readers. So, their writing often is "anchored"—always published in the same spot so readers know where to look. This often is the left-hand column on the section's front page (thus this chapter's title, "In This Corner ...").

Picking a subject and writing angle for a game column is simple compared to your challenge in focusing the type of column we're now discussing. After all, in a game column, you focus on the key play or strategy or the player who won or lost the game.

But what to do when you're deprived of such a spot-news angle?

Well, think of a quarterback reading a shifting defensive secondary, judging whether to go for a quick down-and-out or to toss the bomb. Or a batter wondering whether the outfield sidled enough to the right so that a simple poke over the third baseman's head would bring in a run—or whether to swing for the bleachers.

That is, in this type of column writing, you're surveying the *entire sports scene*, noting subtle shifts in news and reader interests, then deciding whether to "poke" in a quick-hit column or swing for a biggie.

We'll turn first to big-hit columnists who flex their very considerable journalistic muscle on larger issues in the sports world. Then, we'll look at other column forms—the roundup, how-to-do-it column and the outdoor essay.

Writing Tough Stuff

George Vecsey is damned mad—and it shows.

Baseball team owners discuss renting advertising space on players' uniforms, and Vecsey fires his *New York Times* column, "Sports of the Times," like a cannon:

> Everybody was wondering just how baseball might respond to its epic 1998 season. Now we know. The weasels are thinking of renting out the uniforms to advertisers.
>
> What a grand idea. The glorious Redbirds that have festooned the St. Louis uniforms for much of this century will compete for space with pizza parlors. The dignified stripes (not pinstripes, by the way) that grace the Yankee uniform will be cheapened by the advertisements for video games. Or whatever ...

There's more tough stuff. Bemoaning "Major League Baseball's lack of respect," columnist Vecsey fires a second cannon shot at owners:

> They are willing to turn their players into walking billboards next year. They say it would be done tastefully. Of course it would. As tasteful as stadiums being named for corporations that will probably be swallowed up or out of existence in a few years.
>
> The advertising blitz on uniforms would be as tasteful as the shameless pressure on cities to build luxury boxes for people who actually hate baseball but love to ingest shrimp and wine in trendy settings.
>
> George Vecsey
> *The New York Times*[1]

In case those cannon shots missed, Vecsey continues to fire away at "baseball's own crass penchant for uglification," acknowledging there is no such word in his Spell-Check—"but there will be when people get a load of advertisements on uniforms" being suggested by "the grubby marketing gang."

So, it's the wider issue of commercialization of baseball that angers Vecsey. For a *New York Times* colleague, it's violence in sports:

> When Owen Hart, a 34-year-old professional wrestler known as the Blue Blazer, plunged more than 50 feet from the rafters of a Kansas City arena to his death in the ring ... fans thought it was part of the show, the kind of grand entrance they had come to expect. They cheered as his body was carried off. After all, the World Wrestling Federation had billed the nationally televised pay-for-view event as "Over the Edge."
>
> It's easy enough to dismiss the tragedy as a circus accident without much resonance in "real" sports. State athletic commissions conveniently delineate between an exhibition such as pro wrestling and a so-called true competition such as boxing (in which the occasional "accidental death" is actually caused by the purpose of the sport, not by a faulty harness hookup) ... so we think we don't have to care if the bouts are scripted or if the obviously scripted racism, sexism and violence should be investigated.

That's Robert Lipsyte in his column, "Backtalk." He continues:

> Perhaps we should think again. This popular entertainment may be a glimpse of a future toward which most of sports is inexorably slouching. It is getting harder to figure out where "over the edge" begins, and how soon that dangerous territory on the other side will become our home field.
>
> ... I'm filled with strange new questions. Why doesn't my heart jump anymore when a hockey goon slams an opponent's face into the Plexiglas? Do I need teeth spilling out like Chiclets? When the racing car spins into the crowd, will they show replays? Am I ghoulish or just jaded? How soon will Mike Tyson be ready to bite someone's head off?
>
> Are we already beyond Rollerball? Is it time to start getting in line for Christians and Lions in their Garden update?
>
> Lipsyte asks whether sports marketing—the drive for ever bloodier spectacles—is behind "the epidemic of concussions in football, of exploding physicality in basketball, of head-hunting in baseball." ... And, he reasons:
>
> Especially if coach and the market approve. In our ongoing forum on Jock Culture and its effect on common sensibilities, pro wrestling is worth discussion. It may still be a cartoon, but the pressure it puts on other live entertainments to crank up the action is real.
>
> Robert Lipsyte
The New York Times[2]

Note the *thematic thrust* of these columns. Lipsyte and Vecsey both provide big-picture treatment of subjects broadly meaningful to the future of sports— violence and commercialization. And both write without spot-news pegs.

At the *Chicago Tribune* (from his usual perch in the left-hand column of the sports section's front page), Skip Bayless addresses another big-picture subject, and eats a little humble pie in doing so:

A mother calls. What should she tell her NFL-crazy 8-year-old when players are accused of murder?

A father writes. How can he explain a player's racist comments to his baseball-mad 10-year-old?

I feel a little guilty giving them my answer. They should tell their children what they should have from the start, what my parents should have taught me, what my forefathers in sportswriting should have revealed from the earliest days of standing-room-only sports.

What I wish I had written more honestly about over the years, if I hadn't been raised to hero-worship.

Parents should teach their children what my life in locker rooms has taught me: Pro athletes routinely make the worst role models, more often teaching us what not to do. Shouldn't that be predictable considering many pro jocks aren't much more mature than the kids who adore them?

For Bayless the questions continue:

Mix too much money, too many temptations, too much idolatry, too few normal-people rules, too much roaring reinforcement to commit near-murder on the football field, to intimidate hitter with lethal-weapon fastballs, to win at all costs ... and you expect star athletes to set examples for kids?

Where along the way did we confuse athletic ability with exemplary behavior? Legendary athletes with the Nobel Peace Prize? What's wrong with teaching kids to admire the performances and not the performers? Why set them up for disillusionment and rebellion by making them believe the jock-god myth?

Now, an angry accusation—and Bayless focuses on fellow sportswriters and himself:

But occasionally we all sanitized, romanticized and canonized in the tradition of Grantland Rice. I grew up reading the collected works of "Granny," as he was called. Yet outlined against the blue-gray October sky, his lyrical prose and poetry turned athletes into mighty warriors who in their spare time saved damsels in distress and cured the lame. Intentionally or not, Rice and other legendary scribes of his time helped create the Great Sports Lie.

The greater Rice made his subjects sound, the more readers loved ol' Granny and the more these towering "role models" trusted him. He became their drinking buddy, their partner in myth. Grantland Rice, sportswriter, became very rich and famous turning Genghis Khans into invincible Gandhis.

Skip Bayless
Chicago Tribune[3]

Aside from big-picture thematic thrust in this type of column writing, do you see other characteristics emerging? I see two so far:

- The columns we've studied are driven by accumulated emotion—anger, even. These columnists collect, store and then haul out for use their accumulated emotion the way you collect and use facts for a straight spot-news story.
- Sacred cows are slain left and right—Vecsey spears those owners (the "weasels") who want to over-commercialize baseball; Lipsyte shoots dead the assumption that you're not a real athlete unless you commit violence; Bayless goes after grown-up children who pose (and badly) as role models in pro sports; and all three columnists pass around the blame—some of it to fans who support the wrongs as well as rights in sports and sportswriters who create fiction surrounding sports today.

The three columns represent yet another characteristic, which, unfortunately, I don't have room to demonstrate. These columnists *write long*. Bayless carries on for an amazing 32 column inches, Vecsey and Lipsyte for hundreds and hundreds of words. At this level, columnists get the newshole they need to write the way they want to write.

The *Times'* Lipsyte also shows *intellectual* depth in a lengthy column on show-boating by athletes to "put down" opponents. In reporting strong enough to grace *any* story in the *Times* on any subject, Lipsyte interviews psychiatrists and psychologists:

> The psychiatrist says the throat-slashing gestures in pro football may be a positive force, offering vicarious satisfaction to fans and sublimating the players' desire to really hurt someone. The psychologist says the gestures are symptomatic of something much darker and more complicated than end zone posturing: players are acting out the projections of an angry America.
>
> It's a hard gesture to interpret beyond the obvious in-your-face, I'm-the-man message. Why is it necessary for some of the country's richest, best-looking and most admired young men to signify themselves with what seems to be a cheesy, adolescent, retrograde symbol? Isn't scoring a touchdown enough? When did winning become empty? Whatever happened to cool? Analyze that.

One psychologist tells Lipsyte that fans are bored and "look to sports for explosive excitement." And players, "narcissistic and lacking in identity, reflect the fans' anger. There's no authority for them anymore."

Deep stuff! And there's more:

> Dr. (Fred Smith), psychiatrist and psychoanalyst, thinks that "while sports serves as an outlet for aggressive energy, the important question is:

When does it go over the line? The throat slashing is not OK if it undermines the other values of the game such as sportsmanship and respect for opponents. I think the throat slashing can be seen as a descendant of the antics of Jimmy Connors and John McEnroe in tennis."

Now, Lipsyte strikes in another direction, questioning health professionals themselves:

[T]here seems to be a tendency for the psychiatrists, in particular, to either dismiss athletics as beneath their professional dignity or to be such passionate fans that they blur their professional boundaries. Traveling with athletes, befriending them, thrilled by access and confidence, they think of themselves as part of the team.

This can be as harmless as aping jocks. It has been as dangerous as psychiatrists becoming drug connections. Perhaps worst of all, and most common, as evaluators of prospects or counselors to troubled players, some shrinks lose sight of any responsibility to the needs of the individual.

Like many sports doctors in general, they see their job as getting the athlete back in the arena—to win, not necessarily to become healthier. Their allegiance is to the customer—team management—rather than to the patient.

Robert Lipsyte
The New York Times[4]

So, *another* characteristic emerges for this type of column writing: to play in the big leagues of top-ranked columnists you must display intellectual depth in your reporting and writing. You must have wide-ranging interests in more than scores and stats. And, you must possess the professional strengths and expertise needed to report and write on any subject, not just sports, for any of these great newspapers, the *New York Times, Chicago Tribune* and others.

And *courage.* You must have the courage to go where timid journalists refuse to go, courage to write it forcefully as it should be written.

Here's Tom Cushman of the *San Diego Union-Tribune* on a prizefight:

There are only three possible explanations for the scoring of two judges who reduced the convincing victory of England's Lennox Lewis over Evander Holyfield to a draw status:

1. Abject incompetence. 2. Payoffs—either through the promise of other lucrative assignments, or in cash. 3. A gun held to their heads, and I'm not referring to a water pistol.

Tom Cushman
The San Diego Union-Tribune[5]

Stimulate, Explain, Advocate

No single "formula" exists to guide you in writing forceful opinion columns. But basic ingredients needed in such writing *can* be expressed in a formula: Call it the "SEA Formula"—Stimulate, Explain, Advocate.

Actually, opinion writing in any journalism sector—politics and business, for example, must include those ingredients if it is to succeed. Think of this column structure:

INTRODUCTION
state the subject
explain the issue
define the problem

BODY
provide "added value" reporting
flesh out details
quote conflicting authorities
discuss balancing views
outline alternatives

CONCLUSION
express your opinion
suggest/demand action
prompt reader involvement

And, Write!

Following a structured writing formula doesn't guarantee your opinions will be read. You must *write*—and well—to lure readers into even intrinsically interesting material.

Our best sports columnists know that. Here's Thomas Boswell, in Havana, for a look at Cuban baseball:

> HAVANA—Going back to Havana after 21 years is like looking in the face of someone you once loved after their corpse has been exhumed. You cannot believe that something so beautiful can become so hideous while still resembling itself. Rust never sleeps. Neither does decay or decomposition.
>
> Cuba is falling apart one crumbling concrete wall, one unpainted pillar and one dry-rotted '46 Oldsmobile coupe at a time. If a jet flew low and created a sonic boom, would the whole city collapse into a pile of rubble?

With terrific imagery, Boswell's introduction tempts readers to forge ahead. He doesn't stop there, though. Boswell inserts, throughout the body of his *51-column-inch* story, a series of fascinating vignettes that *maintain reading momentum*. Here's one:

> As six of us, all veteran journalists, rode through the city on Friday night after attending Game 1 of the Cuban equivalent of the World Series, our cab wound through dozens of residential side streets—largely lightless, as bleak as some Eastern European blitzkrieged bomb site.
>
> "Have any of you ever seen anything like this anywhere?" I asked.
>
> Nobody even bothered to answer.

Boswell & Co. are in Havana to watch the Baltimore Orioles, who flew in from Miami (which is "90 miles and 40 years away") to play a Cuban team. Deep in his story, Boswell "juices" his writing momentum with another vignette, this one from a game between two Cuban teams, Santiago and the Industriales:

> After a home run, the players in the Industriales dugout stood and formed a conga line, high-kicking in unison. On a close play at first base, one team argued. The whole team. They came off the bench, 25 strong, like a hockey fight. At a real Cuban game, you never know what you'll see. A woman may come on the field in the fifth inning to serve the umpires coffee near third base. Down here, you even have to watch the foul balls. One was caught by a cop in the third base crowd on Friday. With no windup, he fired what must have been a 90 mph strike from the stands right to the third baseman. A blur. A seed. Down here, you even have to put a radar gun on the cops.

> Thomas Boswell
> *Washington Post*[6]

So strong—so *beautiful*—is Boswell's writing that you ingest his message (including "Cuba hates the United States; but Cubans love Americans") without knowing it!

Frederick C. Klein, author of wonderfully graceful sports essays for, of all papers, *The Wall Street Journal*, reports—in irresistible language—that things aren't quite what they seem in Merrie Olde England:

> LONDON—I'll tell you something you might not have suspected about cricket (the sport, not the insect). It's that everything that goes on upon its fields isn't cricket.
>
> "Cricket" has become synonymous with scrupulous fair play, but how, then, do you account for the behavior of the Cambridge University players during their match against Oxford University at Lord's here the Sunday before last?
>
> More than once, Cambridge pitches passed Oxford batsmen unhit and the balls were caught behind them by the wicketkeeper, who held them aloft in triumph while his teammates hurrahed. If the pitches had tipped their bats, the hitters would have been out, but the umpire ruled otherwise and their turns continued.

Now, how to explain to Americans what that means? A real writing pro does it:

> The fielder's gesture was a ruse, like that of a baseball fielder claiming to have caught a ball he really trapped.
>
> Frederick C. Klein
> *The Wall Street Journal*[7]

Do you want to read about people who bet on making money in horse racing? No? Let the *Journal's* Klein change your mind:

> ARCADIA, CALIF.—The lure of the big score draws people into horse racing, but it's elusive there as elsewhere. For every horse that wins a big purse or bet, five or six others munch their oats in anonymity, with their owners gagging down their bills. The excellent advice about not buying anything that eats originated at the ovals.
>
> Frederick C. Klein
> *The Wall Street Journal*[8]

There's something about race horses that moves the writer's muse for some sportswriters. Here's George Vecsey of *The New York Times* reporting on his first sight of Charismatic, great-grandson of the champion Secretariat, as horses emerge from an air-cargo plane:

> Down came the trainer, D. Wayne Lukas, in jeans and boots, a green jacket and white cowboy hat. Then came Lukas' favorite stable pony.

> Then came royalty. The first part out of the doorway was the nose with the white marking, not quite as elongated as that of his great-grandfather, but starting in the same spot, right between the forceful eyes. Seeing Charismatic for the first time, I got the chills.
>
> George Vecsey
> *The New York Times*[9]

That Vecsey jewel was deep in a column—and it kept me reading to the end.

Crusade for Improvement

To write a regular column for a major newspaper is to stand on a high platform visible throughout the sports world and speak with a voice heard by hundreds of thousands of readers.

Don't waste that opportunity to crusade for improvement.

Shirley Povich didn't. He fought to change sports for the better during the *74 years* his column appeared in *The Washington Post* (where, Publisher Katherine Graham said, he was responsible for attracting *one-third* of the newspaper's readership).

When Povich died in 1998, Ira Berkow wrote in his *New York Times* obituary that Povich's column was "literary yet earthy, opinionated yet generous, topical yet filled with historical perspective, and a pleasure to read."...

One of Povich's many crusades was for racial integration of pro football, particularly by the Washington Redskins, and he used his column to make a point when a black player scored against the team:

> Jim Brown, born ineligible to play for the Redskins, integrated their end zone three times yesterday.
>
> Shirley Povich
> *The Washington Post*[10]

In 1962, the Redskins gave in and hired a black player, Bobby Mitchell.

For hockey columnist Kevin Paul Dupont of the *Boston Globe*, violence is a sore point:

> Look, if Player X goes out with the intent to injure Player Y, there truly is nothing anyone can do about that. That's true of every professional sport worldwide ... , just as it is on the playground, in the supermarket, on the highway and anywhere else evil creeps into our society. Hockey only increases the odds for nitwits to take aim because it arms them with the tools of the game, sticks and steel blades. Late-night convenience stores have been terrorized by far less.

What can be done? Dupont:

What can hockey do to prevent it? That's the wrong question. Folks looking to NHL headquarters for the fix are the same ones who call (the weatherman) to answer for the 18 inches of snow in the driveway. The league handed out suspensions, took pay out of players' pockets and can only hope that the current punishment—and the implied promise to increase such penalties—diminishes future crime. What else do you want, handcuffs with official NHL logos?

The frightening truth is that there is no fix. What, ask owners not to sign (brawling players)? OK. But who makes up the cull list? How are potential perpetrators identified? Impossible.

How about this for a preposterous suggestion: *Tell fans to stay away until these goons are gone.* Don't bet on that. In today's society, there's a better chance that crowds would drop if the threat of bodily harm were reduced. Who do you suppose is filling the stands of auto racing tracks around the country? There are more meatheads than motorheads out there, guaranteed.

The only thing that put a stop to intent-to-injure incidents is the conscience that fills the helmet.

Kevin Paul DuPont
The Boston Globe[11]

Note above the emotion in Dupont's writing: "nitwits" playing hockey, owners who hire brawlers, "goons" on skates, "meatheads" at motorways—and fans who lust for violence and, thus, who are responsible for it.

No soft tippy-toe essayish style for Dupont. He's as subtle as a hockey stick in the eye.

Harvey Araton of *The New York Times* is no less direct in a column condemning sexual violence against women by professional athletes and, particularly, men who father—then abandon—children:

You hear about the paternity suits, and ask why can't these guys just use condoms. Anyone who has spent time around famous athletes knows that many regard women in the same vein—easily obtainable, utterly disposable.

Harvey Araton
The New York Times[12]

Sarcasm is the weapon for two columnists crusading against ever-increasing ticket prices fans must pay.

Mark Heisler of *The Los Angeles Times* describes money problems in the NBA following a lockout of players during the 1999 season, then comments: "Not that anyone is in actual trouble, unless you're a fan who would like to take a family of four to a game for less than $500."[13]

Lynn Zinser of the *Colorado Springs Gazette* lays it on team management:

While sitting around this week wondering whether I should sell my car to buy Rockies season tickets, which comes to $8,748 for four infield box seats, or go straight for a second mortgage and a 12-game corporate suite deal ($14,400) ...

OK, so I wasn't doing that. But I have kept my Rockies season ticket brochure around for laughs. In a pinch it also makes a handy coaster.

The economics of sports can be a wonderful source of comedy. And relatively speaking, baseball is the affordable professional sport.

Sunday's NBA All-Star Game might as well be held on Oz, which is far more appropriate than Oakland. The players combine to make more than the gross national product of a small country. Those fans lining the court, they combine to make the gross national product of a large country.

Lynn Zinser
The Colorado Springs Gazette[14]

Lesson: A column is a major soapbox. Use it for a good purpose!

The Roundup Column

Ever notice your own conversational patterns with a friend you haven't talked to for days? You tend to wander over all sorts of subjects, don't you? You're catching up on what's happened since your last chat.

The *roundup column* serves the same purpose—bringing your reader-friends up to date on what's new since your last column.

Boston Globe columnists do this superbly under a "standing hed"—an unchanging headline—variously reading "Boxing Notes," "Baseball Notes" and so forth.

Using personal interviews, news service material and information collected by *Globe* reporters, the columnists range widely across a sport, often in thousands of words that take up nearly a full page.

In "Boxing Notes," Ron Borges leads with a forthcoming welterweight prize fight, then examines recent and future action throughout boxing. The writing includes penetrating analysis:

Well shop-worn at 33, according to experts, (former junior welterweight Vincent Pettway) is not the Pettway who was once junior middleweight champion, and how he became No. 1 contender for the 147-pound title is difficult to fathom, impossible to logically explain, and illustrative of the ills that are eating away at boxing's credibility and moving the sport closer and closer to federal takeover that would be welcome by many who love it.

Ron Burges
The Boston Globe[15]

And, Borges' column contains a section titled, "Short Jabs"—tidbits on other fighters throughout the sport.

In "Baseball Notes," Peter Gammons (also ESPN's major league baseball analyst) structures his column the same way—analysis on the Seattle Mariners' chances in the forthcoming season, then tidbits from around the leagues (such as, "There is a lot of speculation swirling around the Dodgers, from the possibility of Pat Gillick taking the club presidency to Kevin Malone sifting through trade possibilities").[16]

At *USA Today*, Christine Brennan, in her weekly column, "Keeping Score," takes the same chatty approach to figure skating:

> HUNTINGTON, W.VA.—You talk to the promoters and the agents and the marketing people, and they'll tell you, in a whisper, that figure skating is in a little bit of trouble. Not a lot, but a little.
>
> To be sure, skating's TV ratings still beat the numbers of almost any other big-time televised sport, and female figure skaters are some of the most recognizable athletes on the planet. But things are not as they were in the good old days of 1994. No, those dreamy days of scandal-inflated viewership, of tabloid-TV crews falling all over each other on skaters' front lawns, of an Olympic short program actually becoming the sixth-highest-rated show in the history of American TV—those days are now long gone.
>
> Ratings are down. Arenas aren't full. And the next big shot in the arm for the sport is more than two years off, the 2002 Olympic Games.
>
> Christine Brennan
> *USA Today*[17]

At *Newsday*, columnist Bob Glauber is given a *full page* for his bits-and-pieces coverage of NFL action. He opens with detailed discussion of coach Dom Capers of the Carolina Panthers and his "mishandling" of team discipline, then moves smoothly into those tidbits so beloved by fans:

> Here's the scuttlebutt:
> In Chicago, team president Michael McCaskey said he'll evaluate Wannstedt after the season. ...
> In St. Louis, the Rams might try to force Vermeil's hand by requiring that he fire some of his assistant coaches.
> In San Diego ... .
>
> Bob Glauber
> *Newsday*[18]

The tidbit approach is used frequently in roundups on television and radio coverage of sports. Major newspapers regularly assign columnists to comment on news within the broadcast industry and what's available for fans to see and hear. These columnists—Steve Kroner of the *San Francisco Chronicle* and Prentis Rogers of *The Atlanta Journal-Constitution* among them—treat sports broadcasting as serious news requiring thoughtful commentary.

Let Others Speak

Not every column must be filtered through your intellect or reflect your personal views. Occasionally let others use your speaker's platform.

Will McDonough (a superb writer/analyst) steps aside in his *Boston Globe* column. His intro:

> JACKSONVILLE, FLA.—We're down to the Elite Eight in the NFL's postseason tournament, and it's time to analyze what these teams have to do to have the best shot of advancing to their respective conference championship games. As always, commentary from men whose teams have faced both participants ... .

Now, McDonough turns over the entire column to direct quotes from his guests:

> Miami at Jacksonville, analysis by Jets director of football operations Bill Parcells: "There is one important factor here to begin with that should not be overlooked. Miami's preparation time. Jacksonville has been off for two weeks, getting healthy, and with plenty of time to prepare. My guess is that they probably prepared more for Seattle, thinking Seattle would win the game, but they still should have a wide preparation edge on Miami. ...
>
> Washington at Tampa Bay, analysis by Lions coach Bobby Ross: "This should be a great matchup with the Washington offense going against Tampa's defense, which to me is the fastest in the league. They are so quick on defense that if you don't play against them on a regular basis, like we do twice a year, their speed kind of blindsides you." ...
>
> Minnesota at St. Louis, analysis by 49ers general manager Bill Walsh ... .
>
> Will McDonough
> *The Boston Globe*[19]

It's great reading, and columnist McDonough does his readers a favor by letting them listen directly to knowledgeable football veterans chatting about forthcoming games.

How-to-Do-It Columns

Exploding popularity of do-it-yourself sports gives you a major opportunity to reach out to readers with how-to-do-it columns.

Favorites with writers and reader-fans alike are golf and tennis, but all participatory sports—skiing, surfing, skydiving, you name it—are invitations for expert commentary.

Clifton Brown of *The New York Times*, a golf writer, takes readers into the fine art of putting. First, a newsy intro:

The speaker was David Duval. The subject was putting.

As Duval held his trusted putter in his hand during a recent conversation, he was asked about this week's United States Open, which is being played for the first time at Pinehurst's revered No. 2 course beginning Thursday. Duval has never played a tournament at Pinehurst, a course characterized by unusual greens that drop off on all sides, like bowls turned upside down. But when it comes to making putts, Duval believes that some basics never change, that it is important to take the same attitude to Pinehurst in North Carolina, to Augusta National in Georgia or to anywhere else in the world.

"At this level, I'd say confidence would be 96 to 97 percent of putting," said Duval, who is the world's No. 1 ranked player.

Second, Brown passes along how-to-do-it tips from Duval: confidence is born of hard work ... Duval uses a conventional putting style ... other golfers use left-hand-low or cross-handed styles. ...

Third, in a sidebar titled, "Get a Grip," Brown presents—with photos—tips from instructor Dave Pelz on putting grips:

> 1 CONVENTIONAL: A baseball bat-type grip ... most natural and comfortable to most players.
> 2 LEFT HAND LOW: For right-handers, the left hand is below the right ... helps keep the lead wrist from bending ... helps square the shoulder to the target.
> 3 LONG PUTTER: The left hand anchors the club to the chest, eliminating wrist action.
>
> Clifton Brown
> *The New York Times*[20]

In the column, "Tip of the Week," a *Boston Globe* correspondent walks readers through a golfing lesson he gave a reader who wrote the newspaper for help with a "fat" shot—which occurs when the club digs into the ground before hitting the ball:

> We introduced a three-step exercise to help Brian clear his arms from his body and set up to the ball from a better distance. Having him take a stance the width of his shoulders, I asked Brian to hold the clubshaft parallel to the ground at a hip-high level with his arms comfortably stretched and fully extended.
>
> Rick DePamphilis
> *The Boston Globe*[21]

You'll note above the precise instruction passed along by both golf writers. How-to-do-it columns should not be literary exercises that meander over fields of imprecision. Help your readers putt better, swing better!

Note above also that writer DePamphilis slips into the personal pronoun "I" with his golfing tips. Personalizing your writing brings it alive.

An Associated Press writer does that by *running in the Boston Marathon*, then entertaining readers with lively writing:

> BOSTON—Veterans of the Boston Marathon spook race rookies with tales of Heartbreak Hill the way grandparents scare their grandchildren with ghost stories.
>
> And like those youngsters, the rookies listen with a mix of fear and skepticism. How bad could Heartbreak be, they think, even if it is the most famous climb at Boston and comes between the 20- and 21-mile marks of the race?
>
> After running my first Boston Marathon on Monday, I can say this: it can be pretty darn bad.
>
> John Affleck
> Associated Press [22]

The "how-I-did-it" story form is exploited wonderfully by George Plimpton, described by *Modern Maturity* as "America's most celebrated sports jester and journalist" and by himself as "a participatory journalist for *Sports Illustrated*."

Plimpton makes a handsome living by playing pro football (for a few downs) boxing champions, skating in the NHL, then (and this is the man's genius) being properly self-deprecating:

> I am often asked how I survived quarterbacking for the Detroit Lions, playing "power" forward for the Boston Celtics, boxing with light-heavyweight champion Archie Moore, playing goalie for the Boston Bruins and so on—without showing some physical evidence of what I have been through.
>
> "You seem unmarked," my friend said. ...
>
> "What I have suffered is mostly psychic damage," I replied. "A bruised ego."
>
> I explained that in each of my athletic confrontations, I had been humiliated ... losing 29 yards in five plays as quarterback, being busted about in the boxing ring, giving up record-length home runs in Yankee Stadium. The life of a participatory journalist is not an easy one.
>
> George Plimpton
> *Modern Maturity* [23]

Want to have fun? Want *your readers* to have fun? Poke fun at yourself.

The Outdoors Column

> When we reached the west shore of Maine's Salmon Stream Lake, there was only about an hour of daylight left, so we made haste to load our canoe and make the crossing to the family camp on the tip of the peninsula on the opposite shore.

> There was a stiff northeast wind blowing, but the venerable 20-foot Grumman aluminum canoe I leave upside down and tethered to a spruce at the road's end was more than adequate for the half-mile trip. Pushed by a two-horsepower outboard, we traversed the water in less than 15 minutes, putting up a flight of eight Canada geese on the way.

That's Nelson Bryant, outdoor columnist—nay, *essayist*—for *The New York Times*, inviting you to sit back, read slowly to absorb each word, then *feel* that stiff northeast wind blowing and *watch* the geese go up.[24] Bryant's column is an invitation accepted eagerly by *thousands* of his readers who travel vicariously with him through the great outdoors.

And, *listen* to this one:

> There was no warning.
> One moment last September, a friend and I sat on a tree snag deep in the Idaho wilderness, surrounded by 2.2 million of the world's loveliest roadless acres.
> We sipped steaming coffee without talking, contemplating the luxury of aloneness as a thin line of campfire smoke joined the rising sun in trees around the meadow.
> Suddenly, the silence was shattered by a mournful howl.
> There was a second, then another, and another until a chorus of crescendoing echoes drowned the fire's crackling pitch.
> Wolves.
>
> Bill Monroe
> *Sunday Oregonian*[25]

Spot-news *reporting* of outdoors events generally is weak, even though, as discussed in Chapter Ten, more than 73 million Americans fish every year and 20 million hunt.

But, look closely at outdoors *columns*, and you'll find some of the strongest and most entertaining writers in any sports section.

The *Times'* Bryant and writers like him are *stylists*, who draw word pictures that transport readers to woods and stream. They make you *see* and make you *hear*.

Others pragmatically address (often with humor) the question asked by all who hunt or fish: Where do I find the big bucks, how do I catch the big fish?

> What do lawyers, shrinks and sharks have in common? In August, they leave New York and head for New England. We deal here with the sharks: the phenomenal numbers of makos, blue sharks and porbeagle that have ventured here from southern waters the last few weeks.
> Despite talk of stripers disappearing offshore and bluefish changing feeding patterns, this midsummer period seems much like past years—solid, if not frantic fishing, in most waters. The lesson of midsummer, when the fish

do not feed as wildly as in spring, is to be ready to vary methods, baits and lures. If bluefish were on the top yesterday, maybe today you have to put away the surface plugs and rig for deep water.

Tube 'n' worm rigs seem to be effective in most places, with chunked mackerel showing to be effective, and live eels best for deep stripers over rocky bottoms.

> Tony Chamberlain
> *The Boston Globe*[26]

As all strong how-to-do-it journalism should be, Chamberlain's writing is richly detailed on, for example, how to catch flounder ("use a sinker slide to bounce off the bottom") or sea bass ("They've been finicky, but night and early morning anglers are getting them in the boat.").

Writing for *Outdoor Life* magazine, Jerry Gibbs is similarly detailed. Referring to an artist's drawing of a fast-moving trout stream, Gibbs advises, "Shoot a big sculpin fly, plug or spinner here and let it sweep down and close as possible to the undercut bank without snagging. The brown trout version of 'Jaws' will be hiding here."[27]

Writing for all frustrated chair-bound executives who read the *Wall Street Journal*, Michael Pearce says, "Come along!"

> STANWOOD, MICH.—Camouflaged from head to toe, (Fred Smith) and a guest quietly knelt as a guide broke the early morning silence by grinding and slapping two antlers together to simulate the fight of two battling white-tailed deer.
>
> Within minutes it became obvious the deception had worked. The white-tailed buck came steadily, yet cautiously, through the thick timber, ears perked, eyes scanning and nostrils quaking as it searched for sound, sight or scent of whatever whitetails had the audacity to be in its territory. ...
>
> A single well-placed shot from a scoped .44 magnum Colt dropped the buck in its tracks.

> Michael Pearce
> *Wall Street Journal*[28]

Clearly, however, it's not the *killing* that outdoors columnists celebrate in their writing. It's the *outdoors*. Note these leads:

> The sun was falling fast, and the end-of-the-day hues of orange, red and light blue were dancing on the water's surface at Lake Lanier.

> Scott Bernarde
> *The Atlanta Journal-Constitution*[29]

> CHATHAM, MASS.—We were only five minutes out of Outermost Marina when we saw the birds, hundreds of birds, milling above the ocean

like windblown pepper. ... Our guide nudged the throttle forward, and we had to hold our caps in place.

The sun struggled to burn through the overcast. Here and there, bright blue patches of sky appeared beyond holes in the cover, leaving silver puddles on the black seas. It was an eerie morning, and I imagined the late film director Alfred Hitchcock smiling benignly as (the guide) cut the power and the backwash pushed his 18-foot flats boat, the Amberjack, into the flock of shrieking, dipping birds.

Striped bass were breaking water all around us.

Pete Bodo
The New York Times[30]

Hopped abroad the Tracer the other night and woke up at dawn on the other side of Santa Catalina Island.

The ocean was smooth, the air cool and clean. Quite a contrast to the fishermen, who clambered up from below like living dead, wiping sleep from their eyes, making their way to bait tanks brimming with live squid, then reaching in without hesitation, as though this was the way they started every morning.

And what a way to start a morning!

Wearing the same clothes you slept in. Sporting new whiskers on an unwashed face. Still tasting last night's cigar. Slugging coffee as black as the ink being squirted all over your shirt by the squid you're trying to stick on your hook.

This is the essence of island fishing, any fisherman will say. Whatever problems you might have, you've left them back on the mainland.

Peter Thomas
The Los Angeles Times[31]

Question: How many columnists do you see writing such wonderful vignettes out of, say, your state legislature or, as another example, Congress? How many catch the *flavor* of their story the way these outdoors columnists do? Second question: How many stuffy, impersonal columns written in dull, leaden language about politics catch readers the way these outdoors columnists must?

The Moment-in-History Column

Strange thing about sports fans: More than most people, perhaps, they're nostalgic—even for times they never knew, places they never went, people they never met.

You've heard it:

Could Joe Louis in his prime have knocked out Muhammad Ali in *his* prime? Or, would Rocky Marciano have taken both of them?

Who was the greatest quarterback? Hockey player? Tennis player?

Who in the past ran the fastest, jumped highest and threw the hardest?

All to say, you can score *big* with columns that dip into famous moments in sports history. Here's one way:

> LOUISVILLE, KY.—The year was 1950, and your faithful agent had just arrived in Atlanta when he was assigned to cover the Kentucky Derby. I was as green as a truckload of turnip tops. I had never covered a horse race before, and writing on the other side was the *Journal*'s Ed Danforth, a native Kentuckian, who knew horses and horse people, and all the guys around the track called him "Colonel."
>
> I had heard a broadcast of The Hopeful from Saratoga the summer before and a horse name Middleground won it. So, having nothing better to go on, I picked Middleground. Middleground won, beat the favorite and paid a nice price. I blushed when I got home and saw that my paper then, *The Constitution*, had run a box on the front page headlined: "Bisher Picks Derby Winner." Lord, I didn't want to rub Danforth the wrong way. He could write of horses and make it sing.
>
> Furman Bisher
> *The Atlanta Journal-Constitution*[32]

That's Bisher, moved out to the sports section's front page for the occasion, letting reader-fans know he's on duty in Louisville for his *50th* Kentucky Derby.

For Bisher, a horse race unleashes the memories, which make great reading; for Mitch Albom of the *Detroit Free Press*, it's opening day in Tiger Stadium—the last opener before the stadium is torn down:

> DETROIT—It was like climbing to the tree house one last time. Through the narrow turnstiles and dimly lit corridors, then up into the sunlight—like straddling a big branch with your feet dangling happily. That's the feeling. Say what you will about the current state of sports. A ballpark in springtime always makes you young.
>
> Which brings us to the strange juxtaposition of Monday afternoon. How, in one day, can you feel both youthful and ancient? How do you say hello and good-bye? Normally, Opening Day in Detroit is all about firsts. The first home game. The first rush of summer. The first bleacher hot dog. This time, it was also about lasts. Fans stood in the aisles, soaking in the view as if watching a loved one board an airplane. There will be no more Opening Days at the corner of Michigan and Trumbull.
>
> The Ballpark of the Century has begun her farewell season.
>
> Mitch Albom
> *Detroit Free Press*[33]

It's *the moment* that draws Dan McGrath, *Chicago Tribune* sports editor, back in time in his column:

My favorite Montana moment ... The 49ers were in Philadelphia in 1989 and were rather banged up, Joe included, as they prepared to face a Buddy Ryan team with Reggie White, Jerome Brown, Seth Joyner and other bad-intentioned bruisers. And brother, did Buddy turn them loose. Montana went down six times in the first half alone, I believe, tossed around like a rag doll. He wasn't used to such treatment, nor to having someone—Brown, I think it was—stand over him and taunt him after a collar just before half-time.

Bad move. Montana came out for the second half and just lit the Eagles up, throwing for four touchdowns in a 10-point win. He was as tough as he was talented.

Dan McGrath
Chicago Tribune[34]

For a *Sports Illustrated* columnist, writing about today's promising young pitchers reminds him of Charles (Togie) Pittinger, "also known as Horse Face," who threw for the Boston Beaneaters and the Philadelphia Phillies in the early 1900s, and "for one year he was the worst pitcher in the game." There follows a statistical rundown on Horse Face who "became the first pitcher to lead his league in six negative categories—losses (22), runs allowed (196), earned runs allowed (136)" ... the list is long, the percentages and figures dazzling, and all undoubtedly were devoured by baseball fans nostalgic for the "good old days" they never knew.[35]

For Dave Kindred, writing in *The Sporting News*, the retirement of hockey star Wayne Gretzky stirs memories from the 1980s:

I don't know hockey. I understand it only if I think of it as basketball with a thousand turnovers. But I know this: When Gretzky came to town, I never took my eyes off him. To see Gretzky moving with the puck was to see Larry Bird moving with the basketball. Something good would happen. It was almost as much fun to watch Gretzky without the puck. You knew that pretty soon the puck would be on his stick again.

Dave Kindred
The Sporting News[36]

For true nostalgia buffs, *losers* hold equal fascination with winners. To mark opening day in major league baseball, David Margolick finds a loser for a trip into yesteryear (and lands on *The New York Times'* front page):

More than 50 years after the ball was hit, Joe Cleary can still see the bad hop. Coming in for the Washington Senators in his first major league game, with two runners on base and one out, Cleary got the first Boston batter to hit what looked like a perfect double-play ball. Instead, it skipped into the outfield. Then the roof fell in.

Eight more batters came to the plate that day in August 1945, and Cleary got only one of them out: the pitcher. The Red Sox scored 12 runs and though not all were charged to him he ended up with an earned run average of 189.00—the highest calculable e.r.a. in baseball history. When he returned to the dugout, he and his manager nearly came to blows. And "the short, unhappy life of Joe Cleary in the big leagues," as Cleary himself now calls it, was over.

The major league season starts today and ... dozens of rookies will see stardom looming before them. But for all their promise, at least a few will become answers to a trivia question, appearing but once. Something—injuries or fate or their own abilities—will keep them from coming back.

David Margolick
The New York Times[37]

Margolick's story, which jumps inside to cover a *full page*, examines the short, equally unhappy careers of others among baseball's losers—including a seminarian named Aloysius Travers who pitched a complete game for the Detroit Tigers (whose players were on strike) and gave up 26 hits; and a Brooklyn rookie who yielded four hits to the first five batters in his debut in 1918, and was so upset he walked off the mound, enlisted in the Navy and never was heard from again.

As for Joe Cleary, the ultimate loser who opened Margolick's column, he says that when the Red Sox scored 12 runs against him, in his single inning of infamy, his manager was so upset he didn't even come out to the mound to take him out of the game. The manager just disgustedly waved for Cleary to come in to the dugout.

"It was like he'd just found me in bed with his wife," Cleary told the *Times* writer.

Say, did you ever hear the one about ... . (See?)

Summary

—Seasoned—and responsible—columnists can break free from spot news or a game and, instead, critique the wider sports world and even crusade.

—A characteristic of this second-level column writing is the sometimes harsh criticism writers level at such things as commercialization of sports or violence.

—Many columnists are driven by accumulated emotion—anger, even—as they develop big-picture, thematic thrusts for their writing.

—Slaying sacred cows is common for columnists criticizing, say, greedy owners, athletes who are unnecessarily violent or athletes who are poor role models.

—The most successful columnists show enormous intellectual depth in their reporting and writing, ranging far beyond the ordinary in search of topics to cover.

—Courage is a characteristic of great columnists who go where timid journalists refuse to go, and who write forcefully as it should be written.

—No single formula guides you in column writing but think of "SEA"—

Stimulate readers, Explain, Advocate.

—Following a structured writing formula doesn't guarantee your opinions will be read, so you must learn to write well to lure readers into even intrinsically interesting material.

—To write a regular column for a major newspaper is to stand on a high platform and speak with a voice heard by thousands; don't waste that opportunity to crusade for improvement in sports.

—The roundup column gives you a chance to survey a sport and assemble tidbits that bring your reader-friends up to date on what's new since your last column.

—How-to-do-it columns are increasing in popularity with exploding interest in do-it-yourself sports, such as golf, tennis and other outdoors sports.

—Outdoors columns attract some of the best writers in journalism, and the most successful combine imagery of the great outdoors with helpful hints on how to find the big buck and how to catch the big fish.

—Sports fans are nostalgic for the "good old days," even if those days weren't so good and even if the fans didn't know those times, so use your column occasionally to revisit great athletes or games of the past.

Exercises

1. In about 250 to 300 words, outline three columns you could write that critique sports on your campus—how they are played, supported, coached and so forth. Recalling examples in Chapter Twelve, discuss the crusading element and emotion you could put into these columns.

2. Your instructor will select one of the ideas you outlined in Exercise 1. Write that column—in wordage you deem necessary—with strongly reported facts and reasoned logic. Ensure that your writing is balanced and fair, yet strong and, if necessary, hard-hitting.

3. Using the "SEA Formula" discussed in Chapter Twelve, write a column on violence in sports. Take a strong position: Violence is the American way in sports or there is too much violence. This column should fit the crusading mold discussed in this chapter. Let the reader see your logic and how you arrived at your decision.

4. Write a roundup column on sports activity on your campus. Reporting this column will take time, as you must collect tidbits from all corners of the campus. Consult sports information services and the athletic department. Your mission is to inform readers, in about 500 words, generally what's happening in campus sports. View it as an effort to bring reader-fans up to date.

5. Write an outdoors column on a subject of your choice (but with approval of your instructor). Try to catch the imagery—the sound of geese, the smell of campfire smoke—we saw in some of the columns studied in Chapter Twelve. Use wordage necessary.

Notes

1. "Sports of the Times," April 4, 1999, national edition, p. 29.
2. "Backtalk," May 30, 1999, national edition, p. 13.
3. "Romance of Sport Is a Bygone View," Feb. 13, 2000, Section 3, p. 1.
4. "Backtalk," Dec. 12, 1999, Sports Section, p. 13.
5. Drawn from a digest of columnists from around the country, *Los Angeles Times*, March 21, 1999, p. D-2.
6. "Cuba's National Pastime in Despair," March 28, 1999, p. D-1.
7. "On Sports," July 9, 1999, p. W-7.
8. "On Sports," March 6, 2000, p. A-28.
9. "Sports of the Times," June 3, 1999, p. D-5.
10. "Shirley Povich Dies at 92; Washington Sports Columnist," *The New York Times*, June 7, 1998, p. 19.
11. "Pro Hockey Notes," Oct. 10, 1999, p. C-5.
12. "Sports of the Times," Dec. 23, 1999, p. D-1.
13. "Small Ratings Don't Hurt Big Picture," *The Los Angeles Times*, Feb. 13, 2000, p. D-5.
14. "The Buzz," *Columbus Ledger-Enquirer*, Feb. 14, 2000, p. B-2.
15. "Boxing Notes," March 28, 1999, p. C-17.
16. "Baseball Notes," *The Boston Sunday Globe*, Oct. 24, 1999, p. D-17.
17. "Keeping Score," Oct. 21, 1999, p. C-3.
18. "Capers Is Cooked in Carolina," Dec. 20, 1998, p. C-2.
19. "Top Scout Team Has Its Say," Jan. 15, 2000, p. G-1.
20. "Big on Short Game: Putting at Pinehurst Could Be Decisive," June 13, 1999, Section 8, p. 1.
21. "Tip of the Week," Sept. 9, 1999, p. D-12.
22. Dispatch for afternoon papers of April 20, 1999.
23. "Still Standing," May/June 1999, p. 31.
24. "Outdoors," *The New York Times*, Oct. 24, 1999, automobiles special section, p. 1.
25. "Tracking a Lone Wolf's Path to the Future," Feb. 28, 1999, p. C-9.
26. "Fishfinder," Aug. 13, 1999, p. E-9.
27. "So, You Think You Know How to Fish ... ," *Outdoor Life*, April 1999, p. 56.
28. "Where Really Big Bucks Are Easy to Find," Dec. 22, 1994, p. A-12.
29. "Spoon Jigging Can Load Creel With Fish Fast," Dec. 5, 1999, p. E-22.
30. "Outdoors," Aug. 20, 1994, Sports Section, p. 33.
31. "Island Fishing Is Not for Everyone," March 19, 1999, p. D-14.
32. "Derby Handicapper Has His Day," May 1, 1999, p. D-1.
33. Dispatch for afternoon papers of April 13, 1999.
34. "Sports Talk," Dec. 26, 1999, Section 3, p. 16.
35. "Spotlight," *Sports Illustrated*, Sept. 20, 1999, p. 96.
36. "He Knew All the Angles," April 26, 1999, p. 87.
37. "New Season for Heroes and One-Game Wonders," April 4, 1999, p. A-1.

Addendum

AP Style

Most newspapers and many other media use *The Associated Press Stylebook and Libel Manual* or use AP style as the basis for their own stylebooks.

Get your own AP stylebook. It's imperative that you learn style. Not knowing style signals editors that you're an amateur. For readers, it creates confusion if there are glaring inconsistencies in your writing—"eleven" in one graf, for example, "11" in another, or if you use "yards" one day and "meters" another.

Here, with permission from The Associated Press, are selected examples of AP style on sports usage.

Abbreviations—Spell out all but the most common, such as NBA, NFC and NHL.

All-America—AP's football or basketball team. An *All-American* was selected in one of those sports.

AstroTurf—A trademark; otherwise use *artificial grass*.

Athletic teams—Capitalize teams, associations and nicknames, such as Red Sox, Big Ten, Colts.

Auto racing—In qualifying, list driver, country, car, qualifying speed (1. Alain Prost, France, Ferrari, 170.297 kph (107.919 mph)), and for results, list driver, country, car, laps completed (1. Alain Prost, France, Ferrari, 44.)

Backboard, backcourt, backfield—For consistency, AP style varies from some dictionary usage.

Ball carrier—Two words, but: **ballclub, ballplayer.**

Baseball—AP lists 52 usages (line up as a verb, lineup as a noun, for example). Check AP's stylebook. In *numbers* usage, it's *first* inning, *10th* inning; *one* RBI, 10 RBIs; the pitcher's record is 6-5. Final score was 1-0. *Leagues* are American League, American League West, AL West, etc.

Basic summary—List winners in order of their finish, with name, affiliation, time (60-yard dash—1, Steve Williams, Florida TC, 6.0).

Basketball—It's backboard and backcourt, free throw and free-throw line, half-court pass, hook shot, man-to-man and play off as a verb and playoff as a noun and adjective. *Numbers* are first quarter, second-quarter lead, 6-foot-5 forward, but he's 6 feet 5 inches tall. The National Basketball

Association (NBA) subdivisions are Atlantic Division of the Eastern Conference, or NBA East, etc.

Bowl games—Capitalize them (i.e., Rose Bowl).

Boxing—AP lists three major sanctioning bodies, the World Boxing Association, the World Boxing Council and the International Boxing Federation, and 16 weight classes, from junior flyweight (108-111 pounds) to heavyweight (over 195 pounds). Knock out is the verb, knockout the noun and adjective. A fighter is knocked out if he takes a 10-count. If a fighter can't continue, say the winner stopped the loser. There is no "technical knockout" in most of boxing. Summaries: Randy Jackson, 152, New York, outpointed Chuck James, 154, Philadelphia, 10.

Canada Goose—Not Canadian goose.

Coach—Lowercase as a job description (not title).

Courtesy titles—Don't use unless necessary to distinguish between people (Mr. Smith, Mrs. Smith).

Decathlon—Summaries include time or distance performance, points earned, cumulative total points (100-meter dash—1. Fred Dixon, Los Angeles, 10.8 seconds, 854 points).

ERA—Use in all references to earned run average.

Football—Ball carrier, ballclub, blitz (as a noun *and* verb), place kick but place-kicker. For yardage, use figures: 5-yard line; he ran for 6; a 4-yard gain. But: a fourth-and-two play. The team won its fourth game in 10 starts, on a final score of 21-14, and the team record is 4-5-1. Field goals are measured from point of kick, not line of scrimmage. Goal posts are 10 yards behind goal lines. Include that distance.

Fractions—Put full space between whole number and fraction, 3 3/4.

Golf—Birdie is one stroke under par; bogey, one over; an eagle, two under. Numbers: He had a par 5 to finish 2-up for the round; a par-4 hole; a 7-under-par 64; the par-3 seventh hole; for clubs: a No. 5 iron, a 5-iron shot.

Gymnastics—Scoring is by points in individual events: Sidehorse—1. John Leaper, Penn State, 8.8 points.

Handicaps—It's a 3 handicap; he is a 3-handicap golfer.

Hit and run—Is a verb; hit-and-run is a noun and an adjective. (He wanted to hit and run; he scored on a hit-and-run.)

Hockey—Face off is a verb, faceoff a noun and adjective; it's a power play but a power-play goal. Hat trick applies when a player scores three goals in a game. It's the National Hockey League, and for NHL subdivisions, the Wales Division of the Campbell Conference and so forth.

IC4A—Is the Intercollegiate Association of Amateur Athletes of America.

Lacrosse—Is scored in one-point goals, played on a field 110 yards long; goals are 80 yards apart, with 15 yards of playing area behind each goal.

Matches are four 15-minute periods, with overtimes of varying lengths to break ties.

Left hand—Is a noun, left-handed an adjective, left-hander a noun.

Match summary—Is used for one vs. one contests, such as tennis, match play golf, etc. Example: Jimmy Connors, Belleville, Ill., def. Manuel Orantes, Spain, 2-6, 6-3, 6-2, 6-1.

National Association for Stock Car Auto Racing—NASCAR.

National Collegiate Athletic Association—NCAA.

Play off—Is a verb; playoff and playoffs, noun and adjective.

Postseason—Doesn't have a hyphen; neither does preseason.

Racket—Not racquet.

Record—Not "new record."

Runner-up—And runners-up.

Scores—The Reds defeated the Red Sox 4-3; the golfer had a 5 on the first hole and finished with a 2-under-par score. Note comma: Boston 6, Baltimore 5.

Ski—Skis, skier, skied, skiing, ski jump.

Swimming—Score in minutes, seconds, tenths of a second, hundredths (if available): Men's 200-meter Backstroke Heats (fastest eight qualify for Saturday night final) heat 1—1, John Naber, USC, 2:03.25. It's men's 440-meter relay; on second reference, men's 440 relay.

Tennis—Scoring is by points, games, sets and matches. A player wins a point if the opponent fails to return the ball, hits it into the net or out of bounds. A player also wins a point if the opponent is serving and fails to put the ball into play after two attempts (that's a double fault). Player must win four points to win a game. Both players begin at love (or zero), and advance to 15, 30, 40 and game (the numbers have no point value—they're simply terms for 1 point, 2 points, 3 points). The server's score always is called out first. If a game is tied at 40-all (or deuce), play continues until one player has a two-point margin. A set is won if a player wins six games before the opponent has won five. If a set becomes tied at five games each, it goes to the first player to win seven. If two players tie at five games, then at six, they normally play a tiebreaker—a game that goes to the first player to win seven points. Sometimes, rules call for a player to win by two games. A match may be either a best-of-three contest that goes to the player or team that first wins two sets, or a best-of-five contest that goes to the first player or team to win three sets. Set scores: Chris Evert Lloyd defeated Sue Barker 6-0, 3-6, 6-4. Tiebreakers are indicated in parentheses after the set score: 7-6, (11-9).

Track and field—Scoring is in distance or time. Clearly state which, meters or yards: men's 100-meter dash, women's 880-yard run, etc. It's 3-minutes, 26.1 seconds, and in second reference, 3:26.1. For hurdles and relays, it's

100-meter hurdles; in the second reference, 200 hurdles. For field events: 26 1/2 (for 26 feet, one-half inch). Basic summary: 60-yard dash—1, Steve Williams, Florida TC, 6.0.

Volleyball—First team to score 15 points wins, unless game must continue until one team has a two-point spread.

World Series—The Series on second reference (AP's exception to general principles of capitalization).

Yard lines—It's 4-yard line, 40-yard line. He plunged in from the 2; he ran 6 yards; it was a 7-yard gain.

Name Index

Subject Index